Diabetes
without DRUGS

Diabetes
without DRUGS

THE
5-STEP PROGRAM
TO CONTROL
BLOOD SUGAR NATURALLY
——— AND ———
PREVENT DIABETES
COMPLICATIONS

SUZY COHEN, RPh

Author of the Syndicated Column "Dear Pharmacist®"

RODALE

This book is intended as a reference volume only, not as a medical manual. The information given here is designed to help you make informed decisions about your health. It is not intended as a substitute for any treatment that may have been prescribed by your doctor. If you suspect that you have a medical problem, we urge you to seek competent medical help.

Mention of specific companies, organizations, or authorities in this book does not imply endorsement by the author or publisher, nor does mention of specific companies, organizations, or authorities imply that they endorse this book, its author, or the publisher.

Internet addresses and telephone numbers given in this book were accurate at the time it went to press.

Direct edition was published in January 2010 by Rodale Inc.

Printed in the United States of America
Rodale Inc. makes every effort to use acid-free ∞, recycled paper ♻.

Book design by Joanna Williams

Library of Congress Cataloging-in-Publication Data

Cohen, Suzy.
    Diabetes without drugs : the 5-step program to control blood sugar naturally and prevent
    diabetes complications / Suzy Cohen.
        p.   cm.
    Includes bibliographical references and index.
    ISBN-13 978–1–60529–733–0 hardcover
    ISBN-10 1–60529–733–X hardcover
    ISBN-13 978–1–60529–675–3 paperback
    ISBN-10 1–60529–675–9 paperback
    1. Diabetes—Alternative treatment.   2. Naturopathy.   I. Title.
    RC661.A47C64   2010
    616.4'6206—dc22   2009052599

Distributed to the trade by Macmillan.

6   7   8   9   10   11   12   13   14   15   hardcover

4   5   6   7   8   9   10   11   12   13   paperback

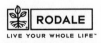

We inspire and enable people to improve their lives and the world around them
For more of our products visit rodalestore.com or call 800-848-4735

I dedicate this book to those of you who are ready for a health transformation. By changing what you "know" about diabetes, you can change the fact that you had it.

Acknowledgments

I would like to acknowledge a few special people who played an important role in my life during the time I was writing this book. First, my supportive husband, who is an amazing, talented man: Sam, I am the lucky one, for my life would be meaningless without you! Why do we waste all that time together sleeping?

My lovely children, Rachel, Michael, and Samara, have filled my life with more joy than I thought possible: My love for you is eternal, no matter where you are, and I want you to know how proud I am to be your mom.

My parents, Helen and Bill, who taught me that there were no boundaries in life and to just keep putting one foot in front of the other: I love you both very much.

Marita and Janet, you two are the most understanding and devoted friends I have. Thank you for always being there when I need you most. Susan Berg and Karen Bolesta: It takes a lot of guts to publish a book that is so unique compared to most in its genre. Thank you for the opportunity, and please know that your decision will impact lives for many years. There is a trickle effect.

Special thanks to Rachel Cohen for your watchful eye upon my work, and for a million brilliant edits to this manuscript. Also Susie Deck: The world needs more teachers like you—thank you for working tirelessly to tidy this up. Alice Feinstein: How wonderful to have you hold my hand as I crossed the finish line. Thank you for your bionic editorial eyes. And Doug Hall: You give doctors a good name with your amazing mind and caring heart. I would be so hungry without my morning breakfast of powerpoints!

Janis Vallely, my agent extraordinaire: You believe in me, and for this, the world is healthier. Kim Pearson: this "kiddo" adores you and rests easy knowing you've always got my back. And finally, Annie Gross, my literary midwife: We did it, and she's beautiful! I think you are a fantastic editor and scientific researcher, and you have a heart of gold. May we always have chocolate and well-running Macs :-)

I am grateful to friends, colleagues, and researchers who offered brilliant insight along the way: Dr. Nan Fuchs, Dr. David S. Klein, Dr. David Perlmutter, Dr. Gregory Johnson, Dr. David Zava, Dr. Patrick Hanaway, Dr. Isaac Eliaz, Dr. Alan Miller, Dr. Mark Stengler, and Virginia Hopkins.

Contents

Introduction

Do you really think that today's healthcare system wants you to know about plant-derived cures for diabetes? Without you, business could crumble. In the meantime, the diabetes epidemic is stealing the life (and limbs) out of people. As the great motivational speaker and philosopher Jim Rohn once said, "If someone is going down the wrong road, he doesn't need motivation to speed him up. What he needs is education to turn him around."

It's a good thing you're holding my book because I'm going to give you the education of a lifetime in the coming pages. The first lesson is this: To get well, you must change your thinking, rather than wait for medicine to change its treatment plan.

I am sure that without you, your family suffers. So I will help you change the way you think about your condition, your meals, your medicine, your kitchen, and, most of all, your ability to heal. You have this power, and you can heal yourself. You just need some guidance to get turned around.

I promise to give you scientifically researched options to help you avoid complications such as nerve pain, heart disease, and vision loss. I have delved into the most remote corners of medicine to find the most incredible studies that support the use of natural herbs, vitamins, and minerals. Why the most remote corners? Because Mother Nature produces plants that give us good "medicine," but no one can expect to make big profits from these. You don't see TV commercials for these holistic items, nor is any money spent on promoting natural products to physicians.

Before I was a syndicated columnist and author, I worked as a retail pharmacist and also a consultant for nursing home residents. What I learned is that our healthcare system is focused on masking symptoms rather than healing people. This is why I've spent many years studying functional medicine principles, which do not advocate the use of prescribed medications, unless necessary.

I pride myself on thinking "outside the pill," and my special educational background allows me to view illness from the perspective of biochemical imbalance—

that illness represents a "glitch" in your system. So I'm less focused on which medications will reduce your blood glucose and more focused on what nutrient you are deficient in, or what hormones you are missing. Conventional medicine offers patented drug therapies attempting to minimize the symptoms of diabetes, whereas functional medicine offers minerals, vitamins, or other nonprescription supplements to restore a deficiency.

If you have diabetes, your doctor has made you focus on lowering your blood sugar numbers, which means you eat a restricted diet, you may have to take medications, and you probably have to poke holes in your fingers to track your blood sugar. Do you realize that measuring blood glucose by itself is fairly useless? Are you aware that some of the foods promoted as "healthy" to patients with diabetes could actually kill brain cells?

If you've been told that you can't make insulin anymore, that might be wrong, too. I've found supplements that regenerate beta cells and help produce more insulin. I want to teach you how to take good care of yourself. Then you can spread the word about how you lost weight and did the impossible—cured yourself of a supposedly incurable disease. It can be done. I can teach you about inexpensive supplements and herbs that reprogram your genes to create better health. I can teach you how to retrain your palate to not crave sweets anymore. The body can heal. Healing begins in your mind first, so believe in yourself.

Do not let anyone tell you that diabetes is not reversible, or that there is no cure. Make a commitment today, to learn more, take healthy supplements, and eat more living, raw foods. With commitment and effort, the abundant health you dream of can be yours. Wrap your mind around thoughts of healing and wellness. You will have taken a crucial first step toward recovery because the body follows the mind.

A WORD OF CAUTION

The information presented in this book is based on the education, training, and professional experience of the author. Any time you make changes to your medication regimen, you should consult your physician. The herbs, vitamins, minerals, treatments, and diet recommendations in this book should not be taken without consulting your physician to be sure that they are right for you, with your particular medical history.

It is essential that you receive appropriate laboratory and clinical monitoring even when using natural treatments recommended in this book. The purpose of this book is to convey information and is for educational purposes only. It is not intended to treat, cure, or diagnose your condition. It is intended to raise awareness of potential natural therapies for health and wellness. Suggested dosages for dietary supplements are intended as general guidelines. Please comply with your treating physician's orders. The publisher and author expressly disclaim all liability for any injury that may arise from the use of the information contained in this book or the supplements that have been recommended.

PART 1
UNDERSTANDING DIABETES

CHAPTER 1

It's Not Science Fiction; It's on Your Plate

Some ingredients in your food have the potential to give you diabetes. Surprised? Well, consider the possibility that you've never been given the whole truth about the ingredients in the foods that you love. You've not been told just how bad they are, or how they contribute to disease.

Relax! This isn't going to be a lecture on what you should or should not eat. This is just a story. Let's go on a journey together . . .

Once upon a time, a crop of wheat spent months growing in a serene field in Kansas. The farmer had taken special care before planting the seeds to make sure the soil was tilled and properly fertilized. He sprayed the field with various pesticides, fungicides, and other chemicals to protect the harvest. And there we have our first problem. It shocks me, but 83 of the active ingredients in pesticides are still in use even though studies have shown that they can cause cancer in animals or humans.

After the Kansas farmer's wheat matured and turned a beautiful golden color, he harvested the grain and placed it in a grain elevator until he was ready to sell it. Any time wheat is placed in storage, workers need to keep an eye on it, making sure it stays cool and dry, because rainy, warm weather promotes the growth of fungus. Of particular concern is *Fusarium graminearum*, a fungus that can infect both animals and people. It can cause vomiting, loss of appetite, diarrhea, staggering, skin irritation, and immune system suppression.

Wheat kernels are typically ground into various types of flour. In my story, the Kansas farmer's wheat is destined to be turned into "all-purpose flour" because demand for this flour is high. And here we have the second problem (actually the third if you count the possibility of fungal contamination).

To make all-purpose flour, wheat kernels must be stripped of their bran and germ layers. This stripping process removes the most nutritious parts of the grain, such as the fiber, minerals, and vitamins. Oddly enough, this flour will probably command a higher price than natural whole wheat flour because it will go through more processing.

The insanity doesn't stop there, though. The flour—which is naturally brown—still needs to be whitened using a chemical that is standard in the flour industry, chlorine gas. The Environmental Protection Agency categorizes chlorine gas as a pesticide and defines it as a flour-bleaching, aging, and oxidizing agent that is a powerful irritant, dangerous to inhale, and lethal. Chlorine gas, when it comes in contact with wheat, also forms another substance called alloxan, which is known to destroy pancreatic function. *Did you catch that?*

ALLOXAN TOXIN: IT'S IN YOUR BREAD

Alloxan is so good at destroying the pancreas that scientists even use it in clinical trials to induce diabetes in lab animals! It is a well-documented fact that bleached white flour is contaminated with alloxan. Who would do such a thing? Someone (and that someone is probably a megacorporation) who makes a living from turning wheat into flour, that's who.

Let's take a closer look at this toxin. As mentioned above, when flour is processed in modern mills to make white flour, it undergoes a chlorine gas bath (chlorine dioxide). Other chemicals are used, too, including benzoyl peroxide, which people apply externally to zap their zits.

Anyway, chlorine gas reacts with some proteins in the flour and produces alloxan as a by-product. Alloxan is anything but pure, and it's never disclosed on labels of products that use bleached white flour. In animals, alloxan destroys beta cells, the specialized group of cells in the pancreas that make insulin. And insulin, as you know, reduces your blood sugar levels.

So in short, the more alloxan consumed, the more likely the development of diabetes, at least in lab animals. This isn't a secret. Scientists routinely use alloxan to destroy the pancreas of lab animals, usually rodents.

Alloxan looks similar to glucose, so it's readily taken up by beta cells, where it sparks tremendous free-radical damage and kills the cells so they no longer produce insulin. When enough beta cells die, insulin production stops.

Researchers inject the healthy animals with alloxan to induce diabetes. When the animal is sick, they test certain drugs to determine drug efficacy. Does this mean that alloxan can similarly destroy the beta cells in the human pancreas, thereby closing down insulin production and causing diabetes? Do you want to find out by exposing your own pancreas to this deadly substance?

Alloxan is in almost all commercial baked goodies made with white flour. Is it just me, or do you feel like a guinea pig, too?

The U.S. milling industry produces about 140 million pounds of flour each day, and the use of chlorides for bleaching flour is considered an industry standard. Alloxan is a by-product of the bleaching process. Since food manufacturers aren't actually adding alloxan to the flour, it's not going to appear on ingredient labels. But usually between 5 and 15 grams per 100 grams of flour could be contaminated. This means that the next soft white bun you reach for is not only void of nutrition but also contains potential poisons.

If you eat *anything* made with white flour, you are probably eating alloxan regularly. Believe me, the average American eats far more pounds of baked goodies per year than fruits and vegetables (which weigh more).

And with that much consumption, I'm guessing you may be one of the people who eats a lot of alloxan without even knowing it. Shocked? I hope so, because I want you to remain motivated to avoid foods that spike your blood sugar and potentially damage your pancreas.

The *Textbook of Natural Medicine* calls alloxan a "potent beta-cell toxin." It's a shame that the FDA sanctions the use of this chemical in products that people eat every day. I honestly don't think you have a death wish, because you are reading my book trying to get well and are clearly willing to make changes. I'm so proud of you for taking this step.

It's a wonder to me that white bread and other products made with white flour can put a person at risk for diabetes and all of its complications, such as diabetic coma, amputation, blindness, kidney failure, nerve pain, and eventual death. A man named Jack used to come to the pharmacy where I worked in the late 1990s, and he had diabetes. I told him to give up white flour goods and gluten-containing foods. He didn't want to. I saw him last year—unfortunately, he had given up his right leg instead. As a complication of diabetes, that leg had to be amputated. I'll never know for sure if my suggestion would have helped him, but I think it could have. I'm going to teach you in subsequent chapters how to cook with flours that are not contaminated with toxins such as alloxan.

Turning naturally dark, nutrition-packed wheat into white, nutritionally empty flour happens as a result of the strong demand from consumers to eat muffins, pastries, breads, and biscuits that are white, not brown. I have always been puzzled at the name "all-purpose flour" because to me, it doesn't even serve the primary purpose of food, which is to provide nutritional value, so I think it should be renamed "no-purpose flour."

Many people buy wheat germ to add to their baking recipes or to supplement

VITAMIN E PROTECTS YOU

The toxin alloxan, which is found in most white flour, can damage the pancreas. But even if you've been eating white flour goodies for decades, there are still things you can do to help minimize the problem. First of all, *stop* eating white flour from this day forward. Whole grain flour is better (so long as you are not gluten intolerant), and almond flour, rice flour, or quinoa flour are even better alternatives. Those are the ones I use in my house.

If you've been eating a lot of white bread, buns, and biscuits all your life, there's something you can take to help reverse the damage—vitamin E. In animal studies, this potent antioxidant protected lab rats from alloxan damage.

I know we're not rats, but we are mammals (just like rats), and I think taking a powerful antioxidant, such as natural vitamin E, could be beneficial for you, especially if you have consumed a diet high in white flour products or you have a history of diabetes in your family. Try taking 400 IU of mixed natural vitamin E tocopherols daily.

their diet. If you buy wheat germ, guess what you're doing? You're paying a lot of money to buy the nutrients that were stripped in the process of making all-purpose flour. You have to realize that wheat germ is where most of the essential nutrients in wheat are concentrated, including vitamin E, folate (folic acid), phosphorus, thiamin, zinc, magnesium, essential fatty acids, and fiber.

HOW SWEET IT ISN'T

Now let's return to the story I was telling you before I went into my rant about white flour. Let's turn our attention to another farmer. This farmer lives in Florida and grows sugar cane in his semitropical fields. His sugar cane will eventually be pressed to produce molasses, a healthy sweetener. There are three grades of molasses: mild or first molasses, dark or second molasses, and the most intense, dark form, blackstrap molasses. And as you guessed, I'm all for your choosing blackstrap molasses, as it contains energy-producing iron, bone-building calcium, and a wealth of other healthy minerals.

Now here comes the real head-scratcher. Most of the molasses that comes from sugar cane does not end up on grocery store shelves as molasses. Instead, molasses is stripped of its life-giving vitamins, minerals, and fiber as it is processed into white sugar crystals, the kind you find in big bags at the supermarket.

So most sugar cane—which can produce nutrition-rich molasses—instead becomes nothing more than an alien substance that is never found in nature. Hey, but it tastes good, right?!

Nutritionally naked sugar crystals are very sweet. They are also bleached because Americans think white sugar is pretty. (I know; it doesn't make sense to me either.)

RECIPE FOR DIABETES

Now let's conduct an experiment. We'll combine the white all-purpose flour with white sugar and add some white table salt. Add a pinch of baking powder, a little baking soda, and some yeast (which is a form of fungus). Now add some liquid, such as cow's milk, which may be linked to diabetes, but more about that in Chapter 4.

Heat this goopy substance to about 350°F. It will rise and expand. When it cools off, we'll deep-fry it in refined vegetable oil loaded with trans fats that don't readily dissolve in your bloodstream and therefore cut off blood flow to your heart. Now let's cool off the deadly time bomb. And to make it attractive we'll paint it pink with a sticky mixture made from red food coloring, white sugar, and some more greasy trans fats. This is a good time to tell you that the red food colorant comes from boiling and crushing cochineals, insects also known as bee-tle bugs. *Ewww!*

Does what we made sound appetizing to you?

Would you eat it or serve it to your kids?

Could I get you to eat it for a hundred dollars?

How about if I serve it with coffee and call it a doughnut?

A PILL FOR EVERY ILL

That story may have been hard to swallow, but if you eat bagels, muffins, hamburger buns, or any other product made from white flour, the story line remains pretty much the same. The American diet is laden with dangerous chemicals that promote diabetes. Even people who think that they eat healthy have kitchens full of canned, boxed, or processed foods.

People think wheat flour is good for them when they see it on the label, but wheat flour it just another way to say white flour. Think of it this way. When a recipe reads "add 1 cup of flour," don't you just automatically pour into your measuring cup regular all-purpose white flour that you buy from the grocery store in those big bags? It probably doesn't dawn on you to use any other kind.

That's what wheat flour is, and though you may think it's healthy, it's really not. As you saw in our story, it has been heavily refined and then bleached white. This type of junk flour looks nothing like the beautiful, nutrient-dense grain it was made from.

We are trained to think that flour comes one way, and we follow our taste buds like zombies in the dark. I promise that in the chapters to follow you will learn all about eating healthy, nutritious, tasty foods *without* compromising your health.

Now do you believe me when I tell you that you are not given the whole truth about the foods you eat? Twenty-five years of nutritional advice from brain-dead health officials has only made us fatter and sicker.

Our life expectancy at birth in America is now estimated to be around 77.9 years. In 1995 it was 75.8, and in 1955, it was 69.6 years, according to a report from the National Center for Health Statistics. So far, it all sounds pretty good, right? But the report also contains the fact that in 40 other countries, life expectancy is higher than it is the United States. By the way, the top place goes to Andorra, a tiny country in the Pyrenees Mountains between France and Spain, whose citizens' life expectancy is estimated to be 83.5 years. Japan is number two. Macau, San Marino, and Singapore rank third, fourth, and fifth.

We have been seriously duped. Ah, but no worries, doctors can prescribe lots of pills to bring your blood sugar level down. And more drugs to lower your cholesterol, some to reduce your blood pressure, and, of course, for all that belching and indigestion, there are acid blockers. You may need insulin shots by now, too. It's the American way, a pill for every ill.

When the medications stop working for you—and eventually they will—you might wind up with a bad infection, so bad that antibiotics fail to help you. Then doctors might need to cut off your limbs, one at a time. You'll have to take more drugs for the excruciating pain, depression, and insomnia. You might wind up in a nursing home because family members cannot care for you any longer.

Gosh, sorry. This story is suddenly taking a dark turn. This doesn't have to be *your* fate, however—not if you carefully follow the dietary and lifestyle advice presented in this book. But unfortunately this will be the horrific fate for many, since 24 million people in the United States struggle with diabetes and an estimated 221 million battle the disease worldwide. Back in 2000, the World Health Organization proclaimed there was a "global epidemic of obesity," and the numbers of people with diabetes have been climbing ever since. It doesn't have to be that way. Open your mind. You *can* heal yourself.

If you were paying attention at the beginning of this chapter, then by now you've realized that you are not given the whole truth about what you eat. Instead, you are awash in colorful advertisements for foods that contain god-awful ingredients, accompanied by advertisements for medications that mask the problems that eating these foods brings about.

THE TIME FOR CHANGE IS NOW

Corporations with the money to call all the shots put lots of unsafe food chemicals into our food supply. Then they try to sell us more chemicals in the form of drugs, as if drugs could miraculously neutralize the damage done by the American diet. Yeah, right. Fast food, fast infirmity.

I have a novel idea for food manufacturers. *Why not change the foods we eat?* It's like the pink elephant in the room, and yet Americans don't want to talk about it. I guess someone has convinced us that our situation can be managed only with drugs or the diet plan offered by the American Diabetes Association, which I happen to take issue with. I'll tell you why in a later chapter. But for now, do make one commitment. Don't eat any more white baked goodies, okay?

In my house, I don't eat or serve my family anything made with white flour. There is no white table salt and no white sugar around here. (The story on salt is in Chapter 9.) If you want to get healthier and save your pancreas, make that your number one rule: NO WHITE.

I want your flour, sugar, and salt to all have some color, and I'll tell you exactly what to purchase and cook with in later chapters. But for now, **no more white**. Go ahead and take your first healthy step toward wellness. Make that commitment today.

DON'T KILL YOUR KIDS WITH KINDNESS

Several generations have been raised on chemically processed, nutritionally void foods with pretty labels on them. Have you ever watched Saturday morning cartoons? There are nonstop advertisements for foods that contain a lot of artificial, dangerous ingredients and preservatives—which will extend the shelf life of the food longer than the life expectancy of the child!

Parents don't want to be mean to their kids, so they buy them all the foods their kids nag them for, foods that they've seen on TV commercials. With brainwashing like this, our children are expected to die younger than their kind parents, who acquiesce to their requests for individually wrapped kiddie-crapola. These foods don't even support life forms like mold!

How do our children benefit nutritionally? Clearly, they don't. The latest statistics I saw in 2009 stated that one person is diagnosed with a form of diabetes every 3 minutes in the United Kingdom. According to another report published in London in December 2007, a study of more than 1,000 British children age 10 to 14 showed that many of them will die at an age a decade younger than when their parents will die! So if their parents live to be, say, 76 or 77, the kids will die at age 66 or 67. And it's all because they are eating too much junk food, are not eating their fruits and veggies, and are couch potatoes to boot. Here are the statistics from the study:

- Sixty-two percent of the kids did not eat the recommended five servings of fruit and veggies per day.
- Nearly 18 percent ate fewer than three full servings of fruits and veggies daily.
- Some 39 percent did not eat breakfast every day.
- Fully 20 percent of the kids said they didn't eat any lunch at least once a week.
- And 63 percent—that's almost two out of every three kids in the study—said that during the week, they ate at least one "takeaway meal." (That's British for fast-food takeout.)

And the deadly white frosting on the toxic white cake here is that these kids in the United Kingdom are relatively sedentary; 48 percent said they exercise for less than an hour a day; 17 percent said they get no exercise at all!

All of this information prompted David Haslam, clinical director of the National Obesity Forum in England (formed in 2000 in response to the alarming rate of obesity in the United Kingdom), to declare the 10-year sentence on these children who, after all, didn't mean to do anything wrong. They are the victims of the crime, and yet they are the ones who won't get the chance to do the time.

NUMBER JUNKIES

It's not just British scientists who pay attention to numbers.

Americans in general are fixated on lowering all kinds of trackable numbers—those for cholesterol, triglycerides, and blood sugar. We are all eating ourselves sick. Yet we've been indoctrinated into a mind-set that we can eat whatever we want, so long as we take this little pill and our blood sugar falls into the "normal" range.

IS IT THE CHICKEN OR THE EGG?

A Harvard study published in February 2009 found that people who ate an egg per day were 58 to 77 percent more likely to develop type 2 diabetes than non–egg lovers. This study was large, analyzing 57,000 people. Eating seven or more eggs per week will increase risk for death by 50 percent if you have diabetes, so go easy on them. Chicken lovers may be on to something, though. A small study done on 28 people found that those who eat chicken (and low-protein diets in general) enjoyed lower cholesterol and reduced serum creatinine, which is great news for your kidneys.

So which is better, the chicken or the egg? If you're not vegan, I say both, just in moderation. Eggs are an inexpensive source of high-quality protein, and they contain important nutrients, such as vitamins, minerals, antioxidants, and good unsaturated fats. So if you like eggs, just limit them to three per week or use them only for baking, like I do. Buy free-range eggs because they have more nutritional value than factory-farmed eggs. And eat freshly cooked chicken or turkey, so long as it's hormone-free, lean, and natural, not processed deli meat.

Americans are number junkies, focusing way too much on what the glucometer reads and not enough on what we eat. Sad but true, the American healthcare system is more concerned with teaching you how to track your blood sugar number than with teaching you how to repair your pancreas, reduce systemic inflammation, and, most important, how to do it without drugs.

Even though drugs put a cap on your blood sugar, they don't permanently solve the problem. In fact, they may make it worse. Think about it. Where does all the blood sugar go when your medicine pushes it out of your bloodstream? It doesn't dissolve. It doesn't go poof and magically disappear! It gets deposited onto your abdomen, thighs, and butt. In other words, the drugs turn the excess sugar into fat, or they force the sugar into surrounding cells against their will. This process kills innocent bystander cells.

The diabetes disease process continues, despite your medication. Innocent cells die as excessive sugar is forced into them. But when your doctor measures your blood sugar level, or when you take your own readings with a glucometer, the sugar levels are fine. People still cheat on their diet—and you know who you are!—but as long as that blood sugar level is in range, you and millions of other number junkies will continue to eat the same dangerous nutritionally void foods.

Other important factors in keeping your blood sugar levels under control, things such as exercise, alternative remedies, and, yes, even medications when

> ## SKIP THE SULFUR
>
> If you enjoy molasses, make sure you get the unsulfured kind, which is made from mature sugar cane without any chemicals. Unsulfured molasses contains extremely low, naturally occurring levels of sulfites. Sulfured molasses, on the other hand, is made from young, green sugar cane, and a preservative, sulfur dioxide, is added during the extraction process. This creates mayhem for people who have sulfite sensitivities! Why would we need more chemicals in something as pure as molasses? I've never understood it either.

appropriate. But first, it will be helpful to take a closer look at diabetes, how it manifests in your body, and what the symptoms and risk factors are. You'll find that information in Chapter 2.

REVERSING DIABETES

Finally, I want to assure you that in many cases it is indeed possible to reverse diabetes. Here are some of the things that can help do just that. We will be looking at all of these in greater detail throughout this book:

- Look inside your medicine cabinet to see if you take a drug that causes hyperglycemia. That may be *all* you need to do. Statins, which lower cholesterol, can cause high blood sugar.
- Exercise to increase your fat burning potential.
- Reduce cholesterol, blood pressure, and inflammatory chemicals in your body.
- Take antioxidants and green supplements to reduce free-radical damage.
- Take supplements that activate the PGC-1 alpha and SIRT1 genes. (I promise, this is not complicated.)
- Spur those powerhouses in your cells (mitochondria) to detoxify you.
- Eat a diet rich in natural organic fruits and vegetables and low in animal fats.
- Eat healthy carbohydrates and fiber-rich foods.
- Quit smoking and reduce alcohol consumption.
- Avoid foods that contain high-fructose corn syrup.
- Find and correct deficiencies of iron (ferritin) and thyroid hormone that lead to diabetes.

CHAPTER 2

The Many Faces of Diabetes: Know Your Risk Factors

All food, including that beef Stroganoff you had last night, must be broken down into its smallest particles so that nutrients can get into your bloodstream. These nutrients include fats, amino acids, and sugars. With diabetes, all eyes are on sugar.

Insulin is a hormone that your pancreas produces. Think of insulin as a bus, and its passenger is sugar. After you eat, certain parts of your food are converted to sugar, which ends up in your bloodstream. The sugar in your blood hops on the "blood sugar bus"—insulin—and gets toted around your body. Insulin drops the sugar off at various stops in your body, such as your brain cells, so you can think; your muscle cells, so you can move; and your heart cells, so it can beat.

Are you with me? There isn't a set schedule for the bus stops. Where the sugar gets unloaded is based on the needs of your body. In a healthy person, all of your cells welcome the sugar delivery. Insulin drives up and unlocks a little door to each cell—the cell's receptor site—so the sugar can get in. Once inside, the party starts, and sugar starts making energy for you. You want sugar *inside* your cells, not loitering outside in the bloodstream.

When you exercise, the blood sugar bus (insulin) drives faster and drops off more sugar (glucose) to your muscle cells to give you an energy boost. When you're reading this book, your cells don't need as much energy, so the blood sugar bus stops delivering the sugar to your muscle cells and drives it over to your liver for later use. The liver is like a parking garage, where the insulin bus stores some of the sugar in the form of glycogen. *Insulin shuttles sugar from your blood INTO your cells.* Got it?

Your body can use only so much sugar at a given time, but it can store any extra sugar from your diet in the form of glycogen to use later. All this takes place under the influence of insulin. In the liver, *excess* sugar undergoes a conversion and gets stored as cholesterol and triglycerides. Isn't that a shocker? *Excess sugar is turned into cholesterol and triglycerides,* yes fat!

If you have diabetes, it simply means that your body's sugar delivery system is out of whack. Either your pancreas is not making enough insulin to meet your needs, or your cells are not able to receive the sugar delivery that your insulin is trying to make. Before we look at the different kinds of diabetes, let's take a look at the warning signs that indicate you may have a problem.

WARNING SIGNS OF HIGH BLOOD SUGAR AND DIABETES

Many people get a surprise when the doctor hands them a diabetes or a prediabetes diagnosis. They go to the doctor for a routine checkup or because of some specific complaint, such as back pain or fatigue, and their lab work comes back with the bad news that their blood sugar is way too high.

If they were really paying attention to their bodies, however, they wouldn't be surprised. As diabetes develops, it announces itself in all kinds of ways, some of them subtle and others really in your face.

FEELING THIRSTY. Your mouth feels dry, and you want to keep your lips planted on the water fountain, despite the line of people forming behind you.

Dehydration is actually about your brain, not your mouth, even though your mouth is dry. Don't believe me? Your brain cells need a steady supply of glucose. When your brain is bathed in overly concentrated sugar water, it will summon fluid from any source to dilute the uncomfortable fluid surrounding each cell. Your brain gets this fluid from other cells, which leads to dehydration. You may have the urge to drink copious amounts of fluid as your body tries to overcome the lack of water.

Soda pop junkies, you're fooling yourself if you think that drinking soda will hydrate you. It never will. Read more about the dangers of soda pop in Chapter 15, where I offer a recipe for healthy alternatives. For now, drink more pure, filtered water. You can do it!

FREQUENT TRIPS TO THE BATHROOM. It makes sense that if you are drinking more water because of constant thirst, then you will be urinating a lot too. You are staring at (or sitting on) the potty more than normal because there is too much sugar in your blood and your kidneys are getting a serious sugar bath.

If your kidneys could speak, they'd say, "Hey, what's the deal here? I'm overwhelmed, so I'm going to pull extra water out of your blood to dilute all this sugar!" Essentially, the floodgates open as your kidneys continuously draw extra water out of your blood in an effort to dilute the sugar bath coming through. All this water fills your bladder, and this sensation causes the urge to pee. Then you become thirsty again, and have to drink more water in an attempt to rehydrate. And the cycle continues.

Your kidneys do their best to eliminate excess glucose. The amount of protein spilling into the urine also increases with time, which interferes with normal kidney filtration. If your kidneys can't filter wastes properly, toxins build up in your bloodstream. The insidious thing is that kidney damage can occur even when blood sugar is controlled by medication. Read Chapter 9 to learn about ways to protect your kidneys.

WEAKNESS AND FATIGUE. Many people feel run down and don't realize that their chronic exhaustion is related to blood sugar problems. The symptoms of fatigue can be easily masked with a mocha latte. Starbucks has a booming business, in part because of the ever-expanding population of tired, weak people with insulin resistance (and no wallet resistance).

When the glucose from your meals can't get into your cells, your cells can't make energy, so you feel tired all the time. Not to mention that exasperating sense of hunger when you just ate a little while ago. What's up with that? If glucose from your meals is locked out of your cells, you never get the energy boost or that satisfying sense of fullness after you eat. Bummer.

NUMBNESS AND TINGLING IN YOUR HANDS OR FEET. This sneaky symptom is really about nerve damage, and can take months or even years to show up. Your doctor terms this pain *neuropathy*. Neuropathy occurs because the bloodstream is overwhelmed with glucose, which is like acid to your nerves. It damages the delicate nerve endings that extend to the hands, legs, and feet. That's when you start to feel the pain, numbness, tingling, itching, and other weird sensations that you may be experiencing. If you have this symptom, you should discuss it with a neurologist in addition to your regular doctor. The good news is that for many people, it can be minimized or managed with several inexpensive, over-the-counter supplements that I'll tell you about in Chapter 10.

BLURRY VISION. If your blood glucose levels remain high, fluid may be pulled from your tissues for dilution purposes—including fluid from the lenses of your eyes. This may affect your ability to focus. Also, teeny tiny capillaries that lead to your eyes become damaged from all the free radicals. Free radicals are damaging molecules that people with diabetes produce in alarming quantities. This is why antioxidants are so important for anyone who has this disease. Antioxidants help neutralize free radicals. I take vision seriously, and if yours is starting to slip, please read Chapter 7 to learn about supplements to help you see the light (and the shadows)! In my opinion, it is never too late to try improving your eyesight, even if you are legally blind.

SKIN PROBLEMS. Some people with type 2 diabetes have patches of dark skin in the folds and creases of their bodies—usually in the armpit, neck, knuckles, and groin. It almost looks like dirt, except you can't wash it off. Sometimes it looks velvety or bumpy. There may be skin tags around these darkened hyperpigmented areas. This condition, called acanthosis nigricans, is a sign of insulin resistance. It means that your body is producing too much insulin in response to excessive blood glucose.

INFECTIONS. Frequent bladder and vaginal infections can be a particular problem for women with diabetes. You would think that taking antibiotics would simply cure a person's infection, but it's not that easy. In the general population, not just among people with diabetes, antibiotic resistance has weakened our ability to defend ourselves against microbes. This resistance is a deadly consequence of many years of indiscriminate prescribing of antibiotics.

Wounds and skin infections are slow to heal in the person with type 2 diabetes, so please read Chapter 10 to learn about wound care and natural skin-savers. I want to emphasize this now because skin infections that cannot be healed could lead to gangrene and ultimately amputation of a foot or limb. It's much easier to prevent a wound than it is to cure it, just as it's much easier to not smoke than it is to cure lung cancer. (Don't worry, I'm climbing down from my soapbox for the moment, but I'll be back.)

LOSING WEIGHT WITHOUT TRYING. Many people with diabetes or prediabetes want to munch all day. Because their cells ignore insulin, which can no longer effectively move blood sugar (energy) into those cells, their muscles and organs feel famished. Improper fluctuations of hormones such as ghrelin (a hunger hormone) and leptin (a feel-full hormone) complicate things and trigger intense hunger. The interesting thing is that you may lose weight without even trying, even though you nosh all day long. Great, right? Wrong!

This kind of weight loss causes you to lose muscle mass. It occurs in part because your body is looking for some energy or fuel (think glucose), and it breaks down muscle cells to get it. Without a constant source of glucose in your cells, your muscle tissues shrink. This is especially noticeable with type 1 diabetes. With type 2, this symptom of weight loss is imperceptible for years because most people with type 2 diabetes are overweight to begin with and the subtle weight loss flies under the radar. Losing weight *is* important if you have diabetes, but I want you to lose fat, not muscle.

THE MANY FACES OF DIABETES

I'm not so hung up on the name of your condition. In fact, I think many people who have been told they have diabetes don't really have certifiable diabetes, but high blood sugar according to lab tests for some other reason, perhaps the result of another medication.

It's easy to get slapped with a label of diabetes when your blood sugar levels come back high after a lab test, but that doesn't mean you have a full-blown case of diabetes. It does mean you have to take action and find a doctor who understands biochemistry so he or she can figure out *why* your sugar levels are up, rather than just putting you in the standard bucket and starting all the standard treatments for diabetes.

Having high blood sugar (hyperglycemia) is the proper term given to people when their blood sugar rises. It's not the same thing as having diabetes, which is a very complex inflammatory disease.

In my opinion, and that of many medical experts, diabetes is a disease that is related to a lot of free-radical damage, high levels of inflammatory chemicals, lazy chemical pathways, and nutritional deficiencies. There are also some rather complicated medical possibilities. It could be related to enzymatic pathways that are tied to your genetic structure (PGC-1 alpha and SIRT1). This may be the single most important reason behind metabolic disorders such as diabetes. But I don't want to get into these complicated pathways here. I'll discuss these in Chapter 3.

The point is that there has to be a *reason* that your blood sugar is abnormal. If you have a good doctor, he or she will take the time to figure out why, rather than quickly dismissing you with a quick diagnosis of diabetes and starting you on the medication merry-go-round. If you know the reason, you may be able to fix it and reverse or at least manage your condition without any negative outcomes associated with unmanaged diabetes.

One of the major reasons people develop blood sugar and insulin dysglycemia (a scientific term that basically means abnormal glucose metabolism) is that they don't exercise. Exercising changes the way your body processes foods and the way it responds to insulin. Another reason people ultimately get diabetes, is that they eat food portions so large that their pancreas gets overwhelmed and initially insulin levels go up. If they stay up, the pancreas eventually tires out. Remember, insulin is like a bus, and eventually the pancreas that fuels the bus can run out of gas. Let me put this in better perspective. (We'll take a detailed look at the pancreas and how to protect it in Chapter 3.)

When you analyze the blood of an individual who has a normal fasting level of glucose, there is about 1 teaspoonful of sugar in approximately 5 quarts of blood. What do you think happens to the blood sugar bus when you besiege it with a can of soda pop, which contains 10 to 15 teaspoonfuls of sugar? Over time your cells reject the sugar that is being dropped off at their doorstep, shouting "ENOUGH is ENOUGH!"

The point I'm trying to make here is that there are all kinds of reasons your blood sugar reading may be too high. And some of those reasons are *not* diabetes. Here's an overview of the various conditions that come under the abnormal blood sugar umbrella.

PREDIABETES

According to the American Diabetes Association, about 57 million Americans have prediabetes, also known as insulin resistance, hyperinsulinemia, or hyperglycemia. Prediabetes is defined as having a fasting blood sugar (FBS) reading of 100 to 125 mg/dl (milligrams per deciliter). This is not quite high enough to give you a diagnosis of type 2 diabetes, but it means you are on your way unless you intervene now.

What's actually going on in your body if you have prediabetes? Let's go back to that blood sugar bus—insulin. Your pancreas manufactures insulin in adequate amounts, and that insulin bus drives sugar to all your body's cells, but your cells won't open their doors. So the homeless sugar has to dilly-dally out in the bloodstream instead of going inside the cells where you need it.

Your cells don't get fed their sugar, so your body makes more and more insulin because it is frantic to GET THE SUGAR INSIDE THE CELL!!! Because your cells are resistant to it, your insulin levels keep rising in an effort to force the sugar out of the bloodstream and into the cells. And the cells keep thumbing their noses at all this extra insulin, which causes weight gain, by the way. At this stage, serum insulin (if evaluated) may be very high, though FBS are only mildly elevated.

TYPE 2 DIABETES

People with insulin resistance (prediabetes) usually go on to develop type 2 diabetes, which is the most common form of the disease. With all those cells thumbing their noses at insulin and refusing to let the blood sugar in, the sugar collects outside the doorstep, in your blood. Blood sugar remains chronically high with fasting blood sugars at 126 mg/dl or higher.

A lot of the excess sugar in the bloodstream gets converted and tucked away as cholesterol and triglycerides. This stuff is what clogs up your arteries. Excessive sugar and the subsequent rise in insulin are also what make a person overweight. Weight gain is not as tightly related to fat intake as it is to sugar intake.

But type 2 diabetes isn't just about high blood sugar. This disorder is also about excessive inflammatory chemicals and low levels of protective antioxidants. Diabetes affects circulation, cholesterol, and other major hormones in the body.

The excess sugar traveling round and round on the insulin bus in your body with nowhere to call home starts to build up in tiny capillaries and arteries that lead to the kidneys, eyes, heart, and nerves. It contributes to the squeezing off of your entire pipeline—blood flow, which equals life. So now circulation is compromised because the blood can't flow properly. Inflammation builds up, so your body is basically on fire at a cellular level.

As if all this isn't bad enough, if you have type 2 diabetes your brain can't properly receive the messages delivered by the feel-full hormone known as leptin. Leptin is the hormone that tells your brain that you need to stop eating. If your brain can't respond properly to leptin's signal, you will keep eating and eating and eating.

These and other factors are what can lead to the devastating consequences of unmanaged type 2 diabetes, such as kidney failure, blindness, heart attack, stroke, and nerve pain.

TYPE 1 DIABETES

According to the Juvenile Diabetes Research Foundation International, as many as 3 million Americans may have type 1 diabetes. Type 1 diabetes occurs frequently in children and adolescents, so it is sometimes called juvenile diabetes. But "juvenile diabetes" is a misnomer, since adults can also be diagnosed with type 1 diabetes, and sadly, many adults are misdiagnosed as having type 2 when they really have type 1. Each year more than 15,000 children are newly diagnosed with diabetes in the United States. That's 40 children per day.

If you have type 1 diabetes, the insulin-producing cells in the pancreas—called beta cells—have been destroyed or are unable to produce insulin. This is usually the result of autoimmune destruction of the pancreas. Amazingly, some research has found an association between consumption of cow's milk and type 1 diabetes, and I'll go into details about that in Chapter 4.

With type 1 diabetes, blood sugar levels stay high because there is no insulin around to deliver the sugar to the cells. In other words, the insulin bus is on strike. In type 1 diabetes, blood sugar will remain elevated unless injections of insulin are given. Thank goodness we have insulin for this purpose, although I promise to give you other considerations that may help regenerate beta cells in Chapter 13.

TYPE 1.5 DIABETES OR LADA (LATENT AUTOIMMUNE DIABETES IN ADULTS)

Unless you're a research nerd like me, you've probably not even heard of type 1.5 diabetes, also called slow-onset type 1 diabetes or latent autoimmune diabetes in adults (LADA). This disease develops in certain people because they make antibodies against their own pancreas. This means that the immune system thinks your pancreas is an enemy invader and dispatches an attack-cell army to go destroy your pancreatic cells.

LADA requires insulin injections, unless you quickly figure out what is causing the immune system to go haywire. LADA takes years to develop and may never even get properly diagnosed unless you are insistent on a specific blood test called a C-peptide assay. This test measures "endogenous" insulin (the insulin that your body produces on its own). This is the definitive test to distinguish between type 1 and type 2 diabetes. It is definitive because people with type 2 diabetes have a normal or high level of C-peptide and people with type 1 diabetes do not.

LADA is not usually associated with insulin resistance because it occurs in slim—even fit—people, whereas type 2 diabetes normally occurs in people who are overweight.

The sad thing is that people who are misdiagnosed with type 2 diabetes (when they really have LADA) initially respond to certain diabetic medications (not Avandia or Actos) because their bodies still make insulin for a while. As a result, doctors think they are showing signs of progress. Autoimmune diabetes must be treated differently than type 2 diabetes or the disease will progress and the pancreas tissue will slowly die until you need insulin. Since casein and gluten (the proteins found in milk and wheat, respectively) can cause some autoimmune problems, please refer to Chapter 4.

GESTATIONAL DIABETES

Gestational diabetes starts during pregnancy, especially in women over age 25. Being overweight is a risk factor. Because of the obesity epidemic, gestational diabetes is on the rise. Certain ethnic groups, such as Hispanic, Native American, African American, and Asian women, have higher rates than others.

Gestational diabetes usually begins in the second trimester and is associated with preeclampsia, a dangerous condition characterized by high blood pressure and excess protein in the urine after 20 weeks of pregnancy. If untreated, preeclampsia can be fatal to infants and mothers. With treatment, gestational diabetes usually resolves after the birth of the baby, although both mother and child will have greater risks for developing type 2 diabetes later in life. Treatment of gestational diabetes also halves your risk for delivering an excessively large baby or developing preeclampsia while pregnant.

METABOLIC SYNDROME

Many people with high blood glucose levels also have high blood pressure and high blood cholesterol. This triple threat, known as metabolic syndrome, is more common than you might think. The three conditions are almost always tied together. It makes sense because high levels of glucose (strike one) damage the lining inside your arteries, so cholesterol rushes to the rescue to patch you up (so you don't bleed to death from the teeny tiny lesions everywhere).

Excess blood sugar gets stored as cholesterol and triglycerides along with all the other accompanying gunk (for lack of a better description) and clogs arteries (strike 2). The plaque causes them to stiffen or harden (atherosclerosis) and then your blood pressure increases (strike 3). That is metabolic syndrome. If some of the plaque falls apart and gets into your bloodstream, you form a blood clot. If the clot goes to your heart, it can cause a heart attack. If the clot prevents blood flow to your brain, it causes a stroke. A blood clot that travels around the body and eventually lodges in an organ can cause an embolism.

None of these situations is pretty. This is why it's so crucial for you to eat better, exercise, and integrate nutritious, healthy supplements and foods into your daily regimen. Don't be a number junkie when it comes to measuring your blood glucose because good numbers alone won't reverse the progression of metabolic syndrome that leads to diabetes. Likewise, assuming you are getting well because you have normal blood glucose doesn't mean that you have halted the progression of the underlying disease.

HYPOGLYCEMIA

If you have hypoglycemia, you're dealing with that bad boy again, glucose. Only this time the levels are way too low, about 60 to 70 mg/dl.

Hypoglycemia can occur if you don't eat for long periods of time, if you eat too many carbs alone without eating protein to balance them, or if you take too much medication or insulin. Your body does everything it possibly can to maintain a normal, steady flow of sugar, which is fuel for the body, but when there isn't enough, your brain senses the lull and sends messages all over your body to make you miserable.

This is not an excuse to eat M&Ms every few hours; however, you could justify a few of them to keep you from fainting as a result of hypoglycemia. An episode of hypoglycemia comes on quickly, sometimes within 5 to 10 minutes.

Symptoms of hypoglycemia are similar to those of a panic attack and include trembling, nervousness, palpitations, faintness, trouble thinking and speaking, and possibly intense hunger. For those with type 1 or type 2 diabetes, supplementation with chromium is known to reduce blood sugar and maybe even help them get off insulin. But the coolest thing is that chromium is also known to help people with hypoglycemia. Take this supplement only with your doctor's blessings. I'll give you more information about chromium supplements in Chapter 14.

TYPE 3 DIABETES

There's a good chance that you've never heard of type 3 diabetes. I believe that it will soon become part of our normal language. In fact, type 3 diabetes could be the new name given to people diagnosed with Alzheimer's disease. Recent breakthrough studies have shown that insulin is produced by the brain, not just the pancreas.

Amazing, isn't it? This discovery validates the work of scientists who have long studied the connection between impaired glucose metabolism and sluggish thinking. It's no secret that people with type 2 diabetes have a significantly increased risk of Alzheimer's disease, by up to 65 percent.

As a person becomes insulin resistant, the levels of blood sugar and insulin both rise in the bloodstream, but insulin in the brain falls below normal levels. Normal signaling and transmission of brain chemicals start to suffer. Proteins known as beta-amyloid accumulate in the brain. These are nasty, destructive compounds associated with Alzheimer's disease. Fewer memory molecules (ace-tylcholine) are produced, and, simultaneously (as if this isn't bad enough), an imbalance occurs with another brain chemical called glutamate, which in excess can behave like an excitotoxin that damages cells.

Researchers have tested intranasal insulin in people with Alzheimer's disease (type 3 diabetes), and it has proven to be beneficial. The discovery of the connec-tion between insulin resistance and Alzheimer's will help millions of people who are losing their memory, whether or not they have type 2 diabetes. The best way to prevent this kind of Alzheimer's seems to be to keep blood insulin levels low (by keeping blood sugar low). And, of course, this is best done by exercising and eating healthy foods as discussed throughout this book.

RISK FACTORS FOR BLOOD SUGAR DISEASE

No matter what kind of diabetes or blood sugar condition you're dealing with, it's natural to want to know how this could have happened. Why you? Why now? Many factors put you at greater risk for developing any of these conditions.

AGE. The older you are, the greater your risk for type 2 diabetes. It doesn't matter if you're slim or overweight—growing older increases your risk. It's because aging has allowed more free-radical damage to your cells, including those in your pancreas. Free-radical damage is a well-known contributing factor, both to diabetes and to many degenerative diseases. It creates inflammatory chemicals, so there would be way more inflammatory chemicals in Joan, for example, than in her younger sister Jessica.

HAVING LOVE HANDLES. It's true. While you might be more wonderful to hug and squeeze than a bony, stick-figure person, being overweight predisposes you to diabetes. It's shocking, but according to the Centers for Disease Control and Prevention (CDC), about one-third of U.S. adults—more than 72 million people—and 17.1 percent of U.S. children and adolescents (age 2 to 19 years) are obese.

Just for the record, let me give you the clinical version of what it means to be obese: According to the CDC, *overweight* and *obesity* are both labels for ranges (yes, *ranges*) of weight for a given height and these weights are more than what has been determined to be healthy. People who fall into or above these ranges have a higher likelihood of developing diabetes or metabolic syndrome.

Nowadays—which is different from when I was growing up and it was all about the number on the scale—this range is determined by looking at your weight and height and calculating your body mass index (BMI). Sounds like a measurement that aliens might use to converse about us: *"Did you determine the humanoid's body mass index?"* You can just hear the sound effects. All kidding aside, the BMI measurement does offer us a good tool, since it provides a range, and for most people, their weight happens to correlate well with the amount of body fat they carry.

Here's the formula to calculate your BMI (and please don't ask me how they came up with this, because the lengthy, convoluted answer is based on many years of research): Determine your height in inches (for example, 5 feet is 60 inches), and square it (multiply it times itself); then divide your current weight (in pounds) by this number; then multiply that number by 703—and voilà!

Here's an example: Suppose your weight is 150 pounds, and you are 5'5" (65 inches). You would multiply 65 × 65, which equals 4,225. Now divide 150 by 4,225, which equals .0355. Now multiply that number by 703. The final answer is 24.95. To determine the significance of that number, you refer to this BMI chart.

HEIGHT	WEIGHT (LB)													
5'0"	97	102	107	112	118	123	128	133	138	143	148	153	158	163
5'1"	100	106	111	116	122	127	132	137	143	148	153	158	164	169
5'2"	104	109	115	120	126	131	136	142	147	153	158	164	169	175
5'3"	107	113	118	124	130	135	141	146	152	158	163	169	175	180
5'4"	110	116	122	128	134	140	145	151	157	163	169	174	180	186
5'5"	114	120	126	132	138	144	150	156	162	168	174	180	186	192
5'6"	118	124	130	136	142	148	155	161	167	173	179	186	192	198
5'7"	121	127	134	140	146	153	159	166	172	178	185	191	198	204
5'8"	125	131	138	144	151	158	164	171	177	184	190	197	203	210
5'9"	128	135	142	149	155	162	169	176	182	189	196	203	209	216
5'10"	132	139	146	153	160	167	174	181	188	195	202	209	216	222
5'11"	136	143	150	157	165	172	179	186	193	200	208	215	222	229
6'0"	140	147	154	162	169	177	184	191	199	206	213	221	228	235
6'1"	144	151	159	166	174	182	189	197	204	212	219	227	235	242
6'2"	148	155	163	171	179	186	194	202	210	218	225	233	241	249
BMI	19	20	21	22	23	24	25	26	27	28	29	30	31	32

An adult who has a BMI between 25 and 29.9 is considered overweight. An adult with a BMI of 30 or higher is considered obese.

It's as simple as that. In the case of our 5'5" person who weighs 150 pounds, she is just on the outside edge of what this chart calls a "normal" weight, with a BMI of 24.95. I calculated mine just for fun, and it is currently 20.3.

The scary truth is that since 1980, obesity rates for adults have doubled, and rates for children have tripled (I think all those Happy Meals should be renamed Hefty Meals). Obesity rates among all groups in society—no matter the person's age, sex, race, ethnicity, socioeconomic status, education level, or geographic region—have skyrocketed to the point where officials finally noticed that we have an obesity epidemic. The CDC also estimates that about 112,000 deaths are associated with obesity each year in the United States.

The bottom line is that obesity is the number one risk factor for diabetes. According to the World Health Organization, more than 1 billion adults world-wide are overweight, and of those, at least 300 million are obese. Talk about a carbon footprint!

And we in America are not the only ones tipping the scale. Sadly, in developing countries, where people don't get adequate nutrition, many become obese because they eat empty calories.

BEING A COUCH POTATO. Lack of exercise goes hand in hand with being overweight. If you become active and start exercising, you will increase the number of muscle cells in your body. That's good because your muscle cells have more insulin receptors on them, so it's love at first sight when the blood sugar bus pulls in. Having more muscle cells means better blood sugar control.

Exercising also makes your insulin more effective because your cells demand more energy (sugar). According to a study published in the *Journal of Clinical Endocrinology and Metabolism*, just 1 hour of exercise per day for 1 week starts to increase beta-cell function and insulin sensitivity.

Of course, there are other reasons to exercise: You'll look hot and your jeans will fit better. Becoming more physically active can only improve your life, unless you're clumsy like Kramer from *Seinfeld*.

If exercising is difficult for you, then start slowly and lean into it. Begin by parking a little farther away from your destination . . . and the destination should not be Dunkin' Donuts. Take a walk around the block and continue to increase your distance. Meet a friend and walk around the park or downtown. There's always a way to get more exercise.

HEREDITY. Unfortunately, if you have a family member who has been diagnosed with type 2 diabetes, you are at greater risk for getting it yourself. But it's not entirely about genetics. Lifestyle habits learned while growing up have a huge impact. In fact, you may learn to eat a certain way from your parents, which, combined with pure genetics, is why diabetes tends to run in families.

If your parents were sedentary or if they smoked, for example, and you do the same, you are all at high risk for diabetes and other chronic or fatal diseases. If you have acquired your parents' bad habits and you have a genetic predisposition to diabetes, then you have a double whammy. You will have to work harder to change your ways.

On the other hand, just because a family member has a diagnosis of diabetes, it doesn't mean you are condemned to the same fate. It's just a risk factor. I believe that getting type 2 diabetes—or not getting it—is completely in your control.

SLEEP HABITS. It's true. Insomnia makes you more prone to diabetes, among other conditions like depression, chronic fatigue, heart disease, and high blood pressure. Research published in the *Archives of Internal Medicine* found that people who sleep 5 or fewer hours each night are two and a half times more likely to develop insulin resistance or impaired glucose tolerance.

THYROID CONDITIONS. It's hard to believe, but thyroid disease can cause diabetes. When your active thyroid hormone levels are below normal, you sort of go into hibernation and feed tired, you can't burn fat, and your insulin rises. You are much more likely to be diagnosed with insulin resistance or full-blown diabetes.

A blood test tells you a lot. If you have elevated thyroid peroxidase (TPO) antibodies in your blood, it suggests either Hashimoto's disease or Graves' disease, both autoimmune thyroid disorders. This means that your immune system is mistakenly attacking your thyroid gland, which it recognizes as an invader, thereby interfering with its ability to make thyroid hormone. It causes inflammation, weight gain, and higher levels of insulin, which lead to hyperglycemia (high blood sugar).

Having yourself tested for thyroid disease is important. If you undergo a thyroid blood test, it's best to do so in the morning right after breakfast. You should not fast before this test because that may alter your results.

Throughout this book, you will hear me repeatedly link thyroid disease to issues of the pancreas, such as insulin resistance, hyperglycemia, and full-blown diabetes. I think thyroid disease is frequently overlooked as a contributing factor to blood sugar disease and is relatively easy to fix if you have a good doctor. Fixing thyroid disease generally means that you must take medication. Prescription thyroid hormones indirectly help lower blood sugar levels and insulin levels.

In fact, if thyroid disease is causing your high blood sugar level, taking medication for it could erase this whole problem of supposed diabetes. Does this sound too good to be true? Let's look at the science.

It's a fact that TPO antibodies have been reported in 80 percent of people who have type 1 diabetes and elevated thyroid-stimulating hormone (TSH) levels, and in 10 to 20 percent of people with normal TSH levels. (TSH is a brain hormone and elevated levels may indicate thyroid disease.)

In one study of 58 patients participating in the famous Diabetes Control and Complications Trial sponsored by the National Institute of Diabetes and Digestive and Kidney Diseases, researchers began following the health and habits of 1,441 teenagers and young adults with type 1 diabetes, starting back in 1981. During the study, 33 percent of the participants developed hypothyroidism, a thyroid dysfunction in which the gland produces too little hormone.

In this specific study, individuals with elevated TPO antibodies were 18 times more likely to develop hypothyroidism than patients who were TPO negative. The majority of study participants were diagnosed with type 1 diabetes 13 years *before* being diagnosed with thyroid disease, at an average age of 33 years. This study shows a connection between thyroid and pancreas problems. I believe that's just the tip of the iceberg. Do you believe me now? Stay tuned for more information on this important connection and what to do about it.

Protecting Your Pancreas from Free-Radical Damage

Let me just tell you straight out, you are going to have to develop a love affair with your pancreas and protect it with your life. The pancreas is the organ responsible for managing your blood sugar. This organ is also important because it releases enzymes that help you digest your meals. Without these crucial enzymes, you might eat, but you wouldn't be able to digest your food. See why the pancreas is so vital to good health and good eating?

The pancreas has not been glamorized, nor has it captured as much media attention as your breasts, your prostate, and your heart have, but it requires the same care as these other vital organs. Most people don't think about their pancreas at all until it stops working properly. Just as the squeaky wheel gets the grease, over time the greasy meal may cause a squeak . . . and by that I mean in your pancreas, when you begin to feel the effects of years of unhealthy eating.

By improving the health of your pancreas, you will enjoy better health for many years, not to mention enjoy more yummy delights.

REPAIRING A DAMAGED PANCREAS

Many physicians think that the pancreas cannot be repaired, but I disagree. Why? So much new research shows that the pancreas can, indeed, be repaired and encouraged to function better.

In 2004, for example, Harvard researchers published a study in the journal *Nature* clearly showing that in laboratory animals, beta cells—the cells that produce insulin in the pancreas—were able to regenerate themselves. Although similar studies have not yet been done on humans, this is a promising development that I believe has huge implications for reversing diabetes without drugs.

In addition, multiple human studies have shown how both weight loss and exercise can increase the body's sensitivity to insulin, thus reducing insulin resistance. And insulin resistance, as we know, leads to excess sugar in the blood and ultimately to diabetes. One study published in the journal *Obesity* in 2008 looked at the effect of exercise on 24 obese adults age 68 to 72 years for

6 months. The researchers concluded that among people who both lost weight and exercised, insulin sensitivity *doubled*. That's pretty amazing, since we're talking about improved beta-cell function here.

As you know, the more sensitive your cells are to insulin, the healthier your body is. When your cells respond well to insulin, your pancreas has an easier job all the way around. The researchers in the 2008 study concluded that weight loss not only increased insulin sensitivity, thereby improving beta-cell function, but also reduced the risk of developing type 2 diabetes.

I'd say that's a pretty good deal: Choose to exercise and eat properly, and your pancreas will thank you by functioning better and reducing your chances of ever developing diabetes. And no drugs are involved, unless you count the feel-good endorphins that your brain releases when you're shaking your booty to the macarena or cycling through the hills of beautiful terrain.

ANTIOXIDANTS TO THE RESCUE

Another overlooked way to help reverse diabetes without drugs is to neutralize and eliminate the damage done by free-radical toxins by using antioxidant foods and supplements. (Free radicals are molecules that damage the body's cells.)

Researchers at University College in London, for example, reviewed studies on the relationship between eating fruit and vegetables and taking antioxidant supplements, and how either or both might affect a person's risk of developing type 2 diabetes.

First they looked at five studies in which participants (167,128 total across all studies followed for about 13 years) ate three or more servings of fruit daily. Then they looked at the results of nine studies in which participants (a total of 139,793, also followed for about 13 years) took antioxidants. What do you think they found? Do you think they found a lower risk of type 2 diabetes in the people who ate three or more servings of fruit, or in the people who were given antioxidants? Raise your hand if you think it was the people in the antioxidant group who had a lower risk of developing type 2 diabetes . . . YES! Great job! You're absolutely right, although I think I gave it away from the get-go.

In fact, the researchers concluded, on the basis of reviewing and analyzing all these prior studies, that people who took the antioxidant supplements of vitamin C and vitamin E had a 13 percent lower risk of developing diabetes than people who didn't take antioxidants. But they found no reduced risk for diabetes in the studies of people eating three or more servings of fruit or vegetables. Their work was published in the December 2007 issue of *Journal of Hypertension*.

I should add here that these researchers didn't feel they could make a "cause and effect" conclusion between lowered risk of type 2 diabetes and taking the powerful antioxidants, since they didn't specifically study the taking of supplements and the risk.

Nonetheless, this association between reduced risk of diabetes and taking antioxidant supplements is a message I would really like you to pay attention to. If you take steps to make sure you get adequate amounts of antioxidants, then you may be able to prevent diabetes.

Along with vitamins C and E, another strong antioxidant that sweeps away free radicals and improves insulin sensitivity is alpha lipoic acid. In fact, a very exciting article was published in the journal *Endocrine, Metabolic & Immune Disorders Drug Targets*. The article was called "A Current Update on the Use of Alpha Lipoic Acid in the Management of Type 2 Diabetes Mellitus," and my jaw dropped open when I read it. Finally! The mainstream medical literature is beginning to reflect what my colleagues and I in the world of naturopathic remedies have been writing about for a long time.

The researcher who wrote this article is Adrian Poh, MBBS (Singapore equivalent of MD), medical officer at the Alexandra Hospital in Singapore. Dr. Poh wrote, "There is growing evidence that alpha lipoic acid (ALA) has beneficial effects on the treatment of T2DM (type 2 diabetes mellitus) and some of its complications." Dr. Poh noted that alpha lipoic acid works within the insulin pathways in the body to reduce oxidative and inflammatory stress on the body, both of which play a major role in type 2 diabetes. Dr. Poh also called alpha lipoic acid "a potent antioxidant and free radical scavenger."

So there you go. He concluded in his article that ALA is relatively safe even in people with renal (kidney) and liver failure, and underscored the therapeutic value of ALA in specifically targeting insulin resistance and diabetic neuropathy—nerve damage due to diabetes. I happen to know about more terrific, natural remedies that can help you, which you will learn about in the coming pages.

FREE RADICALS COULD COST YOU YOUR LIFE

Part of supporting the work of your pancreas and getting well is to reduce the number of damaging free-radical molecules in your body. Most people don't have a clue what a free radical is, so I'll tell you. I'll spare you the discussion of electrons and protons and just cut to the chase. Free radicals are like loose cannons in your body, and they're on a seek-and-destroy mission. They are electrically charged molecules that get into your cells and try to kill them.

Free radicals generally inflict death by destroying the DNA within the cell, and that's a huge loss, because DNA is what carries your genetic code. After enough DNA damage occurs, and a lot of cells die, your organs become diseased.

When free radicals target the skin (the largest organ in your body), you develop wrinkles and look older. Your risk of getting skin cancer increases too. It happens to all of our organs as we age.

People of a certain age—namely seniors—have more free radicals than those who are younger, and these radicals need to be neutralized. Free radicals are known to kill beta cells in your pancreas, which leads to diabetes and pancreatitis (inflamed pancreas), so one of my suggestions is to take antioxidant supplements to neutralize the free radicals. It's like outsmarting them.

Also, having heavy metals in your body, such as cadmium, lead, and mercury, causes a chain reaction and multiplies free-radical damage a hundred- or even a thousand-fold. So another of my suggestions, which we'll get to later in the book, will include natural chelation supplements that come from plants or alpha lipoic acid, which we just talked about.

In addition to heavy metals, other examples of toxins that spawn free radicals include cigarette smoke, alcohol, pesticides, radiation, and even some medications. For now, let's delve deeper into the structure and function of the pancreas because if you think like a pancreas, you can take better care of yourself.

WHAT EXACTLY IS A PANCREAS?

The pancreas is a long, thin gland—well, a gland-organ, really—that hides behind the lower part of your stomach, deep in your abdomen. It pinkish-gray, about 1 inch thick, and 6 to 8 inches long. You have to use your imagination, but it's shaped a little bit like a helping hand. That's a good way to think of it, since it helps you break down (metabolize) carbohydrates, fats, and proteins into substances that you can digest and absorb as nutrients.

Without your helping hand—your pancreas—you wouldn't be able to eat, drink, read my book, or, for that matter, survive! The pancreas is almost like two organs in one. It's an endocrine gland, meaning that it secretes hormones (such as insulin) into your blood, and it's also an exocrine gland, which means that it secretes digestive enzymes into your gut (not your blood).

Your body has two types of glands: endocrine and exocrine glands. Their basic daily job is to secrete various bodily products, such as enzymes, hormones, and metabolites—substances that help you digest your food.

Endocrine glands are the body's hormone-producing structures. In addition to your pancreas, these include your thyroid, hypothalamus, pituitary gland, adrenals, and even fat cells. In the pancreas, the islet cells (called islets of Langerhans) are small islands of endocrine cells inside the larger portion of the organ. Okay, maybe this is more than you wanted to know, but isn't it amazing?

WHAT DOES THE PANCREAS DO?

The pancreas helps regulate blood sugar and helps you digest food. It secretes several important hormones, including somatostatin, the great regulator of endocrine and nervous system function. The pancreas oversees these functions by regulating the secretion of several other hormones, such as growth hormone, gastrin, glucagon (which stimulates an increase in blood sugar levels, in opposition to the work of insulin), and insulin, that much-discussed hormone secreted by the islets of Langerhans.

During digestion, your body uses two primary hormones—insulin and incretin. Both hormones have one primary purpose—to break down sugar and to maintain a steady level of sugar in your body. Incretin is a gut hormone that actually keeps an eye on the amount of insulin released from the pancreas. Incretin hormones also happen to delay stomach emptying, thereby reducing the spike of insulin release. This process puts less demand on the pancreas and ultimately benefits you by reducing fat and cholesterol storage in your arteries and all over your body. So your pancreas and your gut both work to release hormones that affect the levels of blood sugar throughout the body.

From this point on, I may refer to sugar as glucose so that all the diabetes specialists in the country don't e-mail me with a correction. Glucose is just another name for a simple sugar derived from the breakdown of starches and carbs, such as pasta, bread, and doughnuts. The word *glucose* is derived from the Greek word *glykys,* meaning "sweet," plus the suffix -ose, which means "sugar." So when you read about fructose, sucrose, and dextrose, you'll know that by any other name, it's a sugar and could be just as sweet as table sugar. (I share with you the best types of sugar to eat in Chapter 15.)

Aside from balancing blood glucose, the pancreas is also responsible for storing and releasing digestive enzymes, which you need to break down food into teeny tiny particles. The pancreas sits in your gut like a watchdog and waits for

---

HORMONE ALPHABET

The islets of Langerhans is a hard-working area of your pancreas that secretes many important hormones for you. Say hello to the family:

- Alpha cells produce glucagon
- Beta cells produce insulin and amylin
- Delta cells produce somatostatin
- F cells (also called PP cells) produce pancreatic polypeptides
- Epsilon cells produce ghrelin, one of our "hunger" hormones

---

that burrito to come through and then . . . boom! Digestive enzymes and insulin are jettisoned out to break it down into all its food particles, including glucose. Damage to the pancreas is a serious matter and is not to be ignored. Since insulin is the primary hormone that regulates blood sugar, let's get deeper into that.

INSULIN: SUGAR DELIVERY SYSTEM

In Chapter 2 you learned that insulin is a blood sugar "bus" and that it drops off glucose molecules throughout your body. There is great debate over who actually discovered insulin, but one thing is for sure: It is essential to life and it has widespread effects all over your body.

Your body works constantly to keep a harmonious balance between insulin and glucose at all times. Insulin is produced within the beta cells of the islets of Langerhans. Beta cells constitute 60 to 80 percent of all the cells within the islets of Langerhans. These islets are the big shots in your endocrine system. There are about a million islets in a healthy adult human pancreas, distributed evenly throughout the organ. We definitely want to make nice to them!

Insulin's primary role in your body is to move glucose, extracted from your meals, into each cell. But when that doesn't occur, the blood sugar builds up in your bloodstream, and your glucometer starts leaving you nasty messages.

When there is excess sugar in your body, your pancreas works much harder to secrete even more insulin. That's its job, and you want it to do that. But your cells don't always respond. When they consistently ignore the insulin, all that excess sugar gets stored away, some as triglycerides or cholesterol. You may understand now why one way to maintain healthy cholesterol ratios is to cut down on your sugar and starches. Conventional medicine's answer to high cholesterol is a statin medication, but that can actually make your situation worse. I'll discuss that more fully in Chapter 6.

INSULIN RESISTANCE

Think of insulin as a key that unlocks doors on the surface of your cells. When the doors open, blood sugar is allowed inside. This is good because your cells are hungry for energy, and they transform the glucose into energy. In a healthy person, the pancreas has mechanisms to tell it that your sugar levels in the blood have risen. It then secretes just the right amount of insulin to open those cellular doors.

If insulin can't unlock the doors, then all the glucose loiters outside—in the bloodstream—and you develop high blood sugar, or hyperglycemia (as in too much . . . think hyperactive). Pay attention here, because the take-home point is this: You want the glucose *inside* your cells because it's fuel for your cells. When the glucose is engaged in extracurricular activities—or in this case extracellular activities—you're the one who gets into trouble.

In fact, when the fluid surrounding your cells becomes a bath of sugar water, your cells don't function properly, your brain starves, your energy crashes, and basically your whole system begins to run amok. When certain diabetic medication comes along and forces your blood sugar inside your cells, it can kill these cells. After all, cells can only take so much sugar before they pop. Your goal is to maintain steady levels of glucose by increasing the health of your pancreas, not by force.

Your next goal is to reduce the amount of free-radical damage to your pancreas, and your whole body for that matter! The chapters that follow will teach you exactly how to do that.

BREAD GETS STORED ON YOUR BUTT

When your body converts glucose into energy for your immediate needs, some of it gets stored in the liver and muscle cells in a form called glycogen. This gives you energy to draw upon later. But here's the thing—if you eat a lot of carbs and sugary foods, you will then have an excess of sugar on your hands, and in your bloodstream. And guess where else? (Hint: your butt!)

More specifically, your body converts your carbs to energy, and it stores some for future use. But whatever sugar is hanging around after your body uses it to breathe, digest, sleep, and do whatever else is stored as fat. Surprise! You thought eating low-fat meals would shave the weight off, but it's not true because eating low-fat meals usually means eating more carbs, and this can actually fatten you up and promote diabetes.

That's why your diet needs to include good fats, such as avocados, olive oil, walnuts, almonds, and omega-3 fatty acids, along with the right number of carbs and protein for your body. It sounds so complicated, but that's what I'm here for. You can read more about the role of good fats and find out about the healthiest oils to cook with in Chapter 16.

WHAT'S WRONG WITH THE ADA?

In my opinion, following the standard diet recommended by the American Diabetes Association (ADA) is like locking the door on your destiny and throwing away the key. Doctors who rely solely on the information disseminated by their conventional big-pharma–funded seminars also do patients a big disservice. They advocate the use of drugs as if they will prevent organ damage, but this is not the way to protect your organs, I assure you. One reason that I disagree with the ADA diet is their recommendation to snack throughout the day so you can maintain a steady level of blood sugar all day.

The idea behind continually snacking is to avoid a tidal wave of blood sugar and the resulting insulin surge. Snacking makes sense to millions of those who have had long-standing type 2 diabetes who follow this diet and nosh all day. I agree that if these people don't snack, their adrenal glands become fatigued and hormones such as DHEA decrease, making insulin resistance even more severe. People with long-standing diabetes have trouble storing glycogen, and this is another reason that snacking periodically during the day is fine. Snacking also prevents hypoglycemia in this group of people.

So I agree with the ADA that some people need to snack all day, but not everyone. Why? Because this type of diet causes more problems in people who are new to diabetes, who still have time to recover. In the early years of prediabetes and high insulin (termed hyperinsulinemia), noshing all day long will do more damage than good. And the reason for that takes us right back to the pancreas.

In a healthy person, insulin levels rise after you eat to help you digest your food. Then after a few hours, they return to their normal baseline value. Without a snack in sight, your pancreas has the perfect opportunity to do what it is supposed to do, that is, make another hormone called glucagon. This hormone tells your liver to release sugar (which has been stored as glycogen) in order to maintain a steady level of sugar in your blood. This keeps you from becoming hypoglycemic. In other words, your bloodstream gets a snack, but it comes from your liver.

During this glycogen snacking process, a switch is turned on so you can burn up fat (specifically, triglycerides). This is normal. If you snack throughout the day, as many diabetes experts tell you to do, you circumvent the system. You cause the release of insulin (to digest your snack), thereby turning off any production of glucagon that would normally have occurred. Without the pancreas blowing its whistle, you won't release that glycogen from your liver. And without that glycogen "snack" being served, you won't burn up triglycerides as you should.

Triglycerides are the fats that clog arteries. It's your mitochondria (powerhouses) that help burn up those fats, and they work very hard until they get exhausted from having to deal with all the fat and sugar in your diet for so many years. When they're tired out, the triglycerides and cholesterol in your blood rise. Bring in the statins. That's what some doctors do, don't they? So many simply prescribe cholesterol-busting statins without ever checking your insulin levels or insulin-to-glucose ratios.

Statin drugs don't improve the situation. They mask the problem by getting your cholesterol numbers into the "normal" range. The numbers go down, but the arterial damage does not. It's like blowing the smoke out of the house while the fire continues to burn.

But your physician is happy with you. Inside you are still on fire because your insulin may be sky-high and your powerhouses completely spent. Unless you have your insulin levels checked, you are cooking up the recipe for a major metabolic disorder like metabolic syndrome, heart disease, Alzheimer's disease (sometimes known as type 3 diabetes), and even cancer. High insulin is linked to all of those diseases. Reducing cholesterol (and blood glucose) artificially does not reverse the disease process. It reminds me of the eerie retreating shoreline that occurs right before a tsunami strikes.

BEDTIME SNACKS ARE BAD FOR YOU

If you indulge in food before you go to bed (or really any time after dinner), the buildup of triglycerides and cholesterol becomes significantly worse because sleep is a great time to burn fat. I'm not being sarcastic—I really mean that. Sleep *is* a great time to burn fat because glucagon is released during the night and burns up fat, even though you are sedentary and sleeping. It can do that only if there's no food in the gut while you're sleeping.

Bedtime snacks derail you from this process, and as a result, the fat builds up in your liver, leading to a condition known as fatty liver. Eventually, as your liver becomes ever more fatty, it can't store excess sugar in the form of glycogen like it's supposed to.

A fatty, unhealthy liver could cause glucagon to use sugar improperly, causing your blood sugar to rise even though you haven't eaten. This means that fasting blood sugar will rise, and subsequently, insulin will rise too in an effort to reduce the high sugar levels. The whole process behaves in a schizophrenic way and may explain why in some people, fasting blood sugar levels rise even though they are eating small meals throughout the day, doing exactly what their diabetic expert told them to do.

The climbing levels of blood sugar and the cellular resistance to insulin also helps explain why more and more medications are needed to keep glucose levels under control.

So what's the answer? Rather than focusing solely on bringing blood sugar and cholesterol numbers down, you need to correct the metabolic pathways, hormone levels, and rising insulin levels. In other words, you need to be kind to your pancreas.

LEPTIN: THE FEEL-FULL HORMONE

Remember I mentioned leptin earlier in this book? Leptin is one of several hormones your body makes that tell you to stop eating. It's kind of like a stop sign because when leptin is released (picture the stop sign going up), you feel full. It signals your pancreas and says, "Hey, I'm full, so stop making insulin and start burning fat."

Very few doctors are teaching their patients about leptin but it plays an important role in helping people with diabetes lose weight, heal wounds faster, and, surprisingly, protect against infection, too.

Leptin hormone, secreted by your fat cells, is sent to the hypothalamus gland in your brain, where it tells your brain how much fat is being stored from your meal. Sometimes leptin has a hard time delivering that message to the brain, a condition known as leptin resistance.

People who have leptin resistance tend to hold on to their weight, even though they are hardly eating. This is why you may be trying to lose 10 or 15 pounds, and you simply can't do it, even though you are practically starving yourself. In this case, going on a diet won't help much in my opinion. I'll explain why.

When you go a diet, as some diabetes educators suggest, your brain senses that there are fewer calories around, and it goes into survival mode, storing fat and slowing down your metabolic rate to survive what it perceives as a low-fuel crisis. When you go off your diet (and you inevitably will) and food becomes available again, all those calories head straight to your fat cells to replenish any depleted reserves. The message to the hypothalamus is blocked.

If you are overweight (and therefore leptin-resistant), your brain and your pancreas simply can't hear the leptin signal, so your body thinks you are suddenly in starvation mode, even though you are still eating. As a survival tactic, your body slows down your metabolism (the rate at which you burn up food and turn it into energy). It slows down as a protective mechanism so you don't die of perceived malnourishment.

If the voice of leptin were properly heard, it would tell your pancreas to stop releasing insulin and start burning fat. Leptin resistance occurs years before insulin resistance (and metabolic syndrome or diabetes) does. Two supplements can help your brain wake up to the leptin signal—resveratrol and vanadium. I discuss these in Chapter 14. You should also ask your doctors to measure your leptin levels.

MORE PROBLEMS WITH THE ADA DIET

If you eat constantly throughout the day, as the ADA suggests, your pancreas may get bored with the constant leptin every few hours, after every snack. The beta cells in your pancreas will tune it out and keep producing insulin to bring your blood sugar down from each snack.

All this extra insulin can actually trigger dangerous hypoglycemia (low blood sugar). And hypoglycemia makes you crave something to eat so you don't pass out. What's worse, leptin gets tuned out by your brain, too, so you can't feel when you're full. With chronically high leptin, fat cells just keep on expanding.

A lot of research now points to the brain as Command Central in diabetes, and when the brain is resistant to leptin and insulin, then "Houston, we have a problem!" Obese people tend to have high leptin levels, as well as those with diabetes, but despite the high amounts of the hormone, their cells are still resistant to it.

The ADA recommends that people with diabetes follow the USDA Food Guide Pyramid diet, which relies heavily on fruit. I'm not saying that fruit is bad for you but it may contribute to insulin resistance in people with diabetes.

Are you starting to see the problem with the ADA diet? It creates a perpetual need for insulin, which creates more fat in the body and more inflammation. You wear out your pancreas, and it makes your brain resistant to important hormones like leptin and insulin. Over the long haul, it could lead to more complications of diabetes.

All of this is very complex, but I did my best to simplify it for you. I didn't even mention adiponectin levels, but we can go there if you really want to. (If you do, read the sidebar on the opposite page, titled "Adiponectin, I Love Ya!")

EATING TO MAKE YOUR PANCREAS HAPPY

Rather than noshing all day, you are better off eating three meals per day that are low in carbs and rich in antioxidant nutrients. Your pancreas will thank you. Why? Let's take a look at the research that supports this way of eating.

Researchers at Case Western Reserve University School of Medicine in Cleveland, Ohio, looked at what a high-carbohydrate meal did to the levels of leptin release in young, healthy volunteers. They gave the study participants a meal of cornflakes containing 50 grams of carbohydrates or a low-carb meal. What they found is no surprise to me. They concluded that meals lower in carbs (and with a lower glycemic index, which is a ranking of foods by their ability to raise blood sugar levels) promoted a healthier response to food, meaning reduced cravings for carbs.

The researchers suggested that consuming fewer carbs may be helpful in controlling not only obesity but also insulin resistance and type 2 diabetes. I agree. Low-carb meals make you crave fewer carbs and sugary foods. But higher-carb meals make for a vicious cycle: The more carbs you eat, the more you want to eat.

I can't imagine that any of this surprises you. We've all had that experience of making bad food choices—like eating four chocolate chip cookies—and then wanting to eat the rest of the package. That's why, sadly, people who are desperately overweight tend to *stay* desperately overweight—pills won't help them. They need to relocate their natural sense of feeling full. A meal high in carbs will sabotage you like a feuding clan will sabotage the other family's picnic.

ADIPONECTIN, I LOVE YA!

If you have diabetes, you need to love adiponectin. Actually, we all need to love adiponectin. Why? Because lean fat cells (the good ones) produce and secrete this protein hormone that regulates the metabolism of lipids and glucose. Adiponectin also has anti-inflammatory effects on the cells lining the walls of blood vessels. Research has shown that people who have a *lot* of fat cells and are obese have low levels of adiponectin, and a much higher risk of heart attack. For the record, research has also confirmed that high blood levels of adiponectin are associated with fewer heart attacks.

Bottom line: If you keep your weight down, you'll release more adiponectin, which will protect you from diabetes and other inflammatory conditions. It is much more complicated than I've outlined here, and if you want a broader understanding of the scientific background, you should get a copy of Jack Challem's book, *Stop PreDiabetes Now*.

So . . . say it with me, "Adiponectin, I love ya!"

And, for sure, listen to your mother (and to me) when it comes to eating breakfast as well as regular meals. Research has shown that not only is it better for your pancreas (and you) to eat three meals a day, but it's better still to eat three regularly scheduled meals a day. Research definitely supports this.

A study published in the *European Journal of Clinical Nutrition* in 2004, for example, looked at the impact of irregular meal frequency on circulating lipids, insulin, and glucose levels in nine lean, healthy women in Nottingham, England. The researchers compared fasting glucose and insulin levels and found that the women who ate more irregular meals had *higher* levels of both the bad LDL (low-density lipoprotein) cholesterol and overall cholesterol levels. Isn't that something? In addition, the women who ate irregular meals also had higher peak insulin levels after eating than did the women who ate regular meals.

The researchers concluded that eating irregular meals does appear to produce a higher level of insulin resistance and higher cholesterol levels after fasting than does eating regularly scheduled meals. See how sensitive your pancreas is, and how much it wants you to eat regular, nutritious meals? These things are all connected—the release of leptin and adiponectin, insulin resistance, and eating regular, low-carbohydrate meals. In Chapter 16, I will teach you how to construct a healthier kitchen and give you lots of specifics on what to eat and when.

THE LEPTIN SOLUTION

That was a lot of research to digest. What it all means, however, is that by taking a few simple steps you can invite the hormone leptin to work for you instead of against you. Before we get to those steps, let me summarize in simple terms how the hormone leptin comes into play after you eat.

- You eat something.
- Blood sugar rises after your meal. Insulin is released from the beta cells of your pancreas in response to the elevated blood glucose. (So far, so good, everything is going well.)
- Bummer, your cells resist the action of insulin, leading to excess sugar in your blood.
- Excessive sugar in your bloodstream causes your pancreas to release still more insulin because your cells still want sugar inside.
- All this excess insulin stimulates your fat cells to keep releasing leptin.
- Your brain and pancreas start resisting the "feel full" message that leptin is trying to deliver. You keep eating. And your pancreas does not get the signal to stop making insulin.
- High insulin levels from leptin resistance cause insulin resistance throughout the body!
- And your body stuffs more fat into your fat cells.

Remember, high insulin (and subsequent insulin resistance) is thought to spark many metabolic and inflammatory disorders, including diabetes.

Now here's the solution. There are several ways to overcome leptin resistance:

EAT PROPERLY. You need to consume three meals per day, but no more than four, maximum.

SPACE YOUR MEALS. In my perfect scenario, you'd allow 5 to 6 hours between each meal.

EAT SLOWLY. If you wolf your food down, then you don't give your body enough time to release the "feel full" hormone leptin.

DO NOT SNACK. Constant grazing reduces your body's ability to reset its fat-burning thermostat—the feedback loop of insulin, leptin, and glucagon.

DO NOT OVEREAT. Finish your meal when you feel slightly less than full. In 10 minutes, you will feel full, you'll see.

CHOOSE PROTEIN. Eat a breakfast that contains some protein. Nuts and seeds offer good non–animal-based protein.

PULL BACK ON CARBS. Reduce the amount of carbohydrates that you consume. At breakfast, for example, pass on the white-flour bagels and cereal. Instead, have nuts, berries, seeds, and fresh citrus fruit.

FAST AFTER DINNER. After the last meal of the evening, don't snack on *anything*. I don't care how funny Jimmy Fallon is, or how stressed out you are about the news. Your goal is to *never* go to bed on a full stomach. Allow 10 to 12 hours between dinner and breakfast. Generally speaking, finish eating your dinner about 3 or 4 hours before bedtime.

THE BEST-KEPT SECRET

One of the most important theories behind curing diabetes has to do with mitochondria, the little generators in your cells that make energy and help your cells burn up all the fat and sugar. I'll share this for the benefit of physicians, researchers, and healthcare practitioners specializing in diabetes who may not understand why I recommend what I do to help reverse diabetes without drugs.

I've been very choosy about the natural recommendations in the subsequent chapters because they support cellular health, and they spur mitochondria to start working more efficiently, which could be the key to getting well. Physician and researcher Douglas Hall, MD, is an expert in biochemistry and one of those sleuth doctors who stop at nothing to find the underlying cause of your illness.

Dr. Hall began practicing medicine more than 35 years ago. For the past 15 years, he has immersed himself in the practice of functional medicine, which focuses on healing the underlying cause of disease through nutritional means. This is different from conventional medicine, which focuses primarily on symptoms and the drugs that relieve them. With functional medicine, the entire patient is treated rather than a particular symptom.

Now is a good time to tell you that I am also a practitioner who has been a member of the Institute of Functional Medicine (IFM) for many years. This is the type of medicine that I study in order to offer you nondrug alternatives with such confidence.

Currently, many hours of Dr. Hall's workday are devoted to helping men and women overcome metabolic disorders such as diabetes, metabolic syndrome, neurotransmitter abnormalities, hypothyroidism, bioidentical hormones, obesity, and heart disease.

In studying with Dr. Hall, I shadowed him, meaning that I followed him during the day to see how he treated his patients with these serious disorders and to learn more about the pathology of disease. After just 15 minutes, it became clear that the problem with the way that most doctors treat patients with diabetes lies in the fact that they rely primarily on medications.

With Dr. Hall, and any functional medicine–trained practitioner, we are looking at the underlying cause of disease and correcting that, not just medicating for a particular symptom.

Dr. Hall was kind enough to let me spend some time with him. He taught me about the most progressive theories behind diabetes and other metabolic disorders. He summed it up best when he said, "All diseases are silent until enough tissue damage has occurred in that organ to produce a symptom. The problem is that most physicians' power rests in the power of the prescription pad, and they must become a student before they can become a teacher for their patient."

As a healthcare practitioner myself who deals with sick patients firsthand, I can vouch for that truth. So many doctors, well-intended ones, don't know enough to really cure their patients; they just manage them. Now, I'll share with you what I think is the best-kept secret in the development of diabetes.

Depending on your genetic code, it could go something like this: If you are overweight and have hyperglycemia, your mitochondria—which I will call "powerhouses"—get overwhelmed, or they get lazy, or they die. Then your cells stop working for you. You get even heavier and more toxic internally. Your cholesterol goes up, your waistline increases, blood sugar rises, and your insulin levels do too. Fat and sugar build up inside and outside your cells. Your cells can't handle the excessive load of sugar and fat inside of them and surrounding them in the bloodstream free radical damage occurs. Your inflammatory chemicals rise and then everything runs amok. Hello, diabetes!

HELPING YOUR MITOCHONDRIA MAKE ENERGY

One thing that causes you to have healthy mitochondria, with the potential to resuscitate your cells, is a gene known as PGC-1 alpha. (There's a good reason for the letters. They stand for peroxisome proliferator-activated receptor-gamma coactivator 1.) Research has demonstrated that PGC-1 alpha is the master regulator of mitochondrial biogenesis.

In English, this just means that you can achieve a higher degree of fitness without getting off the couch. I'm not advocating that, of course, but the point is that higher PGC-1 alpha activity means better metabolic fitness through improved mitochondrial functioning. I call your mitochondria your powerhouses because these tiny structures inside your cells burn energy for you.

Do you know what suppresses PGC-1 alpha? Stress does, big time. Stress causes high cortisol (your stress hormone) and lowered thyroid (T3, or triiodothyronine) hormone. And this combination leads to a cascade of metabolic events, including insulin resistance and metabolic syndrome.

Do you know what turns on PGC-1 alpha and helps you prevent insulin resistance? Caloric restriction. Keeping your calorie intake under control activates PGC-1 alpha, and this builds more fat-burning powerhouses for you. But here's the great news: There are also a couple of nutrients that do the *same thing*—they activate PGC-1 alpha, which allows your body to think you are on caloric restriction, even though you are not.

Current theories do suggest that stimulating activity of PGC-1 alpha can help improve diabetes.

Two main switches in your body turn on (or turn off) the activity of PGC-1 alpha. They are enzymes:

SIRT1—silent information regulator T1 (also called sirtuin)
AMPK—5' adenosine monophosphate–activated protein kinase

If you stimulate either of those enzymes, a lovely thing happens. Your body gets the signal to switch on activity of PGC-1 alpha. More specifically, turning on either of those switches signals your body to birth new mitochondria powerhouses, and voilà, you start to burn fat.

In essence, by increasing activity of PGC-1 alpha you help your body to burn fat! And you don't even have to break a sweat. It also helps your body's cells to recognize insulin, and this may very well prove to be the way to reverse diabetes in humans, once and for all. Ongoing research is looking at just this possibility.

Two supplements that have activity in these enzymatic pathways include resveratrol and lipoic acid. Abundant healthy levels of active thyroid hormone

(T3) also prod those "lazy" powerhouses to work for you and process insulin. All of this will be discussed in subsequent chapters.

Two amino acids that activate PGC-1 alpha are arginine (found in nuts) and citrulline (found in watermelon). And you can get these two compounds in the form of cheap, easy-to-find supplements. These can help you lose weight without starving yourself and also reduce your risk for insulin resistance.

A good dose for citrulline is 1,000 milligrams two or three times daily; for arginine, it's 700 milligrams two or three times daily. Citrulline and arginine are not recommended for people who have had a heart attack unless they are closely supervised by their physician. In fact, because so many people with blood sugar issues also have heart problems, it would be a good idea to ask your doctor about these supplements before taking them.

THE GOODS ON GLP-1

The hottest topic in diabetes research right now is centered on a hormone known as GLP-1, which stands for glucagon-like peptide 1. It turns out that GLP-1 plays one of the most important roles in metabolic disorders. Why is it such a big deal? It's huge, actually.

The benefits of higher levels of GLP-1 include increased insulin sensitivity, higher insulin secretion, and increased feelings of satiety (so you don't feel as hungry). It could even be the key to reversing diabetes. This is so cutting-edge that researchers are scrambling to figure out ways to increase the body's levels of GLP-1. In some people, giving oleic acid helps increase GLP-1 and therefore improves their diabetic status. Sunflower seeds and sunflower oil happen to be rich in oleic acid. Tulsi tea may increase GLP-1 also. While we're waiting for those research results, it makes sense to include them in your diet three or four times a week. You can also buy oleic acid supplements.

PUTTING OUT THE FIRE

Now, you might be thinking, "This is overwhelming to me; can you just tell me if I can have cake again and enjoy food like I did for so many years?" The answer is yes, it's absolutely possible to enjoy your life again, but understanding this concept is important because it will help you and your physician to treat your diabetes differently. By that I mean you can start to replenish missing thyroid hormone and start to repair and rebirth powerhouses (mitochondria). All of this will help your pancreas function better and help your body to metabolize sugar and fat in your cells. This, in turn, lowers your insulin level, which cools off the inflammation in your body. My hope is that by incorporating the few dietary changes suggested in this chapter, you can enjoy a longer life and, more important, a higher quality of life.

4

Milk and Bread, Cause for Dread

Have you seen those silly celebrities wearing a milk mustache? I'm referring to the Got Milk? ad campaign that began back in 1995. If you live on planet Earth, you've seen these ads and commercials with famous people promoting cow's milk.

The marketing campaign is brilliant. In 2007, each cow in the United States—that's about 9.1 million cows—produced 20,267 pounds of milk (about 2,357 gallons). In 2006, U.S. farms produced about $35.4 billion in milk! Yikes! All that advertising undoubtedly works because currently 83.9 liters (22.2 gallons) of milk are consumed in the United States each year by each person.

They forget to mention one little interesting fact in the Got Milk? ads. Milk contains about 750 million pus cells per liter (related to mastitis ailments). According to April 10, 2004, issue of *Hoard's Dairyman* (the National Dairy Farm Magazine), the number of pus cells (somatic cell count) in milk from California's unhappily diseased "happy cows" has soared to new heights. In 2002, the average liter (about 4 cups) of California milk contained 298 million pus cells. In 2003, just 1 year later, the average liter of California milk contained 11 million more pus cells than in 2002, along with traces of blood, mucus, feces, and dangerous microorganisms. There has been increasing attention given to this issue over the years and improvements in counts have been made, however, some advocacy groups feel the cell count is still too high.

Not to focus exclusively on California, I expect the story can be repeated in dairies throughout the country. If you think about it, humans are the only mammals in the world that continue to drink milk after infancy, let alone drink milk from a completely different species. Cow's milk can be processed and turned into other dairy items, such as cream for your coffee, butter for your bread, cheese, yogurt, and ice cream.

Call me neurotic, but the idea of nasty things in dairy products just freaks me out a bit. And to think I used to consume some cow's milk several times a month. In recent years, I've learned more about the substance, so now I keep

---

MAKING SENSE OF MILK ALLERGIES

Casein is the predominant protein found in milk and cheese. Lactose is the predominant sugar found in milk. Many people are allergic to casein, but they don't know that because they haven't ever thought to have a blood test done to determine this. They sneeze and make mucus after eating meals with dairy products in them, and they assume they are lactose intolerant. That may or may not be the case. A person can have a food sensitivity or full-blown allergy to both lactose and casein. In European foods, casein may be referred to as caseinogen. (Hint: the scientific word for a substance that triggers allergies is *antigen*.)

---

myself on a low-pus diet! I may order a few lattes over the course of the year while traveling in places where the cafés don't offer healthier options for milk, such as hemp, almond, oat, or goat milk.

GOT MILK? MIGHT GET DIABETES

I get annoyed when I see headlines intended to promote the consumption of milk and dairy products. Milk—or should I call it what it really is, cow juice—is portrayed as a healthy drink for babies and adults. Many children-oriented health organizations insist that toddlers drink up cow's milk as if it's going out of style, recommending 2 cups for children ages 1 to 3 years old, 2 to 3 cups for kids ages 4 to 8 years old, and 3 to 4 cups for kids between 9 and 18. A lot of agencies are making recommendations along these lines, so these are rough estimates, but you get the point.

In 2008, the American Academy of Pediatrics changed its recommendation for feeding weaned babies whole milk until the age of 2. They changed it to suggest that kids at risk for being overweight—or whose families have a history of obesity, heart disease, or high cholesterol—should drink reduced-fat 2% milk between 12 months and 2 years of age. The recommendation is also that *all* kids should be switched to low-fat 1% milk, after their second birthday.

Anyway, to further confuse the public, headlines on TV and in magazines tell you "Dairy Consumption Prevents Obesity and Diabetes."

Oh, really?

Do you honestly think milk is good for your waistline and your pancreas? I'm surprised that so many intelligent consumers fall prey to the false conclusions they hear on TV or hear from their doctor. Let's take a closer look at one study published in a respected journal that many physicians parroted to their patients. It was published in *JAMA* in 2002, and concluded that dairy prevents heart disease, obesity, and diabetes.

STRIKE 1: The study was funded in part by General Mills, which owns Häagen-Dazs ice cream, Betty Crocker, and Yoplait yogurt. I see this as a conflict of interest, don't you?

STRIKE 2: The foods in the study that qualified as "dairy" included those that were 100 percent dairy, for example, milk, sour cream, or yogurt. But foods were excluded if dairy was just part of the recipe, in other words a "mixed" dish. To give you an example of how flawed the study was, pizza—which contains a lot of cheese!—was *not* counted because it contains a crust, so it's not 100 percent dairy. Macaroni and cheese was not considered dairy either, because there are noodles in the dish, nor was milk with cereal (because of the cereal), ice cream, cheeseburgers, milkshakes, or cream cheese. How stupid is that? Of course, these meals are dairy, and they will definitely fatten you up, but this was *not* considered in the trial that officially concluded, "Dairy foods prevent obesity." Duh!

STRIKE 3: You're out! In the press release I read from the National Dairy Council, it said, "while the researchers were unable to explain how dairy foods impact IRS [insulin resistance syndrome], they speculate that several components, such as calcium, lactose, or protein, may play a role."

Wait, let me get this straight. Nobody can explain *how* dairy helps alleviate the problems of diabetes, including insulin resistance; they just want us to eat dairy foods? The press release goes on to say that dairy foods can help control weight and reduce the risk of heart disease and type 2 diabetes. But this flies in the face of numerous well-designed, placebo-controlled studies that prove that dairy foods *increase* heart disease and diabetes.

There are studies that implicate the role of whole milk in one of the most tragic conditions in children, type 1 diabetes. In fact, I found no fewer than 11 studies that made this link between whole milk and diabetes. Researchers have found that, sadly, type 1 diabetes is the most common form of diabetes in all parts of the world—at least the parts of the world they had measured by October 2007, when the research was published.

Does it surprise you to learn that the countries where the consumption of cow's milk is the highest also have the greatest prevalence of type 1 diabetes? Leading the globe are Finland, Sweden, Norway, and Great Britain, in that order. If more pediatricians read their medical journals, they would never recommend dairy for babies.

In fact, where cow's milk consumption by infants is the lowest—in China—the incidence of type 1 diabetes is also the lowest—0.1 case per 100,000 people per year. Where cow's milk consumption is the highest—in Finland—the incidence of type 1 diabetes is the highest, at 37 people per 100,000 per year. The evidence couldn't be much clearer, could it?

Here's the real kicker (and too bad they didn't kick over the bucket of milk): One research article, published in the journal *Pediatric Diabetes*, also cited "early introduction of cow's milk proteins" as a risk factor, right up there with C-section delivery, stomach viruses in pregnant women, and preeclampsia. That's not exactly subtle.

By the time 2006 rolled around, Finland's milk consumption went down to about 225 liters (48.6 gallons) per person per year, yet the risk for diabetes is still 36 times higher than in Japan, where consumption is only about 40 liters per year. Ironically, Finland's rate of osteoporosis was also incredibly high, despite the consumption of all that milk. That's probably because humans don't easily absorb the calcium from milk, like we do from plant sources. Remember, cows are getting their calcium from plants, too. They graze all day on grass. We should get our calcium in a similar fashion—from plants.

I don't like to see milk pushed on humans. It's food for calves, not humans. It's designed to bring a calf to 600 pounds in about 6 or 7 months. Don't you think maybe milk puts weight on you, too?

So when you see headlines that suggest how good milk is for you (or your health) think twice. It's not that it hurts everyone, because it doesn't. It only hurts people who are susceptible to it. And children may be more susceptible to pancreatic damage and immune system suppression. Many people with type 2 diabetes could be at risk, too.

As you learned earlier in the book, some types of diabetes (type 1) occur when the immune system attacks the pancreas and destroys the beta cells, which make insulin. This devastating disorder is linked to diet, sometimes directly to dairy products. Several studies have made the link between milk and symptoms of type 1 diabetes, but you won't see headlines like that because there would be a monumental impact on the dairy economy.

THE MILK-DIABETES CONNECTION

How exactly can something as seemingly pure and wholesome as cow's milk end up causing or contributing to a serious disease like type 1 diabetes?

The scenario goes something like this:

- Babies get weaned off breast milk very early and put onto cow's milk, or milk-based infant formula.
- The milk goes to the small intestine, where it gets digested into its tiny fragments. Some of the milk proteins, such as casein, break down into their smaller parts, amino acids.
- In susceptible infants, the milk is not fully digested, so the partially digested food globules squeeze out of the gut and into the bloodstream, where they begin to cause symptoms.
- The immune system says, "Hey, what are you big globules doing in the blood? Get out of here!" and defends the body by attacking and trying to kill these foreign proteins, which should not be in your blood or tissues. But guess what? These protein fragments unfortunately look a lot like the beta cells in the baby's pancreas, and the little one's immune system can't distinguish between the cells from the pancreas and the foreign proteins, so it launches an all-out attack and, unfortunately, destroys both.
- When enough beta cells have been demolished by the well-meaning immune system, an infant can no longer produce insulin. Hello type 1 diabetes for the rest of your child's life.

Do you think this sequence of events can occur in an adult with a compromised immune system or a leaky gut? Do you think that partially digested milk proteins could leak out in the same exact fashion and get into an adult's bloodstream? You bet they can!

You can test yourself or your child to see whether he or she has antibodies to partially digested cow's milk protein. The indicator would be elevated levels of bovine serum albumin (BSA). This protein, found in cow's milk, is associated with Crohn's disease and type 1 diabetes.

Children with diabetes have high levels of BSA, whereas nondiabetic children have normal levels of BSA. One truly remarkable study found that of 142 diabetic children, every single one had BSA antibody levels that exceeded normal. Of the 79 nondiabetic children tested, not one had antibodies that were abnormal. This tightens the connection between cow's milk and diabetes.

If more children were screened early on, like at the first sign of digestive stress, growth failure, or high blood glucose levels, then a dairy-free (casein-free) diet could be instituted, and I believe this could save some children from developing full-blown type 1 diabetes. I also feel strongly that special-needs children, such as those with Down's syndrome, Asperger's syndrome, or autism or those with signs and symptoms of attention deficit hyperactivity disorder, should be put on a casein-free, gluten-free diet.

Why keep banging your head and paying lots of money for medications (that have dreadful side effects) when you can try simple dietary changes, which may produce miraculous results? There are no guarantees, but I've seen it work firsthand in some of my clients and their children.

MILK: FRIEND OR FOE?

Parents who are trying to raise healthy children get mixed messages about milk. Here is a short sampling of the messages and why the issue is so confusing to people:

MESSAGE—DON'T DRINK MILK: In the September 1995 edition of its journal, *Pediatrics*, the American Academy of Pediatrics recommends that parents avoid feeding cow's milk to their babies, based on several Finnish studies that showed a clear connection between type 1 diabetes and infants drinking cow's milk.

MESSAGE—DO DRINK MILK: This same article in *Pediatrics* acknowledged that since 1909, local, state, and federal government agencies had been emphasizing the need for milk in children's diets. Drinking milk was a cornerstone of the National School Lunch Program, administered by the U.S. Food and Drug Administration.

MESSAGE—DON'T DRINK MILK: Just a year earlier, in 1994, researchers in another study, published in the journal *Diabetes Care*, stated that "these new studies, and more than 20 well-documented previous ones, have prompted one researcher to say the link between milk and juvenile diabetes is 'very solid.'"

MESSAGE—DO DRINK MILK: This is what most pediatricians are telling young mothers in a misguided effort to make sure that growing toddlers don't have weak bones. What they don't realize is that the countries with the highest milk consumption have the highest rate of bone fractures, but that's my next book. I'll go into some details shortly about the scientific studies that back up that assertion.

MESSAGE—DON'T DRINK MILK: *The Lancet*, the most revered medical journal in England, in 1996 concluded that "antibodies to bovine beta-casein are present in over a third of insulin-dependent diabetes mellitus patients and relatively non-existent in healthy individuals."

So what's a parent to do? It's likely that most parents will be relying largely on what their pediatrician tells them to do, and some might be influenced by what television commercials and million-dollar ad campaigns suggest. Hopefully your own pediatrician and diabetes educator are aware of these studies that show the dangers of drinking milk and have warned you of this.

POPULAR DAIRY PRODUCTS

Thanks to industry and technological advances, manufacturers derive a variety of interesting products from milk, such as whey protein, powdered milk, kefir, and condensed milk. All of these products contain the milk sugar lactose and the predominant milk protein casein. How concerned do we need to be about all these products?

WHEY PROTEIN. When milk is made into cheese, whey is a by-product. Whey protein is offered as a protein supplement that can be added to smoothies and shakes. Bodybuilders use a lot of whey protein to bulk up. Whey contains the amino acid cysteine, which is actually a strong and useful antioxidant that sweeps away free radicals.

POWDERED MILK. It's just evaporated milk. The powder can be easily transported and used for people in the military, and for others who could use the nutrition. You reconstitute it by adding water. But powdered milk is commonly used in infant formulas. This is alarming to me because powdered milk often contains oxysterols—free radicals that have the potential to cause atherosclerotic plaques (clogging of the arteries).

KEFIR. It's a fermented milk drink that you can buy at health food stores. Commonly used to replenish beneficial bacteria in the gut, kefir is made from kefir "grains," which are essentially just bacteria and yeast. Kefir is fermented, and it turns into a slightly sour, slightly alcoholic beverage. The types of pure kefir not laden with sugar may contain strains of probiotics such as *Lactobacillus acidophilus* and *Lactobacillus kefiranofaciens*.

SWEETENED CONDENSED MILK. This is just cow's milk that has had the water removed and sugar added. It is a sweet, thick product used in dessert recipes, such as key lime pie. It fascinates me that this form of milk can stay fresh—

I guess that's the best word for it—for about 2 years! It was developed by Gale Borden Jr. back in 1856.

WHAT'S IN MILK?
PARENTAL DISCRETION ADVISED

Let's take a closer look at what—in addition to all those pus cells that I mentioned at the beginning of the chapter—is in most commercial brands of milk.

GERMS. Milk has to be pasteurized in order to destroy certain microorganisms. The process of pasteurization heats the milk to about 150°F for about 30 minutes. This kills most of the germs in milk, but it also destroys the healthy enzymes and vitamins in the product. Pasteurization destroys vitamin C and iodine. It also makes the calcium in milk insoluble.

The debate over pasteurized versus pure milk persists. No doubt raw milk is more nutritious for you, but some experts feel that you increase the risk of bacterial infection from such organisms as salmonella, listeria, and whatever else slips in from fecal contamination when you drink it raw. But when you pasteurize, you make the calcium in milk relatively insoluble. Isn't that why milk is pitched to you as a healthy beverage in the first place? For the calcium? And popular commercial brands are all pasteurized. (Some states still allow the sale of raw milk from small, family-owned farms. Those products can be found mainly in health food stores.)

So what does the pasteurization of milk products really mean? Ironically, it could mean a higher risk for weak bones, bad teeth, and infections because pasteurization causes calcium in milk to become relatively insoluble. You can't absorb it as well as you can from clean, raw milk. The point here (and small, authentic dairy farmers know this) is that raw milk contains nutrients that can nourish the body, nutrients that strengthen bones, whereas pasteurized milk is basically dead. In fact, many brands of milk have been pasteurized two or three times to kill off all the potential germs. By the time you get all the bacteria out, you've also taken out all the good stuff. So it's a catch-22.

CASEIN (OR CASEINOGENS). This is the most predominant protein found in cow's milk and cheese. It's also found in many soy products. Casein turns into casomorphin in the body, which then causes the release of histamine. What does histamine do? Think allergies, sinus problems, and possibly asthma, food allergies, and diabetes.

When people sneeze after eating, or get the sniffles after eating foods or sauces containing a dairy product, it will no longer come as any surprise to you. Many healthcare providers have found that for some people, going dairy-free can solve allergy and asthma conditions. If you want to avoid casein found in dairy, to help with allergies or diabetes, you should know its other aliases:

Calcium caseinate   Hydrolyzed caseinate
Sodium caseinate   Milk protein

LACTOSE. Lactose is a sugar found in natural raw milk, and also some tropical flowers. At birth, we have a lot of lactase, an enzyme that helps us break down lactose. Our supply of lactase dwindles quickly as we age. When milk is pasteurized, the process turns lactose into beta-lactose, a sugar that gets absorbed rapidly into the bloodstream, more easily than plain good old lactose. This rapid absorption means that your child may become hungrier faster because he or she is not as satisfied, which could mean weight gain.

Many adults know that they are lactose intolerant, meaning they do not have the enzyme (lactase) needed to break down the lactose in milk. The bacteria in your gut have to multiply like crazy to help your body break down the milk. This can lead to all sorts of digestive troubles, which begin anywhere from 30 minutes to 2 hours after ingestion of dairy products (milk, butter, cheese, yogurt). Those types of dairy products actually have a more concentrated amount of milk proteins/sugars compared with milk. Symptoms of lactose intolerance range in severity and include loose stools, rumbling in the belly, gurgling, constipation, flatulence, bloating, cramps, and nausea.

I have been asked by many people whether lactose-free milk and nonfat milk contain casein. The answer is yes. Nevertheless, people who drink these products in an effort to remain lactose-free still get casein, and may still suffer with medical problems as a result. Lactose and fat content of milk have nothing to do with the protein content.

If you are really planning to go dairy-free (casein-free), then altered milk products are not the answer. Almond, rice, hemp, or oat milk are better choices.

Shocking, but true: Casein is also found in many soy products. It's unfortunate that many people who are allergic to milk go dairy-free and begin eating soy cheese or soy milk, and they don't realize that they are getting the milk protein anyway and their dairy-related problems will persist. If you want to completely avoid casein, or you are vegan, then you need to start reading the fine print on your food products to make sure that you are steering clear of this milk protein.

You can get a blood test to see whether you have a sensitivity to dairy proteins. The test checks for antibodies to casomorphin. Ask your doctor about this test at your next appointment. If you do have the test, make sure you take it between 7 and 8 a.m., when your antibodies are highest. On occasion, these tests have falsely negative results.

EnteroLab also offers an anticasein IgA antibody test that uses stool as the testing medium. The sample can be collected at any time of the day, since most of the body's IgA antibodies are produced in the small intestine. The results are accurate.

MILK WATCH LIST

Even if you do your best to avoid dairy products, it's still possible for a few to sneak in unless you're really vigilant. Look for these ingredients and products that hide the use of milk:

CARAMEL COLOR. Most of the time, lactose (milk sugar) is used to help get the deep, rich color.

NATURALOSE. This is a new sweetener on the market known chemically as tagatose. It's derived from whey, and whey comes from milk. This low-calorie sweetener is found in foods, drinks, candies, energy bars, toothpaste, mouthwash, and many other products.

CANNED TUNA FISH. Many brands—StarKist is one notable exception—contain casein, disguised as hydrolyzed caseinate. Read the label to make sure.

CHICKEN BROTH. Don't ask me why milk is in chicken broth, but it often is. Look for "milk solids" or any other aliases for it. Canned or bouillon cubes also usually have it.

WINE. Casein is sometimes used to remove impurities from wine. This is called clarifying.

CHEWING GUM. Really. Read the label carefully to find milk products.

SO WHAT GOES ON THE CEREAL?

If you're committed to avoiding milk, the big question becomes, what do you use instead?

I don't recommend soy milk because so many people seem to be allergic or sensitive to soy, and besides, soy acts a bit like estrogen. Since it shows activity like a female hormone—meaning it's estrogenic—then it just may fuel the growth of estrogen-driven cancers, such as those in the breast or prostate.

You can drink rice milk if you want. It's sold commercially at health food stores and grocery chains. There are several brands. Rice Dream and Pacific Rice Milk are popular. Almond or hazelnut milk are my own favorites.

Another possibility is coconut milk, sold under brand name So Delicious. Goat milk is yet another choice. I think it's purer and a tad cleaner than cow's milk, but it does have some casein. Casein-sensitive individuals should know that any milk derived from a mammal contains casein protein, although the amino acid chains do differ from species to species. Perhaps this explains why people who are dairy sensitive often do just fine consuming goat milk and goat cheese.

I have a much tastier idea for you in my recipe chapter about making home-made milks out of almonds or hemp seeds. You can make these milks yourself or try store-bought brands that are ready to use. I use these healthy milks in many of my recipes. And, get this, not only are these milks casein- and lactose-free, but they also promote better health by providing your body with essential fatty acids and minerals. You can use these milks in your coffee and any recipes that call for milk, even in baking. See Chapter 17 for details.

GOING AGAINST THE GRAIN

Milk, alas, is not the only food that is cause for concern if you have diabetes or any kind of issue with blood sugar. As I mentioned in Chapter 1, bread can be seriously problematic.

Many health experts feel that dairy-free diets don't matter as much as gluten-free diets. In other words, some experts feel that diabetes is more tightly connected to the ingestion of bread, not milk. Let's take a closer look at why bread crumbs may leave a trail to diabetes.

The alloxan contamination mentioned in Chapter 1 is not the only problem with bread. Just as milk has a problematic protein (casein), so does wheat. The problem protein in wheat is known as gluten. I think of it as "glue-ten" because gluten works like glue: It holds bread together, particularly when all the gases form as bread rises in the oven.

If you are sensitive to gluten or if you have persistent problems with your digestion—diarrhea right after eating, for example—you should do whatever you can to completely avoid gluten in your diet. Some flours contain a lot of gluten,

OATMEAL MAY BE OKAY

Why do health experts often recommend that people who are gluten sensitive stay away from oats? Oats, after all, do not contain any gluten. Alas, most brands of oatmeal are produced in the same facilities or on the same equipment used to process wheat. So gluten contamination happens frequently. Some manufacturers, however, go out of their way to prevent that contamination. McCann's brand of steel-cut oats, for example, should be fine for most gluten-sensitive folks because they are produced in a facility that is exclusively devoted to oats, so there is no risk of cross-contamination. That said, and this is very cutting-edge: *Many people who are supersensitive to gluten are also irritated by oats (even the uncontaminated sort). This happens because they have trouble fully digesting oat proteins in the gut, as well as wheat proteins.*

Bottom line? Go ahead and try one of the noncontaminated oat products. But watch carefully for your typical gluten-sensitivity symptoms. If oats cause problems, avoid them in the future.

and some are 100 percent gluten-free. The most popular gluten-containing flours that you should avoid include wheat, rye, barley, spelt, and kamut. All-purpose flour comes from wheat, so this is also a no-no. Oats are often put on the gluten-containing list because of cross-contamination in the factory, not because they contain gluten. Oats are usually processed on the same equipment as are wheat products.

Gluten is not an essential vitamin, mineral, or nutrient. In fact, you can live a long, healthy life without *ever* ingesting gluten. I personally keep a gluten-free house and have for many years. Being gluten-free does not mean that you can never have bread. It just means that the bread you eat does not have gluten in it because you've used gluten-free flour. Don't be afraid of this concept. All of my recipes in Chapter 17 are gluten-free because I use almond flour, a nut flour that has very few carbs and lots of nutrients.

What does all this have to do with diabetes? Bear with me for a moment. If you happen to have a lot of digestive troubles, I'm saying that you may be gluten intolerant. It's unfortunate that many healthcare practitioners don't know that people with gluten sensitivity can have no problems with their digestion at all, zero, nil, nada! These doctors will not connect bizarre neurologic symptoms that occur when your immune system attacks its own brain because of the gluten. These symptoms include such things as peripheral and autonomic neuropathy, numbness, slurred speech, headaches, lack of coordination, muscle pain (poly-myositis), neurogenic muscle atrophy, and retinal degeneration.

Now here's the diabetes connection: Some of those symptoms are exactly the same as those experienced with diabetes, aren't they? And yes, I believe there is an undeniable connection between gluten and certain types of diabetes, such as autoimmune diabetes. And gluten may well be exacerbating (or triggering) diabetes, as well as other autoimmune disorders, such as rheumatoid arthritis and multiple sclerosis.

GLUTEN TIED TO MANY DISORDERS

Here's another tie-in to diabetes. People with type 1 diabetes and extreme gluten sensitivity (celiac disease) also have a higher prevalence of autoimmune thyroid disease. People with Hashimoto's disease, for example, may be unaware that they have an underlying gluten intolerance or celiac disease. But there is a high correlation between high levels of TPO (thyroid peroxidase) antibodies and gluten intolerance. This is important because as you've learned already, low thyroid hormone is a primary cause for the development of diabetes.

If you can reduce thyroid antibodies (TPO antibodies) by going gluten-free, you may actually get to the heart of this particular thyroid disorder, which is disabling for some. When you do that, I believe you may even reverse the trajectory of diabetes because you're quieting down your whole system. Your blood sugar goes down, insulin levels go down, and the stubborn weight begins to just melt away.

It's my best-kept secret, and it's finally out of the bag. I think that going gluten- and casein-free just might play a big role in fully freeing yourself of insulin resistance, obesity, thyroid problems, intestinal disorders, and even neuropathies. There, I really feel much better having gotten that off my chest. Highlight that sentence, and earmark this page because it's *that* important. Help your friends too, by sharing this information. Traditional doctors and diabetes educators are probably frowning right now, going, "Huh? Where is the proof?" The proof is in the gluten-free pudding.

Stay with me, okay, because this is very important. Gluten-sensitive individuals make antibodies to gluten (technically called gliadin). So they have high levels of antigliadin (IgA) antibodies. When measured in studies, these antibodies are found to be high in people with gluten sensitivity and celiac disease. High TPO antibodies could also be a sign that you have gluten intolerance.

I think there are millions of diabetic people walking around who simultaneously have thyroid problems *and* gluten sensitivity. You can medicate with diabetic and thyroid drugs all you want, but until you put the fire out *by removing the underlying food allergen*, you will continue to suffer.

Celiac disease is thought to be an autoimmune disorder that attacks the small intestine, causing the tiny, fingerlike protuberances (villi) that line the inner wall of the small intestine to shrink and flatten. Everyone has millions of villi in their small intestines. When your villi are normal size and healthy, they are able to do their job. When the villi shrink and flatten, a condition known as villous atrophy, less surface area is available for absorbing nutrients. This, as you can imagine, leads to many problems of vitamin and mineral deficiency, including osteoporosis. You must have a genetic predisposition to celiac disease and it starts when a person becomes intolerant to gluten, the infamous wheat protein.

Without at least one of the two main celiac genes, it is highly unlikely that a gluten-sensitive individual would progress to celiac disease. There are, however, many genes that cause gluten sensitivity as well, which predispose a very large population of the world to problems with gluten. Doctors associate gluten sensitivity or celiac disease with digestive troubles that closely resemble irritable bowel syndrome. When digestive symptoms occur, they may include recurrent abdominal bloating, pain, nausea, gas, mouth sores, skin rash, joint pain, diarrhea, or constipation.

When you put someone who is gluten sensitive, or who has autoimmune celiac disease, or who has autoimmune thyroid disease on a gluten-free diet, the antibody levels come down. Fewer antibodies mean less inflammation and less misery. The thyroid gland is happy, the pancreas is happy, and the waistline is happy too.

Going against the grain can really pay off in terms of health. If you don't believe me, just try my recommended diet for 4 weeks and see what happens to you. I'm betting that you'll start to have better digestion and probably lose some weight.

I helped one of my friends by telling her to go gluten-free when she was suffering with chronic, unbearable joint pain, muscle aches, fatigue, and resulting depression. She had been diagnosed with ankylosing spondylitis, psoriatic arthritis, and asthma. She was injecting herself with Humira, a powerful anti-inflammatory drug known to cause devastating side effects, such as serious infections and neurologic problems. In addition, she took a handful of other medications to help with the pain, anxiety, insomnia, and digestive troubles that also plagued her.

Despite all her medications, my friend was not getting any better, and lived in pain 24/7. When she confided this to me, I recommended that she go off all gluten-containing foods and be very strict about this. I also suggested that she take an over-the-counter anti-inflammatory supplement called Zyflamend. Her doctor approved of the Zyflamend, which she purchased at her local health food store. Within 2 weeks, she felt better and wrote this note to me:

Suzy,

You have given me back my life!!!!! And you can quote me!!!! In the past few years, I suffered so in making Passover dinner for the family; my legs ached, as did my back. I couldn't tell anyone about it, because I was the youngest in the family, and always have a sunny demeanor. My whole body ached like I had the worst case of the flu . . . in fact, that's how I lived my life, in that kind of flu-like, relentless pain. . . . the second I opened my eyes, the pain was there . . . BUT NOT ANYMORE! SUZY—you have given me my life!!!! THANK YOU!!!!!

—Ann

So you see, miracles happen, and I share this account with you because if it happened to her, it could happen to you.

And guess what else I've uncovered for you? Scientific studies now confirm an even tighter connection between diabetes and gluten. That's right! People who can't tolerate gluten also seem more prone to developing diabetes and pancreatitis. Wow, wow, wow! So if you think that slice of white bread on your plate is good for you, think about changing brands to something that is gluten-free.

One study pointing to the connection between diabetes and gluten was published in the *New England Journal of Medicine*. It indicated that there's a common genetic susceptibility to both type 1 diabetes and celiac disease. Researchers from the University of Cambridge (England) concluded that both celiac disease and type 1 diabetes may originate from food-related problems. In this study researchers looked at 9,339 young people with type 1 diabetes and no other diagnosed diseases, and 2,560 people with celiac disease. They found several genetic mutations that were exactly the same in people with celiac disease and people with diabetes. The two diseases apparently have a genetic link and share at least seven chromosome regions.

In another study, published in the *New England Journal of Medicine* in 2008, researchers looked at genetic material (DNA) from about 20,000 people, half of them healthy, nearly half with type 1 diabetes, and 2,000 with celiac disease. The overlapping genetic variants occurred on regions of chromosomes—parts of cells that carry genetic code—that are believed to regulate the gut's immune system.

So am I saying that eating wheat or other gluten-containing proteins contributes to—or even causes—diabetes? I think maybe it does, but there is not a clinical study that confirms this yet. The two previous studies that I just mentioned certainly point in this direction. Will I be proven right? Hopefully soon, but in the meantime, rest assured that all my recipes in Chapter 17 are gluten-free, and most are casein-free too. It's important to learn about ways to nourish your stomach and gastrointestinal tract so you can get past gluten-induced damage. There are many books on the subject, and interesting Web sites. None of the wonderful supplements that you take to support the work of your gastrointestinal tract will be effective, however, unless you completely remove gluten from your diet. *Remove it; don't just minimize it.*

TESTS TO DETERMINE GLUTEN SENSITIVITY

There are many tests that you can take to find out whether you are immunologically sensitive to various foods or their proteins. Twenty years ago, I used to recommend blood testing for antibodies, but I don't anymore. The reason is that these tests are not as sensitive as newer tests available today. I'm going to outline only the ones that I feel are the most sensitive and accurate.

STOOL TESTING FOR GLUTEN. I've written about Kenneth Fine, MD, in my prior books. He has developed a highly sensitive gluten test that requires stool, not blood. Kudos to him because no needles are involved, and his tests appear to be even more sensitive than blood tests and biopsies.

Using his tests, you can do your own test for gluten sensitivity (and a few other foods as well) using a stool sample. This is a great, noninvasive way to determine gluten sensitivity, even years before celiac disease may develop.

Dr. Fine compared hundreds of gluten sensitivity tests done on people with the bowel disease colitis. Just 7 percent came up positive on a blood test, while 76 percent tested positive on the stool test he developed. So if you really, honestly want a definitive test, take the Gluten Sensitivity Stool Panel Complete or, if you want the genetic test too, the Gluten Sensitivity Stool and Gene Panel Complete.

I really appreciate that Dr. Fine has made his test kit available directly to the people who need it, you the consumer. You can take control of your own health and buy the test at www.enterolab.com.

Doctors who want to order test kits for their patients may do so by contacting EnteroLab and requesting a fax order form that can be sent directly to EnteroLab from their clinic. The kit will be mailed to the patient.

SALIVARY TESTING FOR GLUTEN. This test was developed by Aristo Vojdani, PhD, who was also dismayed with blood testing. For this test, all that is needed is saliva. The sophisticated test measures levels of AGA (antigliadin antibodies) and ATTA (antitissue transglutaminase). A positive result for AGA means you have gluten sensitivity. A positive result for ATTA reveals autoimmune disease and suggests type 1 diabetes. A positive result for both AGA and ATTA may confirm celiac disease or diabetes.

Doctors can order this test at www.immunoscienceslab.com.

GENETIC TESTING FOR GLUTEN SENSITIVE AND CELIAC GENES. EnteroLab also offers genetic testing for predisposing genes. Unlike some other labs, which only tell you if you are positive or negative for the celiac genes, EnteroLab will tell you exactly what genes you have that relate to gluten sensitivity or celiac disease. The sample is taken by using a cheek swab, another noninvasive procedure.

According to Phyllis Zermeno, a registered nurse who specializes in testing for immunologic food sensitivities: "It is extremely important for practitioners and patients alike to realize how widespread gluten sensitivity is in our society today and the broad spectrum of symptoms and systems that can be associated with this immunologic condition. Obtaining a definitive diagnosis of gluten sensitivity can help individuals make the choice to change their diets and improve their health before serious damage is done to their bodies."

Are you concerned that these tests aren't something that your doctor knows about, or something that she or he recommends? Don't worry, these tests have made it through my web of critical analyses, and I'm very picky about what I recommend to you. If that isn't persuasive enough, mention that the laboratories involved are licensed by the U.S. Department of Health and Human Services. You can buy this test over the Internet. Any lab that offers direct-to-consumer lab test kits is allowed to sell these tests to anyone, except those living in New York and Maryland because these states do not allow residents to buy test kits via interstate purchasing.

VINO IS A NO-NO

Americans love to drink alcohol in any form—beer, wine, aged Scotch, whiskey, tequila. I'll stop now, but you catch my drift.

BEWARE OF HIDDEN GLUTEN

Avoiding gluten can be a challenge. If you know or suspect that you have gluten sensitivity, you need to do everything you can to keep it out of your diet completely. You probably know to stay away from bread and other products made with wheat. Here's a list of other foods that may contain gluten:

Bulgur

Soy sauce

Orange fish roe served on sushi (the green wasabi eggs and red fish roe are gluten-free)

Pasta, unless it is made from rice flour, mung bean flour, potato flour, quinoa, or corn flour

Many gravies and thickeners

Barley

Einkorn

Farina cereal

Maltodextrin and dextrin

Beer

Anything battered with wheat flour

Many processed meats (Boar's Head is okay)

Wheat germ and wheat germ oil

Most cakes, cookies, and bagels

Regular pasta

Malt

Couscous

Spelt (dinkle)

All-purpose flour

Wheat or durum wheat

In 2004, a staggering 2.23 gallons of pure alcohol, on average, was consumed by each person per year. That's the equivalent of about 50 gallons of Bud or 20 gallons of Shiraz each year. Even though alcohol consumption damages the pancreas, people with diabetes continue to rationalize this habit, perhaps because of the latest information on a potential connection between red wine and heart health. Here's the 64-thousand-dollar question: "Can I drink or not?"

The answer you get depends on whom you ask. According to the American Diabetes Association, alcohol can be ingested if your blood sugar is under control and if you do not suffer from major diabetic complications. I happen to disagree. Sorry to be a party pooper, but those martinis will damage your pancreas and liver, making alcohol the most lip-smacking fluid time bomb of all. Drinking alcohol is a major cause for pancreatitis.

In addition, when you drink, your liver becomes obsessed with clearing the alcohol from your bloodstream instead of what it should be doing, which is releasing glucose to maintain steady blood sugar levels. Because the liver is distracted, the result can be hypoglycemia.

The ingestion of alcohol is particularly dangerous for people with diabetes,

GYMNEMA SYLVESTRE TO THE RESCUE!

It's a funny sounding name but *Gymnema sylvestre* is powerful just the same. This herb, native to India, is sold in health food stores. It has been shown to repair and even promote the growth of beta cells in the pancreas. This means that it may help offset the damage done by alloxan and may therefore work to improve blood sugar control. How sweet is that?! There will be more about amazing *Gymnema* in Chapter 13.

especially if you drink on an empty stomach or take diabetic medication or insulin. Even though it takes a couple of hours for alcohol to leave your system, the danger of hypoglycemia—not to mention pancreatitis—continues long after the toast.

Regardless of the dangers of alcoholic beverages, modern medicine has a love affair with red wine, and many studies have been published proclaiming that drinking red wine (to get resveratrol) can protect your heart. My opinion is that it's far better for you to take a resveratrol supplement and get all the benefits without the damaging effects of alcohol. (Information about that supplement is in Chapter 8.) I like resveratrol, and I also like an occasional glass of red wine, but by no means do I agree that drinking red wine for the sake of your heart is healthy.

Is it just me, or have you noticed the disturbing rise in the numbers of people with pancreatitis and pancreatic cancer? Could it be because everyone is drinking wine every night under the premise that they'll get a healthy heart? What a trade-off! Nothing damages the pancreas and liver faster than alcohol. So make sure you minimize your consumption if you have either diabetes or pancreatitis. And if you would like more information about pancreatitis and pancreatic cancer, I have an e-book on this at my Web site.

PART 2

DETECTION, TREATMENT, AND MONITORING OF DIABETES

CHAPTER 5

Medications: What You Need to Know to Stay Safe

I've been a pharmacist for more than 20 years. How do you think I feel as I count out a patient's pills when the side effect profile includes swelling, trouble breathing, fatigue, rapid heartbeat, dizziness, headache, liver failure, heart failure, and so on?

I can tell you how I feel in three "Fs": frustrated, frightened, and freaked out. I have yet to see one patient—just one—be cured from diabetes thanks to any medicine I have dispensed to them. It just doesn't happen. On the other hand, I've seen miracles worked with people who exercise, eat right, and take natural supplements.

The last decade has been very exciting in terms of the development of medications for diabetes. We've seen new types of medications arrive, not just "me too" drugs. Because every person is different, it's nice to have various medications in our diabetic arsenal to allow a doctor to tailor-make your regimen.

Some—not all—of the new meds on the block have advantages over the oldies, because they come in extended-release formulas or combination formulas, or are newly formulated to have milder side effects. However, the older drugs are still effective and often less expensive because they are also available in a generic equivalent.

I believe it would be ideal if most people with diabetes tried to reverse their condition with diet, exercise, and supplements before trying medication. However, medicine has pretty much become the first-line method for dealing with diabetes, and I am aware of that.

You probably don't realize that most FDA-approved diabetic medications sold in the United States are intended and approved for use along with diet and exercise, which means that they are *not* approved for use in people who don't diet and exercise. Unfortunately, many diabetic customers who come to the local drugstore don't adhere to a healthy diet, nor do they exercise. I know because they confess to me, or to the cashier, that it is difficult for them to make these lifestyle changes. Pharmacy clerks routinely ring up their diabetic medications along with candy bars, soda, beer, and just regular old junk food, such as cookies, cakes, or chips.

The American mind-set is that you don't have to do any work if you can just pop a pill and control a number, such as a blood sugar number, or a cholesterol number. Obviously, that's not how *you* think, though, or you wouldn't be reading my book.

NUMBERS MAKE DOCTORS HAPPY, NOT PANCREASES

Medications are effective at reducing blood glucose numbers. This pleases pharmaceutical companies, which raked in $12.5 billion in 2007 for diabetic treatments, up from $6.7 billion in 2001. Using medications also pleases your doctor because it gives him or her a false sense of progress. And they may well please you, too!

One of my concerns is that you'll cheat on your diet because with the help of medications your blood sugar numbers are fine. "Yes, I'll have fries with my Big Mac, and would you supersize it too?" Don't even think about it! Stick with a whole plan to get well. Don't become a number junkie and take a slurry of drugs to chase down your numbers.

Controlling your blood sugar vigorously is not any more beneficial than lowering it to regular levels, according to a study published in the *New England Journal of Medicine*. The Veterans Affairs Diabetes Trial followed 1,800 veterans with type 2 diabetes. After 6 years, the group with tightly controlled blood sugar showed no difference with respect to heart attacks or other dangerous cardiac complications compared with the group that used standard targets for blood sugar.

It's important to understand that medications may play a role for the short term, but they only keep your blood sugar within a specific range. Does this cure diabetes? No, because diabetes is not just a disease of high blood sugar. It's a metabolic disorder that affects all the organ systems in your body, so it's a systemic disorder.

Do keep in mind that diabetes has been reversed in many cases, and I'm going to tell you how throughout this book. Lowering blood sugar with pills is like dumping buckets of water from a sinking boat when you should be plugging the hole.

AVOID THE MEDICATION MERRY-GO-ROUND

If you have high insulin levels or an elevated glucose-to-insulin ratio, then you have prediabetes or diabetes. Even if you do not yet take medications, please do all that you can to avoid them. Once you start medications, it's very hard to get your doctor to agree to discontinue them. It's certainly not impossible, especially since there are plenty of natural solutions that reduce blood sugar and insulin.

And there are many other ways to rebuild pancreatic tissue, but it can be difficult to wean yourself off medications—under your doctor's supervision, of course—once you start taking them. It seems so much easier to take medication. But as you know by now, I don't believe that "easy" is the best choice for your health.

There are inherent risks with drugs. Diabetic medications bring on the risk of hypoglycemic episodes. When blood sugar drops rapidly it can be extremely dangerous. In fact, drug-induced hypoglycemia is the number one drawback associated with insulin and oral medications. People at the highest risk for this problem include those who:

- Take more than one diabetic medication
- Combine prescribed medications with herbal formulas
- Exercise vigorously
- Have stomach problems, kidney damage, or heart damage
- Skip meals

Here's the problem: Once your physician orders medication, you will start on what I call the medication merry-go-round. And as you know, a merry-go-round doesn't take you forward. You wind up where you started with each go-around, and sometimes you get dizzy. In the case of diabetes, a medication merry-go-round looks like this: You start with one medication, and it sparks side effects because it is stealing your nutrients—a condition I call drug mugging. Simply put, your new drug mugs your body of vital nutrients. The supposed side effects—really due to nutrient depletion—will then be diagnosed as new diseases, so you will receive more drugs to deal with all your new "symptoms." Then you have to switch medications because of intolerable side effects.

Years may pass as you sit on this merry-go-round, taking you in circles and never moving you forward. And you never get to fix the underlying problem. Many of my patients have said that over the years they've constructed a miniature pharmacy in their bathroom cabinets.

Going in circles on this unnecessary merry-go-round is exasperating, and it can even be dangerous. See why it's important to manage your condition aggressively, *before* beginning medications?

OUR CURRENT MEDICAL SYSTEM IS WHACKED

Sure, drugs can bring your blood sugar numbers down. But if you're taking medications without changing your diet, your pancreas continues to die, one cell at a time, while free radicals—dangerous chemicals—are spawned. These free radicals destroy your pancreas and create inflammatory chemicals that cause more damage and pain, all while your blood sugar is in perfect range and your doctor is pleased with your progress.

Progress? It's a disgrace that so many people are losing their eyesight, losing their limbs, and losing their lives to diabetes. Our popular medications don't address the cause of the disorder. That's putting it mildly (for publication purposes). Some of these medications actually scare me! Most drugs—aside from insulin, which is useful if you have type 1 diabetes or severe type 2 diabetes—are what I call Band-Aid drugs.

BAND-AID DRUGS

Band-Aid drugs cover up symptoms, just as Band-Aids cover up wounds. However, unlike Band-Aids, these drugs have dangerous side effects. For example, the plethora of drugs prescribed to treat diabetes are Band-Aid drugs because they only lower blood sugar, so you think you're getting well. When you take the Band-Aid off, the "wound" has not healed. It is still oozing. I cannot think of one prescribed medication that reverses diabetes, or even reduces free-radical damage and inflammation. They're all Band-Aids. Remove the Band-Aid (stop the drug) and the wound is still there (blood sugar climbs).

The consequences of untreated diabetes, the emotional implications of these consequences, not to mention the constant health struggles that must be endured, spark such a deep level of frustration within me that I am determined to motivate you to take your health back into your own hands and heal your body. You can do it. You just need to be given the truth about foods and about natural treatment options. You will need to make a commitment right now to change your eating habits and to exercise. You should speak positive affirmations about feeling well. Only then can the healing begin. So let the healing begin today, right now.

Let's affirm. "I have abundant health and feel great."

SOME MEDICATIONS ARE DEADLY

In case you haven't paid attention to the news, or in case your doctor hasn't told you, some drugs given for diabetes actually put the nail in the coffin given the right set of circumstances. One example is Avandia, a popular diabetes drug that is suspected of causing heart failure. As if that weren't bad enough, Avandia and its sister drug Actos appear to double a woman's risk of bone fracture. Why did the FDA allow the makers of Avandia to rake in billions of dollars annually when reports of injury had been trickling in for years? Good question.

In 2008, after enough people checked into the morgue, the FDA decided to issue a "black box" warning to doctors that informs them of the serious dangers of thiazolidinediones—the class of drugs that Avandia and Actos belong to.

Some diabetes drugs cause you to gain weight. They have been blamed for dangerous swings in blood sugar and could possibly kill you. I'm not kidding. The results of the ACCORD trial (Action to Control Cardiovascular Risk in Diabetes) in 2008 found a 22 percent increased rate of death in diabetic patients who were treated aggressively versus those who were given fewer drugs and combinations of drugs. In fact, the study was halted early in February 2008 for ethical reasons.

The situation still had not gotten much better by December 2008, when the *New England Journal of Medicine* published more gloomy results about diabetes drugs. In a nutshell, the study proved that aggressive use of blood sugar-lowering medications to prevent heart disease was a complete and utter failure. Even the American Diabetes Association guidelines are emphasizing a more personal approach to setting goals for blood glucose control. This is because recent evidence has found that intensive treatment with medications does not improve cardiovascular function, and get this, it may cause a *higher* mortality (death rate) in people with type 2 diabetes.

USING YOUR MEDICATIONS SAFELY

I want to help you learn how to use medications safely if you have to take them. *Whether* you have to take them is between you and your physician. After all, he or she is your physician and has your personal medical history at hand. All I'm trying to do is plant new seeds in your head for healing so that you can discuss my alternative suggestions with your physician. If you absolutely have to take medications, then read on, because I'm also going to give you suggestions for natural vitamins and minerals that will offset those nasty side effects that occur from the drug-mugging effects of medications.

I've developed some categories to help you learn about the most popular medications on the market right now. I've made up catchy names for these, but I've included the technical term for these meds in parentheses so that healthcare practitioners who use my book as a reference can also follow along.

MUSCLE MAGNETS (BIGUANIDES)

WHO CAN USE THEM. People with type 2 diabetes or metabolic syndrome.

HOW THEY WORK. Biguanides are extracted from the French lilac plant. They were created after researchers found an active ingredient—isoamylene guanidine—in the French lilac. The initial attempt at creating drugs from the lovely blooms resulted in catastrophe, and a drug known as phenformin was totally withdrawn from the market.

Fortunately, researchers developed a relatively safer version called metformin. Metformin has become the drug of choice for people with diabetes since its introduction in 1994, with nearly 35 million prescriptions filled in 2006 for generic metformin alone.

Muscle magnets make your body more sensitive to insulin. These medications cause your muscles to act like a magnet and attract more sugar, which is good, since you don't want sugar in your bloodstream irritating and inflaming your blood vessels. These muscle magnets put a clamp on your liver and prevent it from dumping out too much sugar (glycogen), making it ideal for overweight people.

Aside from working on both the liver and muscle cells, metformin has several advantages over other prescribed medications. It has a reduced risk of causing weight gain and reduces the risk for dangerous blood sugar lows. Plus it's a better choice for someone with mild-to-moderate heart disease. Emerging studies show that metformin can relieve polycystic ovarian syndrome, a condition tied to insulin resistance.

Medication names

Metformin tablets (Glucophage, Glucophage XR, Fortamet)
Metformin liquid (Riomet)
Metformin and Rosiglitazone (Avandamet)
Metformin and Pioglitazone (ActoPlus Met)

HOW TO TAKE THEM. These medications are best tolerated when taken with food, usually with the evening meal, or, if ordered twice daily, then with breakfast and dinner. If you miss a dose, take it as soon as you remember, or skip it if your next dose is approaching soon. Never double up on doses.

THESE MEDS COULD BE DRUG MUGGERS OF: *Coenzyme Q10, folic acid, vitamin B$_{12}$, and probiotics.* Reductions in these nutrients can lead to liver damage, confusion, depression, neuropathy, muscle cramps, memory loss, depression, mouth sores, diarrhea or constipation, yeast infections, fatigue, high blood pressure, and higher risk for heart disease and stroke. Supplementation to offset the drug-mugging effect of biguanides should include:

Coenzyme Q10—50 to 100 milligrams twice daily (or ubiquinol, 100 milligrams daily)
Folic acid—400 to 800 micrograms daily
Methylcobalamin—250 to 1,000 micrograms daily
Probiotics—one or two capsules daily

POSSIBLE SIDE EFFECTS. Hypoglycemia, abdominal cramping, bloating, nausea, diarrhea, headache, and a funky, metallic taste in the mouth are all possible. Lactic acidosis (buildup of lactic acid in the bloodstream) is another rare but extremely dangerous complication that can occur. Lactic acidosis is associated with a very high mortality rate, especially in people over the age of 80, or those with other major health problems. The buildup of lactic acid in the bloodstream can cause shortness of breath (fast, shallow breathing), muscle aches, weakness, cramps, fatigue, sleepiness, and feeling cold. Discontinue the drug if these symptoms occur and call your physician immediately, as hospitalization may be necessary.

CAUTION. Do not crush, chew, or break extended-release formulas or combination formulas. People who have lung disease, kidney/liver problems, or congestive heart failure should be extremely cautious when taking (or should completely avoid) metformin because the risk of lactic acidosis is greater. Alcoholics, binge drinkers, or anyone who drinks more than 2 ounces of alcohol per day should not take metformin because alcohol in the bloodstream along with metformin can trigger fatal lactic acidosis.

Certain acid-blocking drugs used for heartburn may increase problems from metformin, as can cephalexin (Keflex), an extremely popular antibiotic. Biguanides are not advised in seniors over the age of 80 or those scheduled to receive contrast dye for magentic resonance imaging or other imaging procedures. Metformin should not be used by people with LADA, an autoimmune form of diabetes.

ALLERGY PRECAUTIONS. Do not take this medication if you are allergic to metformin or any ingredients, fillers, or binders in the tablet or capsules. It's okay for people with sulfa allergies.

INSULIN DRIVERS (SULFONYLUREAS)

WHO CAN USE THEM. People with type 2 diabetes or metabolic syndrome.

HOW THEY WORK. These oral medications help stimulate your pancreas to make more of its own natural insulin. Sulfonylureas also increase your risk of hypoglycemia since they drive up insulin, which lowers blood sugar. They won't work well in people with type 1 diabetes because their beta cells don't really produce insulin.

Insulin drivers have kept many people with type 2 diabetes off insulin injections. Older, first-generation drugs were introduced in the United States in 1955, but today's newer, second- and third-generation drugs are more effective and have fewer interactions. Newer drugs also spark less weight gain than first-generation drugs.

Insulin drivers are often used in combination with other medications by people with type 2 diabetes. Of the bunch, Glimepiride is the least likely to cause hypoglycemia and may be the best choice for someone with kidney disease (elevated creatinine levels).

Medication names

First generation:
    Chlorpropamide (Diabinese)
    Tolbutamide (Orinase)
    Tolazamide (Tolinase)

Second generation:
    Glipizide (Glucotrol, Glucotrol XL)
    Glipizide and metformin (Metaglip)

Glyburide (Micronase, Diabeta)
Micronized glyburide (Glynase)
Glyburide and metformin (Glucovance)

Third generation:
    Glimepiride (Amaryl)

HOW TO TAKE THEM. Take these medications by mouth about 15 to 30 minutes before a meal, usually once daily before breakfast. Taken this way, they are effective while you are eating. Some physicians order these drugs to be taken twice daily. If you skip a meal, *do not* take your medication. If you miss your dose while eating, take it as soon as you remember (with a snack), but if it's close to the next normal dosage time, just wait. Never double up on dosage.

THESE MEDS COULD BE DRUG MUGGERS OF: *Coenzyme Q10, folic acid, vitamin B_{12}, and probiotics.* Reductions in these nutrients can lead to liver damage, confusion, depression, neuropathy, muscle cramps, memory loss, depression, mouth sores, diarrhea, constipation, yeast infections, fatigue, hypertension, and higher risk for heart disease and stroke. Supplementation to offset the drug-mugging effect of sulfonylureas should include:

Coenzyme Q10—50 to 100 milligrams twice daily (or ubiquinol, 100 milligrams daily)

Folic acid—400 to 800 micrograms daily

Methylcobalamin—250 to 1,000 micrograms daily

Probiotic—one or two capsules daily

POSSIBLE SIDE EFFECTS. Hypoglycemia, nausea, upset stomach, heartburn, bloating, sun sensitivity, metallic taste in the mouth, easy bleeding, dark urine, mood or personality changes, and seizures. These medications can cause sudden weight gain, which is usually the result of fluid retention (edema).

CAUTION. Do not take these medications with alcohol or blood-thinning drugs or herbs, such as warfarin (Coumadin), clopidogrel (Plavix), heparin, prasugrel (Effient), or aspirin, unless your doctor approves. These medications may not be safe if you do not eat regularly or if you have adrenal or pituitary gland problems or kidney or liver disease. These medications pass through breast milk, so they will affect a baby's blood glucose levels; therefore they are not suitable for pregnant or breast-feeding women.

Never crush these medications without first asking your pharmacist. Some medications have special time-release coatings on them.

ALLERGY PRECAUTIONS. Watch out if you have sulfa allergies. Some people with a mild sulfa allergy can tolerate second- and third-generation drugs, including this class. However, if you have a severe sulfa allergy, I would not recommend this class of drugs at all.

SUGAR BUSTERS (MEGLITINIDES)

WHO CAN USE THEM. People with type 2 diabetes or metabolic syndrome.

HOW THEY WORK. These quick-fix drugs blunt the normal spike in blood sugar that occurs after eating food. Sugar busters get in and out of your body quickly. You take them 5 to 30 minutes before eating, and they stop working within hours. Their goal is to rapidly raise insulin levels while you're eating, when glucose levels peak. That's good; you want your blood sugar bus (insulin) to work hard for you and drive all the glucose into the cells. Because they are in and out of your system quickly, there is less risk of hypoglycemia.

There are currently two sugar busters on the market—Prandin and Starlix. Prandin is derived from benzoic acid, a common preservative in our foods that inhibits the growth of mold and fungus. Prandin has been approved in the United States since 1997. The other sugar buster, Starlix, is a patented drug that is morphed out of an amino acid called D-phenylalanine, which you may recognize as the artificial sweetener aspartame.

Medication names
    Repaglinide (Prandin)
    Nateglinide (Starlix)
    Metiglinide (Glufast) [Launched in Japan, not available in United States]

HOW TO TAKE THEM. Take these medications 5 to 30 minutes before meals, since they work while you are eating. If you skip a meal, don't take your medication. If you miss a dose, take it as soon as you remember or skip it if your next dose is approaching soon. Never double up on doses.

THESE MEDS COULD BE DRUG MUGGERS OF: There are no documented nutrient depletions; however, I suspect that the B vitamins and probiotics could be depleted, so my professional advice is to supplement with:

    Probiotics—one or two capsules daily
    B complex—every morning

POSSIBLE SIDE EFFECTS. Hypoglycemia, weight gain, and gastrointestinal disturbances, such as nausea, vomiting, and diarrhea. Muscle aches, back pain, arthritis, and, oddly, cold, and flulike symptoms may also occur.

CAUTION. Do not take sugar-buster medications if you drink alcohol. Chronic use of nonsteroidal antiinflammatory drugs such as ibuprofen, naproxen, or aspirin may also interact with these medications. Use these sugar-busting meglitinides cautiously, and make sure you tell your doctor if you also take acetaminophen, beta-blockers, blood thinners, thyroid medication, cold medicine that contains pseudoephedrine, or monoamine oxidase inhibitors.

These drugs are primarily processed in the liver, so they are contraindicated (not advisable) in people who have liver damage or a history of alcohol abuse. However, prevailing knowledge suggests that sugar busters can be relatively safe to use in people with kidney failure. Of course, this all depends on your physician's opinions.

ALLERGY PRECAUTIONS. Do not take if allergic to any ingredients, fillers, or binders in the tablet or capsules. These medications are okay for people with sulfa allergies. Because Starlix is derived from phenylalanine, don't take it if you have the hereditary disorder PKU (phenylketonurea) because that condition prevents you from safely processing phenylalanine.

GLUCOSE GOBBLERS (GLITAZONES OR THIAZOLIDINEDIONES)

WHO CAN USE THEM. People with type 2 diabetes or metabolic syndrome.

HOW THEY WORK. The glitazones or thiazolidinediones are the most notorious of all the diabetic drugs on the market. By that, I mean that they are always in the news (especially Avandia) because of increasing concerns about safety. Generally speaking, these drugs help make better use of the insulin you have, so that the doors on your cells unlock, and gobble up any glucose that may be hanging around. They also tell the liver not to release any of its stored glucose.

The glitazones or thiazolidinediones, which typically work optimally within 2 months, are particularly useful in people with insulin resistance. What I like about this class of drugs is that they help lower dangerous low-density lipoprotein cholesterol and levels of inflammatory chemicals, such as TNF-alpha (tumor necrosis factor alpha) or CRP (C-reactive protein), thereby lowering one's risk for heart disease and pancreatic damage. To be clear you want some TNF (it protects you from cancer) but you don't want excessive amounts.

These drugs are almost always used in combination with other medications. Women with polycystic ovary disease sometimes take these medications to lower their blood sugar and increase fertility. Glucose gobblers only reduce blood sugar by about 15 percent and are powerful drug muggers, potentially leading to some eye-popping side effects.

Medication names
    Rosiglitazone (Avandia)
    Pioglitazone (Actos)
    Troglitazone (Rezulin) [Withdrawn in the United States in 2000 after
        hepatitis and liver fatalities]

HOW TO TAKE THEM. These medications can be taken without regard to meals. If you miss a dose, take it as soon as you remember or skip it if your next dose is approaching soon. Never double up on doses.

THESE MEDS COULD BE DRUG MUGGERS OF: *Coenzyme Q10, folic acid, vitamin B$_{12}$, and probiotics.* Reductions in these nutrients can lead to liver damage, confusion, depression, neuropathy, muscle cramps, memory loss, depression, mouth sores, diarrhea, constipation, yeast infections, fatigue, high blood pressure, and higher risk for heart disease and stroke. Supplementation to offset the drug-mugging effect of glitazones should include:

Coenzyme Q10—50 to 100 milligrams twice daily (or ubiquinol, 100 milligrams daily)
Folic acid—400 to 800 micrograms daily
Methylcobalamin—250 to 1,000 micrograms daily
Probiotic—one or two capsules daily

POSSIBLE SIDE EFFECTS. Hypoglycemia, severe loss of appetite, muscle weakness, fatigue, fluid retention (swelling of ankles or legs), weight gain, respiratory infections, headaches, muscle aches, and toothaches. Liver damage is also a possibility. In fact, baseline liver function tests are supposed to be performed before treatment begins and repeated every 2 or 3 months during the first year of therapy. Tea-colored urine or yellowing of the eyes and skin could be the first clue of liver destruction.

CAUTION. Do not use if you have type 1 diabetes, are pregnant, or have liver damage or heart failure. Do not use if you take insulin, because the combination increases fluid retention and the risk for heart failure. Do not use if you drink alcohol.

At least one large prospective study has shown that Actos may decrease the overall incidence of cardiac events in people with type 2 diabetes who have already had a heart attack. Avandia came under fire in 2007 when an article in the *New England Journal of Medicine* reported that data pooled from dozens of studies suggested that this medication caused a 43 percent higher risk of heart attack than a placebo.

Back in 2000, Rezulin—a similar drug that was popular—was recalled because of liver fatalities. In October 2008, the consumer group Public Citizen petitioned the FDA to ban Avandia because of life-threatening side effects. Both the American Diabetes Association and the European Association for the Study of Diabetes advise against using the drug. People with type 1.5 diabetes, hallmarked by low levels of insulin (rather than resistance to insulin), are unlikely to benefit from a glucose gobbler.

ALLERGY PRECAUTIONS. Do not take if you are allergic to glitazones or thiazolidinediones or any ingredients, fillers, or binders in the tablet or capsules. These drugs are okay for people with sulfa allergies, however.

STARCH STALLERS (ALPHA-GLUCOSIDASE INHIBITORS)

WHO CAN USE THEM. People with type 2 diabetes or metabolic syndrome.

HOW THEY WORK. These drugs act like starch blockers. (Think defensive line in football.) If you eat carbohydrates or starches, the drugs will keep your intestinal enzymes from fully breaking down the starch into glucose. This slows the rate at which blood sugar enters your body, blunting the typical blood sugar spike after eating.

Starch stallers suppress a starch-eating enzyme called amylase, which is normally released by the pancreas. I'm as unhappy as a cat in the shower over this (have you ever seen a cat in a shower?) because amylase is a natural IgG histamine inhibitor, which stabilizes mast cells and basophils that otherwise release histamine as part of your inflammatory response. Translated to English, this means that starch stallers might increase histamine-related problems, such as allergies, inflammation, pain, and food sensitivities. That's strike one.

Strike two is that these drugs are not very effective by themselves, so they are prescribed with more powerful drugs.

And strike three, I don't agree with the notion that it's okay to only partially digest your foods, because this taxes your gastrointestinal tract and triggers inflammation, an issue that people with diabetes have to overcome to begin with. I'm not overjoyed that carbs in your meal won't get broken down adequately into glucose, but that's how these drugs work. When you leave carbs partially undigested in your intestine, bacteria and yeast start to eat them and ferment them, which produces a lot of fizziness from the carbon dioxide gas that results. You can get serious gastrointestinal side effects, especially gas—and I mean the explosive sort. It's better to consume natural startch stallers. Natural amylase inhibitors include maitake mushrooms, kidney beans, lentils, and peas.

Can the drugs help you lose weight the way that over-the-counter starch-blockers are advertised to do? No. The only reason I can think of to use these drugs is to allow you guiltless indulgence once in a while, like when you just can't resist a slice of birthday cake or Thanksgiving pie.

Medication names
   Miglitol (Glyset)
   Acarbose (Precose in the United States, Glucobay in Europe)
   Voglibose (Basen in Japan)

HOW TO TAKE THEM. You are supposed to take these drugs with every meal, so if you skip a meal, skip the drug. Take the drug with your very first bite of food. Start with the lowest possible dosage and climb up as directed. Do not take these medications within 4 hours of taking digestive enzymes.

THESE MEDS COULD BE DRUG MUGGERS OF: *Iron.* A deficiency in iron can cause one to feel cranky, tired, depressed, and confused. It could also cause a sore tongue, brittle nails, pale skin, and a racing heart, even with very little exertion.

Iron is the only nutrient depletion that is well documented at the time of this writing; however, minerals stick together the way loving families do. I have a feeling that most of your minerals are being mugged by starch stallers, even if I can't prove it right now. Read more about the importance of minerals in Chapter 14. It's likely that selenium, potassium, calcium, and zinc are also depleted. Accordingly, my recommendation for supplementation includes two options.

Iron is famous for irritating the gut and causing constipation and harmless discoloration of the feces.

Option one (my first choice) is for you to take spirulina, which is a marine-derived superfood packed with minerals and a lot of iron. This could increase your health and well-being in so many ways, with few if any side effects. Information on spirulina is on page 240.

Option two would be to supplement with traditional iron tablets or capsules. The best-tolerated form of iron is iron polysaccharide (Nu Iron or Niferex). Take one capsule (150 milligrams) on Monday, Wednesday, and Friday of each week for 3 months, along with a capsule or tablet of trace minerals each day. The iron and trace minerals may be easier to handle if you take them with meals, so long as you do not consume dairy, eggs, cereal, tea, coffee, or antacids.

POSSIBLE SIDE EFFECTS. Hypoglycemia, bloating, nausea, diarrhea, severe gas, abdominal pain, and cramps. Less common, but occasionally seen, is jaundice—yellowing of eyes and skin and tea-colored urine.

CAUTION. Do not use these drugs (unless under the advice of your doctor) if you have liver disease, bowel problems, intestinal blockages, or any digestive disorders. Do not use starch stallers if you take activated charcoal (such as CharcoCaps), a popular over-the-counter remedy for gas. Do not take if you drink alcohol.

ALLERGY PRECAUTIONS. Do not take if you are allergic to any ingredients, fillers, or binders in the tablets or capsules. Starch stallers are fine for people with sulfa allergies.

INCRETIN INCREASERS (INCRETIN ANALOGS)

WHO CAN USE THEM. People with type 2 diabetes or metabolic syndrome.

HOW THEY WORK. The most famous—or should I say infamous—drug in this class is Byetta (exanetide), made by Amylin and Eli Lilly pharmaceuticals. The makers were forced to put a black-box warning on their drug in 2008 after growing rumblings of drug-induced pancreatitis occurred. (Ye gads!)

Byetta exhibits the same effects as the human incretin hormone called GLP-1. See Chapter 3 for info on GLP-1. Without getting too complicated, these drugs help you digest your foods. The interesting (but gross) thing about Byetta is that it is derived from lizard spit. Seriously, it comes from the saliva of Gila (pronounced *heela*) monsters. Researchers who didn't mind getting chummy with the giant lizards extracted their spit and found a hormone called incretin. It's about 50 percent identical to our own incretin hormone (GLP-1), so it can mimic effects of that hormone. GLP-1 helps you increase insulin sensitivity, thereby helping you lower blood sugar, lose weight, and feel better.

A cleaned-up, powerful drug dribbled onto the market in April 2005. (I'm still stuck on how they got the Gila monsters to salivate. Do they just dangle juicy rats in front of them?)

Anyway, without enough incretin you wouldn't be able to produce enough insulin, and your blood sugar levels would stay high, resulting in chronic high blood sugar and nasty diabetic complications.

Drugs in this class also keep the pancreas from giving up too much glucagon—the hormone that tells your liver to dump sugar into the bloodstream. Incretin drugs will make you feel fuller for a longer period of time.

The brand-name drug Victoza may hold some advantage over Byetta because it will be dosed daily instead of twice a day, so hooray for fewer needle sticks.

And in preliminary studies, Victoza does not appear to cause pancreatitis, and it may be able to lower triglycerides. The drug is now available in the United States, even though its chances were not looking so good—the FDA had refused to approve it because of concerns about thyroid cancer that arose from animal studies. It was approved in Europe in 2009.

An oral version of this drug is in development by Oramed; as of December 2009, studies in patients with type 1 diabetes showed positive results. Studies in patients with type 2 diabetes are under way in South Africa.

Medication names
    Exanatide (Byetta injection)
    Liraglutide (Victoza injection, pending FDA approval)
    Albiglutide (Syncria, pending FDA approval)
    Exendin-4 (another Gila-derived drug that is still in the testing stage)

HOW TO TAKE THEM. Take the medication within 60 minutes before eating. If you forget to take your medication and start eating, then just skip the dose.

THESE MEDS COULD BE DRUG MUGGERS OF: unknown at this point. These drugs are relatively new on the market, so there is as yet no documentation of nutrient depletion. I can still take an educated guess because you all depend on me to think these things out. Exanatide (Byetta) has been associated with life-threatening and sometimes fatal pancreatitis. And low circulating levels of antioxidants can contribute to pancreatitis. Clinical research has proven that when you administer antioxidants to people with pancreatitis, free-radical damage slows down and pain subsides. Does it make sense, then, that Byetta (and possibly all drugs in this class) could be depleting our body of antioxidant minerals and vitamins? On the basis of this theory I would recommend supplementing with several of the following antioxidants.

- Plant-based oral antioxidant: One that contains cranberry, pomegranate, pycnogenol, resveratrol, and green tea extract. You can find these in green drinks.
- Other oral antioxidants, such as vitamins A, C, E, and D; selenium and ubiquinol or alpha lipoic acid. See Chapter 3 for more about antioxidants and how they can prevent or relieve pancreatitis pain.

POSSIBLE SIDE EFFECTS. Hypoglycemia, dizziness, flulike symptoms, nausea, vomiting, diarrhea, and headaches. Also soreness, redness, and itching at the injection site may occur. Pancreatitis is a possible serious complication that has been tied to Byetta. For information about signs and symptoms of pancreatitis, read Chapter 3.

CAUTION. *Do not use incretin drugs if you take insulin.* If you experience abdominal pain (especially on your left side), nausea, fever, or yellowing of the skin, this could mean pancreatitis, and you will require medical attention. Do not take if you drink alcohol.

ALLERGY PRECAUTIONS. Do not take if you are allergic to any ingredients, fillers, or binders in the tablets or capsules. The incretin analogs are safe for people with sulfa allergies.

INSULIN EXTENDERS (GLIPTINS OR DPP-4 BLOCKERS, DIPEPTIDYL PEPTIDASE-4 INHIBITORS)

WHO CAN USE THEM. People with type 2 diabetes or metabolic syndrome.

HOW THEY WORK. Gliptins are a new class of therapeutic diabetic drugs with a method of action similar to that of Byetta and its brothers. They are hardly ever used by themselves because they don't work well. The gliptins, when used alone, reduce hemoglobin A1c by about 1 to 2 percent, depending on whether they are used alone or in conjunction with metformin.

The first gliptin introduced to the United States was Januvia in 2006. This drug and its relatives block the actions of an enzyme called DPP-4, and this slows down the destruction of GLP-1. Long story short, these drugs keep incretin hormones alive longer, which extends the action of insulin. You may experience lower fasting blood glucose levels, but unfortunately there is little to no effect on blood pressure, cholesterol ratios, or weight.

Medication names
   Sitagliptin (Januvia)
   Sitagliptin and metformin (Janumet)
   Vildagliptin (Galvus)
   Alogliptin (investigational; Takeda Pharmaceuticals)
   Saxagliptin (Onglyza)

HOW TO TAKE THEM. Take gliptins without regard to meals, unless your doctor instructs otherwise. If you forget a dose, take it as soon as you remember. If it is almost time for your next dose, then skip the forgotten dose altogether. You never want to double up on doses.

THESE MEDS COULD BE DRUG MUGGERS OF: There are no documented nutrient depletions for sitagliptin or vildagliptin at the time of this writing. The combination drug called Janumet contains metformin, so please refer to page 73 to see what the drug muggers of metformin are—those apply if you take Janumet.

POSSIBLE SIDE EFFECTS. Hypoglycemia, pancreatitis, nausea, abdominal cramps, diarrhea, anxiety, blurred vision, depression, dizziness, nightmares, rapid heartbeat, and headache. Stranger than fiction, but you can also get nasopharyngitis (which is basically a bad cold, complete with labored breathing or other breathing problems), muscle aches, cough, sneezing, sore or dry throat, stuffy/runny nose, loss of voice, fever, and cold sweats.

CAUTION. The disadvantage I see with gliptins is that you need DPP-4 in your body because this enzyme slows the development of cancer. To be fair, no studies to date show increased incidence of cancer in people taking these drugs, but it still concerns me because some studies show increased infection rates and inflammatory chemicals among users, indicating a suppressive effect on the immune system.

If you have allergic conditions, immune system disorders, or a history of cancer, ask your physician for something different. On a more positive note, some intriguing studies suggest that these drugs can preserve and possibly regenerate beta cells. Gliptins are probably a safe choice for people who have serious concerns about hypoglycemic reactions. Do not take this class of drugs if you drink alcohol.

ALLERGY PRECAUTIONS. Do not take gliptins if you are allergic to any drugs within this class or to inactive ingredients used in the formulation.

PANCREAS PUSHERS (AMYLIN ANALOGS)

WHO CAN USE THEM. People with all three types of diabetes (types 1, 1.5, and 2).

HOW THEY WORK. Amylin is a natural hormone made in the beta cells of your pancreas (the same cells that make insulin). Amylin deficiencies are more common in people with type 1 diabetes who have lost their beta cells. When the pancreas cells die or become damaged, amylin levels go down right along with insulin.

TROUBLE WITH LANTUS

Lantus (insulin glargine) is a special "basal" insulin that was FDA approved in 2000. Basal release of insulin means a slow and steady continuous release. Currently, Lantus is the number-one prescribed form of insulin. With Lantus insulin, you can take one shot and have it work all day. There are no ups and downs with Lantus. It provides a steady release of insulin over 24 hours, so you don't have to worry about peaks and troughs, or about eating snacks when you don't feel hungry. This comes as a terrific surprise to many people with diabetes, who otherwise must stick themselves three to six times a day with insulin.

With 24-hour coverage and once-daily dosing, Lantus makes a great form of insulin for people who are needle shy or prone to hypoglycemia. It's been first on the list for many doctors prescribing insulin for their patients because it is less likely to cause dangerous blood sugar lows.

The problem is that several preliminary studies suggest an increased risk of cancer among users of the long-acting Lantus. The FDA is investigating this and is in discussions with the manufacturer to conduct more research about the safety of their medication.

One German study of more than 127,000 diabetic patients taking insulin found that malignancies were more common in people treated with Lantus compared with old-style human insulin. And in a Swedish study involving almost 115,000 insulin-treated patients, those taking Lantus alone were almost twice as likely to be diagnosed with breast cancer. But is it the medication itself causing these problems, or the fact that chronically elevated levels of insulin give rise to tumors? Nothing is conclusive, but if found to be true, the effect could change the face of diabetes treatment and have a cataclysmic effect on Sanofi, the manufacturer. People in the United States are being advised to continue their medication until told otherwise by their physician. I would make sure that you speak openly to your physician about the continued use of this medication, particularly if you have a history of cancer or high family risk. For more information about the drug, you can visit www.lantus.com.

Amylin slows the passage of food through your digestive tract so you feel full, thereby reducing your appetite. You can possibly lose weight without breaking a sweat. I completely disagree with using these drugs for overweight people or for those who remain hungry after eating, although they are sometimes prescribed for these reasons. Pancreas pushers put a clamp on your liver, suppressing the release of stored blood sugar (glycogen), which occurs after eating. The release of glycogen maintains steadier blood glucose levels after eating.

ESSENTIALS FOR PEOPLE WITH DIABETES

It's good to be on the safe side and wear some kind of identification tag or jewelry alerting people that you are diabetic and that you take hypoglycemic agents (even natural ones). Today, there are many options that are stylish, including bracelets, sports bands, necklaces, charms, watchbands, wallet cards, even rubber glow-in-the-dark shoe tags. Your local pharmacy staff can show you their selection, but if you want to see hundreds of different, unique choices, check out the Web site www.medids.com/DiabeticBracelets.html.

Pancreas pushers are often prescribed in combination with insulin or other medications. These drugs are injected subcutaneously, in a manner similar to that used for insulin, but they are not insulin. These drugs are synthetic versions that mimic our own natural amylin.

Medication names

Pramlintide (Symlin, by injection with prefilled pens)

HOW TO TAKE THEM. Symlin should be injected by itself, not with insulin. The injection should be administered right before eating. You need to check your blood sugar before injecting it, as well as after your meal. If you miss a dose of, Symlin at a meal, wait until the next meal. Do not take this medicine if you skip a meal. It should be used only when you eat.

THESE MEDS COULD BE DRUG MUGGERS OF: *Vitamin D.* This is a fat-soluble vitamin that many Americans are deficient in. It boosts immune function. From this information, I'm going to extrapolate that in time, we will learn that these drugs deplete other fat-soluble nutrients, such as vitamins A, E, and K. Accordingly, I would recommend that you take the supplement cholecalciferol (vitamin D_3), about 5,000 IU every morning. You should also take daily supplements of about 15 milligrams (25,000 IU) of beta-carotene (which supplies vitamin A) and 200 to 400 IU of natural vitamin E. Finally, make sure you eat plenty of green leafy vegetables, which supply vitamin K.

POSSIBLE SIDE EFFECTS. Hypoglycemia or nausea and vomiting (especially with high dosages) can occur. Other possible side effects include appetite loss, abdominal pain, dizziness, and indigestion. Pain, itching, or redness may also occur at the injection site.

BLOOD SUGAR ALERT: CHECK YOUR MEDICINE CABINET

Hundreds of medications and herbs can affect your blood sugar—either raising it and causing hyperglycemia, or lowering it and causing hypoglycemia. I've created a list for you so you can see whether you are taking a drug that can affect your blood sugar.

I've also posted a comprehensive list of more than 200 medications on my Web site (www.DearPharmacist.com) and I will update this list for you as it changes.

The following is a list of some of the most popular medications and their side effects on hyperglycemia or hypoglycemia. This list is not intended as medical advice (nor is any of my advice to you technically intended as "medical" advice). I am not suggesting that you stop any of your medications should you find one or more on the following list. Always talk to your nurse, doctor, and pharmacist to approve changes to your medication regimen.

Also note that some natural supplements can alter your blood sugar. You'll find that list below as well.

MEDICATIONS THAT CAUSE HYPERGLYCEMIA

Abilify

Armour thyroid

Asthma medicine containing steroids or albuterol

Baclofen (Lioresal)

Candesartan and hydrochlorothiazide (Atacand HCT)

Carvedilol (Coreg)

Cold medicine containing pseudoephedrine (these sometimes end in D, such as Claritin D or Zyrtec-D, but read labels to find pseudoephedrine)

Estrogen-containing drugs (Premarin, Vagifem, Estring, birth control pills/patches) and hormone replacement drugs

Diuretics (water pills like furosemide or hydrochlorothiazide, also called HCTZ)

**Fluoxetine (Prozac, Sarafem)

HIV medications (Norvir, Invirase, Epivir)

CAUTION. This medication is not recommended for people who have gastroparesis, a condition in which the stomach holds on to food longer than it should. High dosages can cause severe hypoglycemia, so always start with the lowest effective dose. This medication should not be taken if you drink alcohol. A hypoglycemic reaction is more likely to occur if insulin doses are not reduced several days before Symlin is introduced. As weight loss occurs, lower dosages will be

Levothyroxine (Synthroid, Levoxyl)

Nadolol (Corgard)

Niacin (Vitamin B$_3$)

Modafinil (Provigil)

Pantoprazole (Protonix)

Risperidone (Risperdal)

Seizure medicine (Depakote, Phenytoin, and others)

Seroquel

Sotalol (Betapace)

Steroids such as prednisone (Sterapred) and methylprednisolone (Medrol)

MEDICATIONS THAT CAUSE HYPOGLYCEMIA

All medications used to treat diabetes

Alcohol

Aspirin

Beta-blockers for high blood pressure

Bisoprolol (Zebeta)

Clarithromycin (Biaxin)

Diltiazem (Cardizem)

**Fluoxetine (Prozac)

Insulin and other diabetic medications

Levofloxacin (Levaquin) and other antibiotics

Monoamine oxidase inhibitors for psychiatric problems

Metoprolol (Lopressor)

Morphine and other pain relievers

Nifedipine (Procardia)

Phenytoin (Dilantin, Phenytek, Epanutin)

Selegiline (Eldepryl)

Theophylline (Theo-Dur, Theo-24, Slo-bid, Uniphyl)

Verapamil (Calan, Isoptin)

NATURAL SUPPLEMENTS THAT INCREASE BLOOD SUGAR

Licorice root: People take it for stomach ulcers, sore throat, viral infections, and bronchitis.

Fish oils (only very high dosages): People take it for hypertension, atherosclerosis, depression, and constipation.

Glucosamine: People take it for arthritis and chronic venous insufficiency (varicose veins, leg swelling).

**Can cause both hyper- and hypoglycemia

needed. Do not take Symlin if you also take acarbose (Precose), or any other drug that is an alpha glucosidase inhibitor.

ALLERGY PRECAUTIONS. Do not use Symlin if you might be allergic to any of the ingredients in the formula, including the preservative metacresol, D-mannitol, or acetic acid.

> ### INSULIN GROWS ON TREES
>
> Plant-based insulin may hit the market in 2010 because the Canadian-based firm SemBioSys Genetics has figured out a way to use the safflower plant to make a form of insulin that exactly matches human insulin. One acre of safflowers yields 1 kilogram of insulin (about the weight of a small bag of sugar) and will supply about 2,500 patients for a year. The product, known only as SBS-1000, is bioequivalent to Eli Lilly's blockbuster Humulin R insulin.

INSULIN

WHO CAN USE IT. People with type 1 diabetes, those with type 1.5 diabetes, and occasionally people with type 2 diabetes.

HOW IT WORKS. You make insulin in your body, and it is secreted by the pancreas. When the pancreatic beta cells are damaged or destroyed completely, your natural insulin levels decline. The insulin that you inject subcutaneously gets absorbed by your bloodstream, where it detects rising levels of blood sugar.

If you recall from Chapter 1, insulin is a blood sugar bus. It picks up passengers (glucose) and shuttles these sugar molecules to your cells, so your cells can receive the glucose and convert it to energy. The first medications created for use by people with diabetes contained insulin that was extracted from pigs or cows, but many people had allergic reactions to the animal-derived proteins, so the medications no longer contain insulin from these animals.

Although this may sound no more appealing than insulin from pigs or cows, today we use big vats of bacteria to grow insulin. Thankfully, we are able to create a bioidentical form of human insulin, so there are fewer allergic reactions. This is actually a medical marvel for pharmaceutical companies worldwide and also for the many people who need high-quality insulin to survive.

Today's insulin is categorized by how fast it works, something we call onset of action. The table "Insulin Types" on the opposite page outlines the types of insulin available today. One disadvantage of injecting insulin is that it goes hand in hand with weight gain. And while insulin has saved many lives, it is still difficult for many people to overcome their fear of needles. This drug currently requires subcutaneous injection, with the preferred site of injection being the abdomen.

Medication names

INSULIN TYPES			
TYPE	**ONSET**	**PEAK**	**DURATION**
Rapid-Apidra, Humalog, Novolog	<15 min	60–120 min	4–5 hours
Regular U-100, and U-500	30–45 min	2–4 hours	6–8 hours
NPH	1–2 hr	6–8 hours	18–26 hours
Levimir	1–2 hr	Nearly done	18–26 hours (dose related)
Lantus	1–2 hr	Nearly done	22–26 hours

Source: US Food and Drug Administration

HOW TO TAKE IT. Regular insulin or long-acting insulin is generally taken 15 to 30 minutes before your meal. Humalog and other kinds of lispro insulin are taken less than 15 minutes before eating. See the table "Insulin Types" above for more information.

THESE MEDS COULD BE DRUG MUGGERS OF: No nutrient depletions from insulin have been documented at this time.

POSSIBLE SIDE EFFECTS. Hypoglycemia is the most common side effect that occurs with insulin therapy. It can happen fast because the drug is injected directly into your body. Symptoms of hypoglycemia include confusion, nausea, perspiration, headache, heart palpitations, and loss of consciousness. Skin reactions at the site of injection can occur, as can worsening eyesight (retinopathy) and general body swelling. Unfortunately, weight gain is also a very common side effect of insulin.

CAUTION. Insulin vials remain stable and fresh when protected from excessive light and heat. If you forget a dose, do not double up on your next dose. Rotate the sites of injection so you don't erode the fat layer beneath your skin (a condition called lipodystrophy).

Many medications enhance insulin's effect in the body, particularly beta-blockers and angiotensin-converting enzyme inhibitors (medications used for blood pressure and kidney disease), aspirin, and monoamine oxidase inhibitor

---

EVER FELT THE URGE TO BE A GUINEA PIG?

If you've ever wanted to be part of a clinical trial, you can. I can't promise what the outcome will be, or whether you will sprout an extra ear, but if you want to be a guinea pig and get your medicine paid for, there are ways. Some clinical trials actually pay you to participate in medical research. Go to a Web site sponsored by the National Institutes of Health (www.nih.gov), which is part of the U.S. Department of Health and Human Services. If you type in key words (for example, "Diabetes and Florida,") you will get an instant listing of ongoing clinical trials and recruitment information. This site also explains what types of people qualify (for example, "type 2 diabetics only," "type 1 diabetics," or "healthy volunteers"). You can click on the "health" button on the home page, and find "clinical trials," or go to straight to www.clinicaltrials.gov.

---

drugs. Also, alcohol—which is basically the only non–FDA-approved drinkable drug sold over-the-counter—is a big no-no with insulin, and all diabetes drugs for that matter. Even one glass of wine can interact with meds to cause dangerous hypoglycemia.

Diagnostic Tests to Monitor Your Progress

Would you ever drive your car without getting the brakes tested or the oil checked? Consider that you have only one body—and you can't buy another or trade it in. So you'll want to do at least the equivalent of having your brakes checked and using that dipstick to see if you're running on empty. That's what your doctor does when you go in for a routine checkup.

But please don't stop there. Monitoring your progress while taking supplements or medications is one of the best ways to take care of yourself. All the tests that I will share with you in this chapter are useful because besides pinpointing problems, they may also help you determine whether your medication and dietary supplements are working. That's important because the complications of diabetes can damage you behind the scenes. Proper testing can show you—without a doubt—that all your hard work is paying off, and that you're not in danger of kidney disease, infections, ketoacidosis, or dangerous dips in blood sugar.

As you've already learned, your blood sugar is affected by medications, supplements, diet, injury, stress, and infection, among other factors. With your quality of life ultimately at stake, you're harming yourself if you don't consider at least some—if not all—of the tests I suggest in this chapter.

Not to scare you (okay, maybe to scare you a little), people with diabetes die 7 years earlier, on average, than people without diabetes. The good news is that you can control those aspects of your health that contribute to this risk by lowering your blood pressure and cholesterol levels and by closely monitoring your blood sugar to keep it steady and even.

Here are the tests that I think you should have.

FASTING BLOOD SUGAR

This is one of the most popular blood tests that doctors order for their patients, but it's not terribly important in my book in terms of diagnosis. Your blood sugar (and cholesterol) number changes from hour to hour, depending on the time of day and consumption of food, drink, or medications and supplements. "Fasting" just means that you have not eaten, so a fasting blood sugar (FBS) test measures blood glucose after you have not eaten for at least 8 hours. This makes sense, right? Because if your blood sugar is high when you haven't eaten for 8 hours, that's a pretty good indication that you have insulin resistance.

The drawback is that many people with a normal blood glucose reading slip through the cracks and don't get diagnosed with diabetes properly. Why? It is entirely possible to have a perfect FBS level simply because your poor, over-worked pancreas is on overdrive pumping out insulin like crazy to maintain those normal blood glucose levels. So the FBS can be quite normal, while the insulin levels are sky high. Individuals in this state are already in trouble. These people will be told they are fine and can maintain a false sense of security for years or even decades before their diabetes is suddenly discovered. Trust me, diabetes doesn't happen overnight!

People with chronically high insulin are in trouble, regardless of their FBS, so *always* have serum insulin levels measured as well. You'll have to ask your doctor to do this because most don't call for this test as a matter of routine. Now, I hope you see why testing blood levels of insulin, which we'll discuss momentarily, and improving your diet make good sense and can help you to prevent diabetes.

From now on, think of a fasting blood sugar level as a glucose measurement that is a snapshot in time, sort of like a photograph. The FBS is more of a screening device than a predictor for who will actually develop diabetes.

WHY THIS TEST IS IMPORTANT. The FBS is an easy, inexpensive, and nearly painless way to measure glucose.

Of course, it's also possible to get quick results derived from a home glucose testing device, which you are not likely to have on hand unless you already have diabetes. These devices are especially useful if you need a quick measurement of glucose—for example, if you feel symptoms of hypoglycemia coming on or if you want to track how well you are responding to pharmaceuticals or dietary supplements. We'll discuss home monitoring devices later in this chapter.

HOW FREQUENTLY TO MONITOR. The FBS test, done at your doctor's office or a lab, should be performed annually or as often as your doctor recommends it. (The need to test with a home glucose monitor varies from several times a week to several times a day, depending on your health status and your doctor's recommendation.)

NORMAL RANGE. 70 to 100 mg/dl

SERUM INSULIN

Diabetes does not begin when blood glucose (FBS) climbs above normal. As I've said, I think it's more important to measure blood insulin than blood glucose. I realize that flies in the face of current recommendations for lab testing, so I want you to understand why I feel this way.

The problem with diabetes begins when insulin rises. Yes, insulin, not sugar. Insulin levels typically climb right after you eat in order to reduce blood glucose, and then level out a few hours afterward. Insulin rises in response to high blood sugar, and the insulin system, even when it's set on overdrive, can work effectively for many years. That's why many people who may be on the path to developing diabetes still have blood sugar readings in the "normal" range. They may be secreting insulin like crazy, but these prediabetic individuals slip through the cracks until they develop insulin resistance and their FBS numbers go up. As long as they still have normal FBS numbers, these people are told they are fine. They are anything but fine, because high insulin levels are linked to many major disorders.

This serum insulin test is not frequently ordered, but it should be at the top of your list. It can help you discover whether you have prediabetes many years before complications such as kidney damage occur. Shocking, isn't it? But elevated insulin tells your doctor that your beta cells are on overdrive and tiring out. This shows up in a blood test long before insulin resistance develops.

WHY THIS TEST IS IMPORTANT. Chronically elevated insulin causes a cascade of inflammatory chemicals and high levels of cortisol hormone, a condition that can lead to major diseases, including diabetes and cancer. High serum insulin levels can shed light on a prediabetic state, despite normal blood glucose levels. That's a good thing because it gives you years to make dietary and lifestyle changes and to exercise so you can bring the insulin levels down. The ratio of glucose to insulin gives you the very best picture, so when your FBS is measured, your insulin should be measured as well. This ratio is *far* more important than either measurement alone. The ratio of glucose to insulin should be greater than 10 to 1.

HOW FREQUENTLY TO MONITOR. Have this test done every time you monitor your blood glucose levels at the doctor's office, and that should be at least once a year. This way, you can see the ratio.

NORMAL RANGE. Optimum insulin level is 5 to 10 microunits/ml. If your levels are higher than 10, your risk for developing diabetes increases. Above 25, you're looking at a slam dunk for diabetes unless you make some changes quickly.

Ideally, your doctor will measure glucose and insulin simultaneously. Again, the ratio of glucose to insulin should be greater than 10 to 1.

2-HOUR POSTPRANDIAL BLOOD SUGAR AND SERUM INSULIN TEST

The word postprandial just means "after a meal," so this test measures blood glucose exactly 2 hours after you have eaten. Doctors usually don't make you eat before they test. Instead they give you a sugary (Glucola) drink. This test is useful because it shows how well your body processes sugar and starches after a meal and how high your insulin levels rise as a result. A healthy body will be able to return blood sugar and insulin to normal levels 2 or 3 hours after a meal. As you know, blood glucose that remains chronically high can damage your eyes, kidneys, heart, blood vessels, and nerves. The 2-hour postprandial test is sometimes done right after the FBS test.

WHY THIS TEST IS IMPORTANT. It tells you whether your body is producing and using insulin correctly and how you respond to a high sugar/carbohydrate load. A person can be quite normal in the fasting state but have trouble with insulin resistance. If you don't do the 2-hour challenge test, you wouldn't know whether you have this problem because the test done during the fasting state would have registered as normal. I've seen this happen many times.

Now, there's one catch here, so pay attention: After you've had diabetes for a few years, your pancreas may have tired out, leaving you insulin depleted. In a person with type 2 diabetes who is nearing the stage of insulin dependence, the measurement for insulin may be normal. That happens because you simply don't have enough insulin to secrete anymore. So doctors need to routinely test and watch for this pattern.

HOW FREQUENTLY TO MONITOR. If you do not have diabetes, the test should be done annually or at the first sign of symptoms. If you have type 2 diabetes, you should have the test every 4 to 6 months or as often as your doctor recommends.

NORMAL RANGE. 70 to 145 mg/dl for blood glucose. A level of 145 to 200 is too high and will increase your risk for diabetic complications. For insulin, it should be less than 25 microunits/ml. A higher number indicates insulin resistance.

RANDOM. This is the kind of test you can perform whenever you feel funny—too full or too hungry, or when you just want to check what your blood sugar levels are with your glucose monitoring kit. Depending on when you test (how soon after eating, or whether you have eaten properly or fallen off the food wagon), the number should be somewhere between 70 and 125 mg/dl.

You'll find a summary of all the optimum blood glucose test results information in the table below. And I'll go into more detail about home glucose monitoring toward the end of this chapter.

SUGGESTED BLOOD GLUCOSE LEVELS	
Fasting blood glucose	70–100 milligrams per deciliter (or less than 5.5 millimoles per liter)
2 hours after eating (postprandial)	70–145 mg/dl (or less than 7.9 mmol/L)
Random (casual)	70–125 mg/dl (or less than 7.0 mmol/L)

ORAL GLUCOSE TOLERANCE TEST (OGTT)

This test involves a series of glucose measurements that are performed at a lab or at your doctor's office after you drink a sweet liquid beverage that contains glucose. The OGTT requires repeated blood samples taken over the course of 1 hour, or sometimes 2 hours. The measurements track how well you tolerate glucose, hence the name "glucose tolerance," and how you process the glucose after consuming it.

Normally, blood glucose peaks 1 hour after you eat and then drops off in a steady fashion. The OGTT is commonly used to test women for gestational diabetes or for polycystic ovary disease. One study found that people whose 1-hour glucose tolerance test levels exceeded 155 mg/dl and who had signs of metabolic syndrome, such as a spare tire on the gut or high blood pressure, were more likely to develop diabetes.

WHY THIS TEST IS IMPORTANT. It's a more reliable test to determine whether an individual has prediabetes or diabetes because it measures glucose levels over the course of time.

HOW FREQUENTLY TO MONITOR. Every 2 or 3 years, unless you have other risk factors, such as obesity or signs of diabetes, or your doctor recommends it more often.

NORMAL RANGE. Typically, the sweetened drink (usually Glucola) contains 75 grams of glucose (50 grams for pregnant women who are being screened for gestational diabetes).

Here are the normal ranges for 75 grams of glucose:

After 1 hour: less than 200 mg/dl

After 2 hours: less than 140 mg/dl

After 2 hours, if the number is 140 to 200 mg/dl, it means your body isn't handling glucose efficiently and you are prediabetic and at a higher risk for developing diabetes. If the test shows a number higher than 200 mg/dl, it means you have diabetes.

HEMOGLOBIN A1C (HBA1C)

This test is usually done at the lab, but home-testing kits have now been developed (see opposite page). This is one of the best tests to measure how your blood sugar is doing because a single blood test measures your blood sugar average over the 3 previous months. In August 2009, this popular test was recommended by a worldwide scientific committee to become the new gold standard for diagnosing diabetes. This means that doctors will begin using it for this purpose. It also means that many people with prediabetes could slip through the cracks if doctors rely solely on this test. I don't think that A1c is the best diagnostic marker, so please make sure that you still have your insulin and glucose levels measured.

WHY THIS TEST IS IMPORTANT. Because it accounts for all the hills and valleys of blood glucose spikes and troughs, the hemoglobin A1c test is a better indicator of your overall status than the FBS. Hemoglobin, for the record, is a substance inside your red blood cells that carries oxygen to all the cells in your body. Glucose adheres to hemoglobin, so the more glucose you have in your bloodstream, the more glucose you will have sticking to your hemoglobin.

Hemoglobin loves glucose and doesn't want to let it go. As red blood cells containing hemoglobin age, they attract more glucose, a phenomenon that scientists term *glycation*. (It sounds like glucose on vacation!) Hemoglobin holds on to the glucose for its entire life, usually 2 or 3 months. So when you measure the hemoglobin in the blood that has glucose molecules attached to it, that provides the A1c number and tells you whether the glucose content of blood has been too high.

Here is the most compelling finding of all, it seems to me, for making sure you keep your A1c number low. British researchers reported in May 2009, in the British peer-reviewed journal *The Lancet*, that diabetic patients who lower their A1c number by just 1 percent over 5 years can reduce the overall rate of heart

HOME TEST KITS FOR A1C

Measuring your A1c at home is a great way to take control of your health. Home test kits come complete with collection instructions and require a finger prick to get a blood drop sample. They come with a prepaid mailer so when you have completed the test, you drop the sample in the mail to a certified laboratory to be read. Your doctor may have to sign the paperwork ordering this blood test. Your results are sent back to you within 7 to 10 business days.

These products are FDA approved and are considered highly reliable and 99.8 percent accurate. You can't beat the convenience of home testing because you do it when you want to and there are no trips to the doctor or to the laboratory. Also, home test kits may be more affordable than a traditional test taken at the laboratory, combined with a doctor's visit. Always discuss your results with your doctor.

Here are two test kits currently on the market:

Appraise A1c Test: www.appraisetests.com or (888) 764-2384
CardioMetabolic Profile: www.zrtlab.com or (866) 600-1636

Besides measuring A1c, this test measures so much more using just a finger stick (blood spot):

Hemoglobin A1c
Fasting insulin
Fasting triglycerides
Total cholesterol

LDL (low-density lipoprotein) cholesterol
High-sensitivity C-reactive protein

---

attacks by 17 percent and fatal and nonfatal heart attacks by 15 percent. That's pretty amazing, and it seems well worth it to me to forgo that sugary pastry for the moment to savor life longer.

Other scientific studies have shown additional reasons to keep those numbers down. The Diabetes Control and Complications Trial, a major clinical study conducted from 1983 to 1993 and funded by the National Institute of Diabetes and Digestive and Kidney Diseases, showed that people with tighter control on their A1c had a 76 percent reduced risk of eye disease, a 50 percent reduced risk of kidney disease, and a 60 percent reduced risk of nerve disease. This information certainly keeps me on the straight and narrow with my eating habits.

What I like best about the A1c, other than its sensibility, is the fact that you can conduct the test without regard to meals. Doctors sometimes do this test from their office, and home test kits have now been developed if you prefer to do your own assessment. See page 97 for some brand names of home test kits that measure A1c.

HOW FREQUENTLY TO MONITOR. Twice a year if you have diabetes and four times a year if you take diabetic medications or insulin, or whenever your doctor feels the test is necessary.

NORMAL RANGE. The American Association of Clinical Endocrinologists recommends a goal of less than 6.5%. The American Diabetes Association recommends that your A1c be 7 percent or less. Anything above 7 percent means that diabetes is poorly controlled. I feel strongly that diabetic patients should make their goal 5 percent or less.

THYROID PROFILE AND FERRITIN LEVELS

A proper thyroid panel should include tests for a number of thyroid hormones—TSH (thyroid-stimulating hormone), free T4, free T3, TPO (thyroid peroxidase) antibodies, and reverse T3 (rT3). People with low thyroid hormones may have chronic fatigue, dry skin, puffy eyelids, cold hands and feet, constipation, weight gain, swelling of the ankles (edema), hair loss, pale lips, weakness, and, yes, diabetes.

As you age, the number of thyroid receptors on your cells and the ability of those receptors to latch on to active free thyroid hormone is lowered. This means that many older people have underactive thyroid function, whether or not they are diagnosed with it.

You may not think that's a problem, but in fact, it's huge. For many people with diabetes, adequate thyroid function may be the key to controlling progression of the disease, and it's so terribly overlooked. What I'm saying is that a person who has "normal" levels of thyroid hormone at age 50 may still have all the symptoms of low thyroid.

So ask your doctor to treat your symptoms, not your numbers—you may have good thyroid numbers, but because you have fewer receptors, you may need more thyroid hormone. Also, you can have normal thyroid hormone, but if your level of the hormone cortisol is low, your thyroid hormone won't work for you. (Your cortisol level needs to be checked, too. It's a simple test.)

Speaking of simple, I know that all of this sounds complicated, but if I didn't care for you, I wouldn't work so hard to educate you about these critical facts that

I believe make the difference between vibrant health and continued suffering.

Unfortunately, when it comes to thyroid lab tests, many individuals are not tested adequately, so some of these diagnostic measurements are not taken. Doctors may even have told you that you were fine because your TSH level was normal. Doctors with expertise in thyroid conditions maintain that it's old-school thinking to measure *just* the TSH because that number can be in the normal range even when you have low free T3. TSH is a brain hormone not a thyroid gland hormone. Your free T3 hormone tells you a lot more than TSH, because it's in the blood. In fact, free T3 hormone is your active thyroid hormone, and measuring *that* is your best clue for thyroid activity.

You also have to measure your level of rT3. Why? Because a person can have perfectly normal levels of TSH and still have a hypothyroid (low thyroid) condition because they have a lot of rT3. By the way, rT3 goes up with inflammation and the use of conventional thyroid medications, such as Synthroid (levothyroxine). You need to be aware that rT3 is your hormone of inactivity, so if you have too much rT3, you're basically hibernating. Again, if your doctor is old school and looking only at your TSH number, you will be told that you are normal. Well, you're not.

I may be one of the few people writing about this now, but believe me, in 5 years measuring rT3 will be the latest craze. Reverse T3 *blocks* the action of active thyroid hormone, so it needs to be measured. High rT3 indicates you have clinical hypothyroidism.

Why should all this discussion of thyroid hormones matter to a person with diabetes? Because thyroid hormone is needed for fat loss, that's why. It also protects against heart arrhythmias—a frequent problem for people with diabetes—and it gives you energy. Normal levels of thyroid hormone prevent diabetes in most people because thyroid hormone improves insulin levels.

The ferritin portion of the tests that I'm recommending here is a measurement of the levels of iron in your blood. I'm mentioning it here because you should have it measured at the same time you have your thyroid hormones tested. If the ferritin (iron) level is low, then you are not going to be able to make enough active T3 thyroid hormone. Then you will be hypothyroid and feel very tired and/or depressed.

When you have the thyroid panel done at your doctor's office or at the lab, make sure you set your appointment for the morning. Ideally, eat something for breakfast beforehand. This is a nonfasting test. If you go on an empty stomach, it could cause false elevations in TSH and rT3.

WHY THIS TEST IS IMPORTANT. Producing too little thyroid hormone is one of the primary reasons a person develops diabetes. That's because low thyroid levels lead to insulin resistance and weight gain. When you have low thyroid levels, your fat-burning ability slows down because your metabolism is sluggish. You hold on to weight and put it on around your belly. Your insulin levels increase. With high insulin levels, you pack even more weight on.

This is a never-ending cycle, and an underactive thyroid may explain why you can hardly even eat during the day but still can't lose a few pounds. If this description fits you, it's possible that your thyroid gland is malfunctioning, causing your cells to hold on to fat and sugar and not burn it off. Thyroid function goes hand-in-hand with diabetes, so your thyroid function needs to be closely monitored and properly measured.

If your thyroid is malfunctioning, medical treatment should set things right. As your thyroid levels improve and become normal, your insulin and blood sugar levels should too. You will feel better within weeks, and the weight will probably start to come off as well.

HOW FREQUENTLY TO MONITOR. If you feel you are gaining weight without changing your eating habits, or feel particularly sluggish and tired for no reason you can think of, ask your doctor to get your thyroid function tested. Otherwise, have it evaluated annually.

NORMAL RANGE. The complete thyroid panel will reveal several numbers that show your levels for many hormones. The relationship of the numbers to each other is important, and your doctor will interpret those to determine whether you need medication.

You should be aware that the optimum level for T3 hormone is somewhere between 230 pg/dl to 420 pg/dl. (Note that some labs may use different measures.) You can certainly get by on lower levels, but your body functions at an *optimal* level within this range. Excess thyroid hormone will cause heart palpitations, muscle twitching, and insomnia/agitation.

HOME TESTING. You can also conduct an easy home test to help determine your thyroid hormone status, and I have to say this method is pretty valid. Your body temperature tells the story.

There are many ways to take your body temperature. One simple and reliable method is to take your afternoon temperature around 2 or 3 p.m. It should be 98.6°F. If it's less than that, you probably have low thyroid function. Take your temperature every day for a week to get an average. You want it to be exactly 98.6. If it's lower, I suggest that you talk to your doctor about building up thyroid hormone. You can also take a morning basal body temperature. When you first wake up; put the thermometer in your armpit for 5 minutes. Register the reading. Basal temps should be higher than 97.8.

Frequently I hear people say, "I've always had a low body temperature. It's never 98.6, and that's normal for me." I beg to differ. The human body is supposed to be 98.6. So if your temperature normally measures at 97.9, then talk to your doctor about building up thyroid hormone. When levels of this hormone are normal, you will feel more energetic and will be less likely to develop diabetes.

URINALYSIS

Affectionately referred to as "peeing into a cup," this test is a relatively simple, inexpensive way to check for diabetes. If you have too much glucose in your system, your kidneys can't filter it all out, and it "spills over" into the urine. This test consists of a relatively simple analysis of your urine sample—thus *urinalysis.*

WHY THIS TEST IS IMPORTANT. As you know by now, the complications from diabetes come in large part from extra glucose circulating in your bloodstream. For starters, your kidneys are as overworked as two hospital nurses on a hall with 60 beds.

The urinalysis test also looks for a tiny protein in the urine called microalbumin, one of the smaller proteins the body produces. If your kidneys are in trouble, they allow larger and larger proteins to pass into the urine. That's why you want this test done routinely so you can find any extra sugar in the urine ASAP, while your kidneys still function properly.

HOW FREQUENTLY TO MONITOR. Do it annually, as part of your routine labwork.

INSULIN-TO-GLUCOSE RATIO TEST

Getting what's known as a ratio may be the best way to assess health status and track your progress. You want to have a ratio of insulin to glucose of about 1:10.

WHY THIS TEST IS IMPORTANT. As insulin levels rise above a certain level, fat is then pushed into your cells—otherwise known as gaining weight. If your insulin levels continue to rise, more and more fat is deposited into your cells—you gain more and more weight—and pretty soon you feel out of control.

Once the ratio of insulin to glucose climbs above 1:20, you're in trouble.

Don't you think an ounce of prevention is worth more than a pound of fat? You want to keep the fat out of your cells and get your eating habits under control as early as possible before you suffer complications like kidney damage and neuropathies. Both of these complications of diabetes often begin before people even get diagnosed with the condition. I tell you all of this scary stuff because you need to know it. Maintaining your weight is not about beauty—it's a matter of life or death, especially for your kidneys, pancreas, eyes, and life and limbs.

VITAMIN D

The hormone vitamin D (yes, researchers are now referring to it as a hormone) can help you with insulin resistance, nerve damage, immune function, and bone strength. If you don't have enough vitamin D, then your body may produce excessive amounts of inflammatory chemicals, such as tumor necrosis factor alpha (TNF alpha), which increases your risk for pain and autoimmune disorders.

In the August 2009 issue of *Pediatrics*, researchers noted a significant link between vitamin D levels and blood sugar in adolescents. They concluded: "Low serum vitamin D in U.S. adolescents is strongly associated with hypertension, hyperglycemia, and metabolic syndrome, independent of adiposity." In other words, low vitamin D is linked to all these conditions regardless of whether the youngsters were overweight. If this is true for young people, imagine how a vitamin D deficiency can affect someone over 40.

A 2007 study published in *Diabetes Care* concluded that vitamin D can reduce your risk of developing type 2 diabetes by up to 40 percent. In this 17-year study of more than 4,000 people, 187 were diagnosed with diabetes. The 187 also registered the lowest vitamin D levels, regardless of age or gender. Conversely, the beneficial effect of having adequate vitamin D was revealed even after accounting for other variables, such as smoking, body weight, blood pressure treatment, and exercise. In fact, numerous studies in the past few years have confirmed similar benefits from vitamin D for people with both type 1 and type 2 diabetes.

The take-home point here is that you can ask your doctor for a blood test to determine whether your vitamin D levels are adequate. If you need a supplement, your doctor will advise you about how much to take.

WHY THIS TEST IS IMPORTANT. Low levels of vitamin D have been associated with insulin resistance, metabolic syndrome, nerve damage, and a higher risk of cancer and autoimmune disorders.

STATINS CAUSE DIABETES

Statins are popular cholesterol-lowering drugs. They work in the liver by preventing your body from making cholesterol. When you eat meals that have starches and sugar, some of the excess sugar goes to the liver, where the liver stores it away as cholesterol and triglycerides.

Now—stay with me—when you have a statin on board, it's like a message to your liver saying, "No! Don't make any more cholesterol; please stop." So your liver sends the sugar back OUT to the bloodstream. Many statin users come back to see their doctor for a routine visit and find that their cholesterol may be better, but now they have high blood sugar.

It's entirely possible that some physicians mistakenly diagnose their patients with diabetes when in fact they just have hyperglycemia, the result of a medication that was prescribed to them months earlier. See why I told you way back in Chapter 1 that you may not have diabetes?

It's entirely possible that what you actually have is a known side effect of your cholesterol medication. Millions of people take statins. It's one of the most widely prescribed classes of medications in the world, and I personally think that this is one of the reasons now that millions of people think they have diabetes. Read Chapter 8 for natural ways to protect your heart and lower cholesterol. Here are the statin medications and their generic names:

Atorvastatin (Lipitor, Advicor)   Pravastatin (Pravachol)

Simvastatin (Zocor, Lipex, Vytorin, Simcor)   Rosuvastatin (Crestor)

Lovastatin (Mevacor)   Fluvastatin (Lescol)

HOW FREQUENTLY TO MONITOR. Annually. This is a quick nonfasting blood test. There are home test kits available, too.

NORMAL RANGE. 60 to 90 ng/ml

BLOOD LIPIDS

This test checks the levels of fats in your blood—total cholesterol, triglycerides (the major form of fat in our bodies), as well as your LDL (low-density lipoprotein; bad cholesterol) and HDL (high-density lipoprotein; good cholesterol). These fatty globules can narrow or constrict the flow of blood in your blood vessels.

People with diabetes often have low levels of HDL and high levels of triglycerides, adding to their risk for complications. The good news is that it's relatively simple and inexpensive to correct lipid ratios, and I'm not thinking of using powerful prescribed drugs, either.

I've not been shy about my contempt for the indiscriminate prescribing of statin medications to everyone and their brother. Statins can cause high blood sugar. You know these drugs by their brand names such as Lipitor, Mevacor, Zocor, and their generic names, atorvastatin, lovastatin, and simvastatin, respectively. Nowadays, they are even prescribed to overweight children. It's just gotten crazy, hasn't it?!

There are excellent natural ways to reduce your total cholesterol, triglycerides, and LDLs, which I will tell you about starting on page 137.

WHY THIS TEST IS IMPORTANT. Knowing your blood fat numbers is important because if they're high, you can take the steps to reduce the fatty buildup and lighten the load on your arteries, liver, pancreas, and heart. The first step is to reduce carbohydrate/sugar intake because it gets stored as cholesterol and other bad fats.

Having high cholesterol increases your risk for diabetes and heart attack. Not only that, but if you have diabetes, your risk for stroke triples compared to that of people without diabetes, especially if you're in your 50s and 60s. Also note that there are 40 percent more people with high blood pressure among diabetics than among those who don't have diabetes.

HOW FREQUENTLY TO MONITOR. Once or twice a year, or as often as your physician feels it's necessary.

NORMAL RANGE.

Total cholesterol: Less than 225 mg/dl (for age 40 to 49 years; this increases with age)
LDL: Less than 100 mg/dl
HDL: Men—higher than 40; women—higher than 50

Your triglycerides should be below 150 mg/dl, depending on your age, as shown in this chart:

Triglyceride Target Ranges Based on Age

Age in Years	Target Triglyceride Range
10–29 years	53–104 mg/dl
30–39 years	55–115 mg/dl
40–49 years	66–139 mg/dl
50–59 years	75–163 mg/dl
60–69 years	78–158 mg/dl
70 years	83–141 mg/dl

BLOOD PRESSURE

Blood pressure is the force the blood exerts against the walls of the arteries as it's pumped through the body when your blood pressure is high, it is termed hypertension. Blood pressure is recorded as two numbers. The first, or top, number, called the systolic pressure, is the pressure generated when your heart contracts. Obviously, the faster your heart beats, the higher the systolic blood pressure. It may go up with stress, exercise, and caffeine.

The second, or bottom, number is called the diastolic pressure. To remember that it is the bottom number think of *d* for down, as the diastolic number is the one recorded down under the systolic number. The diastolic number is the blood pressure generated when your heart is relaxed. Think of it as your resting pressure. If the diastolic pressure is high when you're resting, that's a red flag that something is squeezing off (or clogging) in your pipeline—with your heart or your blood vessels.

It's ideal to get an average of your blood pressure numbers taken during various times of the day, and in various positions—sitting, lying down, and standing. Taking a blood pressure once during the day, in the same position, doesn't really give you more than a snapshot.

I think it's a good idea to buy one of those digital machines from your local pharmacy to check your blood pressure levels. If your pressure is too high, you may not even know it because you won't be able to feel it. High blood pressure doesn't really have any overt symptoms, which is why it is called the silent disease. Some clues to high blood pressure include headaches or feeling stressed, weak, bloated, or just plain "failing." If your blood pressure is too low, you might feel weak, tired, dizzy, or faint.

WHY THIS TEST IS IMPORTANT. Hypertension is associated with heart attack and stroke.

HOW FREQUENTLY TO MONITOR. Check with your physician to see how often he or she wants you to monitor your blood pressure. Check it at every medical appointment or on a monthly basis. Most chain pharmacies offer this service for free in their waiting rooms.

NORMAL RANGE.

Normal blood pressure: 120/80 mm Hg
Borderline high: 140/90 mm Hg
Borderline low: 90/60 mm Hg

Modern medicine has also devised a scale, which looks at systolic pressure only—remember, that's the top number. Following are the stages of high blood pressure, with any number beyond stage 1 being dangerously high:

Stages of High Systolic Blood Pressure

Stage	Systolic Number
1	140–90 mm Hg
2	160–100 mm Hg
3	180–110 mm Hg
4	210–120 mm Hg

INFLAMMATORY MARKERS

These blood tests measure how much inflammation is in your body. Knowing this gives you a good idea of the kind of damage that may be taking place.

WHY THIS TEST IS IMPORTANT. When inflammation is high in the body, there is usually a lot of free-radical damage to innocent cells and tissues. Inflammatory markers are often elevated if you have heart disease, diabetes, obesity, arthritis, thyroid disorders, chronic fatigue syndrome, and many autoimmune disorders, such as lupus, multiple sclerosis, or Crohn's disease, all of which are localized autoimmune disorders. These tests could include any or all of the following:

TNF alpha (tumor necrosis factor alpha)
CRP (C-reactive protein)
High-sensitivity homocysteine
IGF-1 (insulin-like growth factor 1)

KIDNEY FUNCTION

These tests indicate how well your kidneys are working. Early signs that your kidneys are in trouble are so vague that they might go unnoticed, or you may not connect the symptoms to your kidneys. For example, you may develop low back pain. You may experience swelling in the feet, ankles, legs, or hands, or you might just feel chronically fatigued. You may itch, too. See how easy it is to overlook signs of kidney damage?

Another vague sign of kidney problems is bad breath or a foul or strange taste to your food. By far, the most common early symptom of kidney problems is with urination. You may feel as if you have to go, but only a few drops come out. The color of your urine may darken or you may have to go more frequently at night.

I've written more about how to protect your kidneys in Chapter 9, but what's important here is that you get your kidney function tested. And it's easy. All that is required is a morning urine sample, no needles, no probing. The reason I want you to have a kidney function test is to prevent dangerous toxin overload. The test is easy to perform. It usually requires a little urine to check for a protein called albumin or blood that may be spilling into your urine. Also, a small blood sample will allow your doctor to check for levels of creatinine—a substance that provides another fairly reliable measurement of kidney function.

WHY THIS TEST IS IMPORTANT. The symptoms of early kidney damage often go unnoticed, so it's important to actually test the health of your kidneys with a simple urine test. If you cannot clear and eliminate toxins very well with your kidneys, they will build up in your bloodstream, leading to dangerous—and possibly fatal—consequences.

HOW FREQUENTLY TO MONITOR. Once or twice a year, or as frequently as your doctor suggests.

NORMAL RANGE.

Creatinine: Men—0.6 to 1.2 mg/dl; women—0.5 to 1.1 mg/dl
Microalbumin: less than 30

EYE EXAM

If you have diabetes, your ophthalmologist (and, in some cases, your optometrist) can perform an eye exam. It's best if it's a "dilated" exam in which the pupils are widened with eye drops so your doctor can check for signs of diabetic retinopathy.

In case you didn't know this sad fact, diabetic retinopathy is the number-one cause of blindness in adults under the age of 65. It's sad for anyone to go blind. It's tragic for someone to go blind if it can be avoided, especially with some simple monitoring. Read Chapter 7 to learn about supplements that can protect your retina.

WHY THIS TEST IS IMPORTANT. Without proper testing of the eye, you risk losing your eyesight.

HOW FREQUENTLY TO MONITOR. Once or twice a year, or as your doctor suggests. If you experience any changes to your eyesight, you should make an appointment immediately. Timely intervention can save your precious sight, so you should have your eyes checked by an ophthalmologist at regular intervals, even if you aren't experiencing any noticeable problems, because damage can be taking place internally long before your vision is impaired.

FOOT EXAM

People with diabetes have two primary issues with their feet—poor circulation and neuropathy. With circulation problems of the foot, any infection will heal more slowly, leaving you prone to more complications and even possible amputation. If your feet—and even hands—constantly feel cold, you could have circulation problems (or low thyroid). With less blood flowing to your feet, it is harder for your body to fight infection in that area.

The second biggie is diabetic neuropathy. This condition affects your nerves and can lead to loss of sensation in one or both feet. There may or may not be pain, numbness, or tingling. The problem is that if you don't have proper sensation, you may not sense problems or infections in your feet early enough to avoid complications.

You should develop a routine of caring for your feet and inspecting the top and bottom, as well as between your toes. You are looking for sores, blisters, ulcers, or any type of redness or break in the skin that might suggest infection.

WHY THIS TEST IS IMPORTANT. It reduces your risk for painful complications, such as infections and amputation.

HOW FREQUENTLY TO MONITOR. If you have diabetes, see your podiatrist twice a year. See your doctor immediately if you notice a sore on your foot that is not healing quickly. Learn more about your feet in Chapter 10.

KETONES

Ketones are simply chemicals that form when your body breaks down fat for energy. The body breaks down fat when it can't use glucose. This can occur for a number of reasons; for example, when you haven't taken enough insulin to help shuttle glucose into your cells or when you haven't eaten enough to provide glucose for energy, as happens when you get sick and have no appetite.

HOW TO THROW OUT USED INSULIN NEEDLES

In a given year, about 9 million people will use syringes and will self-administer about 3 billion injections. These shots are needed to treat type 1 diabetes, as well as hepatitis, HIV infection, arthritis, multiple sclerosis, lupus, and other conditions. In the United States, the laws require that you dispose of your used needles by placing them in a plastic container called a sharps box. Ask your pharmacy to order one of these for you, or ask your doctor where you can get one. I searched the Internet, and found many sites that sell sharps boxes online. I even found some on eBay.

What do you do when your sharps container is filled up? There are agencies that pick up and dispose of the containers once you've filled them up with your used needles. Ask your physician's office if you can bring the needles to them so that they can dispose of them for you. Whatever you do, never, ever throw used needles in the trash. You can visit www.safeneedledisposal.org for some information about your particular state laws.

People who go on the Atkins diet (or similar diets where carbs are restricted) deliberately put themselves into a state of ketosis, which is different from keto-acidosis. When your body is in ketosis, you are breaking down fat (instead of carbohydrates) for energy, and you are making lots of ketones.

When diabetic patients have too many ketones circulating in the body, however, this can cause a major diabetic emergency called diabetic ketoacidosis, so it's important to track ketones. (I'll describe what happens during diabetic keto-acidosis shortly.)

You can have ketones measured at your doctor's office with a simple, inexpensive blood test. Many new blood glucose monitoring devices can test for both ketones and blood glucose. Or you can measure ketones at home with a urine test strip.

Two over-the-counter products for measuring urine ketones at home are Ketostix and Clinistix, which are sold at many pharmacies. These are clever little strips that require a urine sample. You can collect the sample in a cup and dip the stick, or you can urinate directly on the strip.

The color change indicates the level of ketones that you are spilling. You'll find a description of what the colors mean on the label. *One thing, though— urine ketones always lag behind blood ketones, which is why blood measurements are more accurate than urine measurements.* Simply put, your blood levels will always be slightly higher than your urine measurements.

If your urine ketone level has been high, and you have taken enough rapid-acting insulin to bring your blood sugar down, then you will probably feel better, although your urine ketone measurement may still be elevated for 2 to 4 more hours.

WHY THIS TEST IS IMPORTANT. If your ketones are high, it's a sign that you do not have enough insulin to control ketone production and that no matter what your weight is—even if you are very overweight—your body is malnourished. The consequences of developing ketoacidosis are dangerous, so frequent testing is recommended.

HOW FREQUENTLY TO MONITOR. People with diabetes should keep urine test strips at home, or use a blood glucose testing device to measure ketones once a week *and at the first sign of any symptoms.* For a list of symptoms see "Early Warning Signs of Ketoacidosis" on the opposite page. If you buy ketone testing strips, I suggest you get the individual foil-wrapped ones because they're more stable. (If you get the bottle of strips, they will probably expire quickly, within 3 months.)

NORMAL RANGE. A negative urine result is normal.

BLOOD TESTS. Normal is less than 0.6 mmol/l.

LET'S TALK ABOUT KETOACIDOSIS

Ketoacidosis is the word used to describe a life-threatening complication that can occur in people with diabetes, especially type 1 diabetes. Most often it occurs because of nonadherence with insulin injections, infection, or prolonged periods without eating. Blood glucose concentrations can climb to 250 mg/dl, although if you are in ketoacidosis, they usually spike much higher. (In a hospital setting, doctors will often measure beta-hydroxybutyrate to get an idea of the situation rather than measuring blood levels of ketones.) Nevertheless, ketoacidosis is a serious and potentially fatal condition.

If you experience ketoacidosis, you need immediate help to increase insulin levels and to replenish heart-friendly minerals, such as potassium, phosphorus, and magnesium, via intravenous infusion. The sad truth is that many adults die because they are mistakenly thought to be drunk when in fact they are dealing with a life-threatening complication of diabetes.

One of the hallmark signs of ketoacidosis is "fruity" breath, which is also what people in an alcoholic stupor exhibit. The scariest part is that you—and

EARLY WARNING SIGNS OF KETOACIDOSIS

Memorize these early signs and symptoms of ketoacidosis so you can recognize a true emergency if you are faced with one:

Fruity breath odor (smells a little like nail polish remover, or acetone)

Fatigue

Extreme thirst despite drinking lots and lots of water

Frequent urination

Thick coating on the tongue (oral thrush)

Persistent vaginal yeast infections or jock itch

Muscle wasting

Confusion

Agitation or aggression

Nausea and occasional vomiting

Pain in the neck, chest, or shoulders

Later and more dangerous signs that require immediate attention:

Breathing problems*

Flulike symptoms

Loss of appetite

Sluggish movements

Vomiting

Unconsciousness or coma

*I'm talking here about the kind of breathing that is referred to as Kussmaul breathing. It begins with hyperventilation—literally breathing too much, thus reducing the amount of carbon dioxide in the blood—and may progress to labored and very deep breathing. It's best described as being "hungry for air."

those around you—may not realize that diabetes is the problem. That's because diabetic ketoacidosis may be the first sign that an individual has diabetes. The diagnosis is made at the hospital after the patient collapses on the street.

Your risks of ketoacidosis go up if your body is low on insulin or uses glucose inefficiently. Another precipitating factor is increased gluconeogenesis—meaning that your liver converts everything you eat into glucose, even noncarbs and proteins.

In fact, if you have diabetes and are currently taking the medicine metformin, this is exactly what metformin was developed to do—stop this excessive creation of glucose from all substances, including proteins, and help shuttle whatever glucose is in your body into your cells to give you energy instead of leaving it circulating around your bloodstream, which is harmful.

High levels of stress hormones such as cortisol also create a higher risk for ketoacidosis. When I say stress, I don't just mean that you are stressed out, although that does matter. I really mean that your body is taxed and dealing with

POTASSIUM MATTERS

Having low potassium can increase your risk for ketoacidosis. Ketoacidosis is not the only condition encouraged by low potassium levels. Another concern is hypokalemia—a condition in which you don't have enough potassium to help your heart beat, your muscle contract, and your nerves to conduct signals properly. Do you realize that many medications in your medicine cabinet actually steal potassium from your body? It's the drug-mugging effect that I've mentioned several times in this book. There are some popular drug muggers of potassium in your medicine cabinet, including aspirin, furosemide (brand name: Lasix), hydrochlorothiazide (HCTZ) (brand names: Hydrodiuril, Ezide, Hydro-Par, Microzide), and steroids (such as prednisone in any form, and other steroids). Iodized salt can steal potassium, too. A complete list of drugs that mug potassium is on page 142. If you take one of the medications on this list, talk with your doctor to see if you would benefit from taking a prescribed potassium drug or an over-the-counter potassium supplement. Generally speaking, the dosage is 300 to 1,000 milligrams per day.

Potassium-rich foods include acorn squash, which for example, provides about 900 milligrams of potassium in one cup. One banana provides about 450 milligrams.

some other huge burden, like pneumonia, the flu, a severe urinary tract infection, major stomach upset, or another major infection such as sepsis. (Sepsis is a bacterial infection that gets into your bloodstream or the tissues of your body. Having surgery is one of the major risk factors for sepsis.)

Other risk factors include inflammatory conditions, such as appendicitis, cholecystitis (gall bladder inflammation), or pancreatitis. I am going into details about ketoacidosis because I want you to understand the dangers of this condition. The threat of ketoacidosis is a good reason to always remember to take your prescribed insulin. Ketoacidosis *is* scary—and usually avoidable if you stick to your insulin schedule.

ADVANTAGES OF MONITORING BLOOD GLUCOSE

Now that we've taken a fairly thorough look at all the tests I think you should have if you have diabetes, I'd like to circle back and take a closer look at one of the most important tests the fasting blood glucose (FBS) test. There are any number of reasons why you need to pay special attention to what your blood glucose levels are and you can purchase these home devices at pharmacies nationwide.

IT PUTS YOU MORE IN CONTROL OF YOUR DRUG AND SUPPLEMENT REGIMEN. If, for example, you are taking new supplements and your blood sugar is coming down, you will not have to argue with your doctor when you ask to discontinue one of your medications. You can show your doctor your numbers in black and white. So there is a degree of empowerment that comes from self-monitoring.

IT ALLOWS YOU TO EAT CERTAIN FOODS THAT YOU LOVE. For example, if you test before and after a particular meal, you can see if that particular meal affected your blood levels adversely. Being able to test gives you the choice of eating something you love to eat—every once in a while—as long as it doesn't dangerously shift your blood sugar levels.

YOU SHOULD BE ABLE TO REDUCE YOUR MEDICATION DOSAGE IF YOU EXERCISE. The more active you become in your exercise routine, the less medication you need. Testing can prove that, and it enables you to reduce your medication dosage as you lose more weight. This is important because you never want to experience a hypoglycemic (blood sugar that is too low) effect. Never reduce your medications without your doctor's approval.

The only thing that I want you to promise me is that you will not become a number junkie and just obsess over your numbers. It's more important to improve the health of your pancreas and other affected organs like your eyes and kidneys than to just chase your numbers down. With that said, let's take a look at some of the most important features that home-monitoring devices have to offer.

GLUCOMETERS MONITOR BLOOD SUGAR

Blood glucose meters (glucometers) are little computerized devices that measure the amount of glucose in a sample of your blood. The levels are displayed on a screen.

To get a sample of your blood, a small needle called a lancet is used to poke the skin (usually on a finger or on your forearm) to get one drop of blood. The drop is placed on a testing strip that goes into the glucose meter, and the blood glucose reading appears on a screen within a few seconds. When choosing a machine, you should keep in mind the following.

COST. My concern here is not so much the cost of the glucometer itself, because most insurance plans will cover the cost of meters, and sometimes there are terrific rebates. It's really about the strips. They are the most expensive part

YOUR INSURANCE MIGHT PAY FOR GLUCOSE MONITORING

Just as with razors (it's not the razor that's expensive, it's the blades), so it is with glucose monitoring devices. Many companies will give away the monitoring devices for free, just so you will buy the test strips they make. It's the test strips that are costly, not the device. Certain insurance plans will pay for your blood glucose monitoring system, testing strips, or lancets. Sometimes all they require is your doctor to write a prescription for it. Call the toll-free number on the back of your insurance plan card and ask about your coverage or look it up online. Don't be shy about doing this. It could save you hundreds of dollars each year. If you're not sure about the answer, check with your local pharmacist and ask for assistance. After all, you know that we pharmacists are in a lifesaving profession.

of testing. Check with your insurance plan about your coverage of glucose test strips and the number the plan covers. If you and your doctor feel you need more test strips than are covered by your insurance, you could ask your doctor to call your insurance plan to tell them why you need additional test strips.

BRAND. It's important to use the glucose test strips that match the brand of your machine. Using a strip that is not exactly calibrated to your machine can alter your glucose results, and if you use your results to determine your insulin dose, you might overdose on insulin. This could cause dangerous, even fatal, drops in blood sugar, so don't try to save money on strips. Use the ones that go with your machine and make sure they are not expired. A variety of blood glucose testing strips are sold at pharmacies nationwide.

SIZE. Pick meters that are light and portable that can fit in your purse or pocket. Newer machines are small and easy to use. Even though you want the meter to be small, make sure that the digital display is large enough for you to see easily, even if you can't find your glasses.

SPEED. New meters on the market take only seconds to display the results of your test; however, some take more than a minute. When it comes to getting a blood sugar number, faster is better, I think.

COMFORT. New meters come with lancets (needles) that are more comfortable to use because they allow for adjustments. This means that you can adjust the depth at which the needle enters your skin. Some meters allow you to draw blood from the forearm, which makes it less painful than a fingertip for some people.

LIP BALM FOR YOUR FINGERTIPS

If you put some lip balm on your fingertips after the test, it immediately soothes the tenderness from all the finger pricks. Just to make sure, I did this on my own finger so I could feel the needle stick, and then feel the effect of the lip balm. I used a brand called Carmex, which is cooling because it happens to contain menthol. Sure enough, there was no ouch and the relief was almost instantaneous. You can buy moisturizing, cooling lip balms at any health food store or pharmacy.

CONVENIENCE. Wearable devices that measure blood sugar levels every 5 minutes are available. These include the GlucoWatch made by Glucon, and the Glucoband made by Calisto Medical. Then a computer printout of your blood sugar profile can be downloaded for you or your doctor to evaluate. If you just want to handwrite your blood sugar and bypass all the techie stuff, ask your diabetes educator or doctor for a free blood sugar diary. You can also find these diaries for free online. Just do a Web search for "free blood sugar diary," and you'll get many Web sites that allow you to download your own form and print it out.

SOMETIMES MORE IS BETTER

Check your blood sugar levels more frequently than usual if you:

- Change your diabetic medicine
- Begin taking a new medication or dietary supplement
- Add a new food to your diet
- Have exercised more than normal
- Change your normal level of activity
- Become sick

PART 3
STAYING WELL ABOVE THE WAIST

7

Protecting Your Precious Eyesight

One of the most frustrating potential complications of diabetes is vision loss and other problems that threaten your eyesight.

Did you know that glaucoma is a major complication of diabetic eye disease that leads to blindness? Also, people with diabetes are twice as likely as those without diabetes to develop cataracts. Cataracts, glaucoma, and diabetic retinopathy all contribute to the high rate of blindness in people with diabetes. (Later in the chapter I'll describe all of these diseases.)

According to the American Diabetes Association, diabetes is responsible for 8 percent of cases of legal blindness, making it the leading cause of new cases of blindness in adults 20 to 74 years of age. About one in five people with type 2 diabetes already has retinopathy when first diagnosed with diabetes, and most will eventually experience some degree of retinopathy. Some 24,000 people will go blind this year as a result of diabetic retinopathy, and 120,000 people will become blind from glaucoma as well.

True, laser surgeries can help certain individuals with some visual problems, but in my book, it's better to protect your vision and take supplements to try to reverse the damage rather than undergo surgery on your eyes.

The most powerful vision-saving supplements are actually the pigments—as in dyes—that impart color to fruits and vegetables. Many of the natural colorants that make fruits and veggies so bright and appealing can also help you see more colors. That's easy to remember, right?

Think of the color that makes blueberries blue. This blue pigment does wonders for your eyesight. Also, think of the color that makes carrots orange. It has impressive benefits for your eyes, too. And while this may sound weird, the red dye that turns flamingos pink is yet another pigment that enhances vision. (Although eating blueberries and carrots is all good and well, please stay away from the flamingos.) We'll get to talking more about these supplements and a few other eyesight boosters shortly, but first let's delve a little deeper into how the eye functions. When you know about that, it will be clear to see why Mother Nature's medicine cabinet is best.

> ## MAKING SENSE OF THE THREE "OS"
>
> **Opticians** create lenses of specified strengths and dispense eyeglasses.
>
> **Optometrists** perform eye examinations and in some states are able to diagnose you. They can prescribe glasses or contact lenses.
>
> **Ophthalmologists** are physicians. They diagnose and treat diseases of the eye. Some offer vision examinations and prescribe glasses or contact lenses.

THE MIRACLE OF VISION

The human eye is nothing short of miraculous. It adapts to light within seconds. Everything you see is because light passes into your eye through the pupil, which is the black dot in the center of your colorful eye. The image is focused through the lens.

In a healthy eye, what you are looking at becomes an upside-down image on your retina, at the very back of your eye. The retina is really a membrane with a lot of nerve cells. The nerve cells convert light to electrical impulses and send them to your brain via the optic nerve. The optic nerve—which begins at the base of your brain, in the back of your head—sends a message to your brain about the picture. While it sounds crazy, you actually get two different pictures, one from each eye. Your brain puts both images together, and turns them right side up instantaneously.

To see images correctly and clearly, you must have adequate amounts of blood flowing to all the parts of the eye. To have proper blood flow, all the blood vessels and capillaries that surround the eye have to be wide open and clear of plaque—the same gunk that clogs up arteries. This is why antioxidants are so good for the eye. They remove all the garbage that collects and damages delicate eye tissues and surrounding blood vessels.

PROBLEMS OF THE EYE

On the next page, you will see that I have pulled together a list of some common eye diseases and disturbances. These visual problems can occur in anyone; however, these particular problems seem to occur most frequently in people who have diabetes. I believe that the supplements I mention later in this chapter can help you retain, and possibly regain, your precious eyesight. In the meantime, here is a brief description of the problems that occur within the eye.

DIABETIC RETINOPATHY. This condition can cause blurred vision, floaters, flashes of light, and sudden loss of vision. This happens when blood vessels in the retina weaken and slowly leak, causing pressure on the macula—the part of the retina responsible for sharp, clear vision. Vision gets blurry at first and can eventually lead to blindness. The longer you have high blood sugar, the more it damages the eye.

MACULAR DEGENERATION. The macula is the central part of the retina. When the macula degenerates, you lose the central portion of your vision. Signs of macular degeneration include blurred vision (especially when reading), faded colors, and distorted vision (seeing wavy lines). This is the most common cause of blindness in the elderly.

FLOATERS. This condition involves tiny spots or squiggly lines that drift over the visual field. As the liquid gel part of your eye (called vitreous humor) shrinks and recedes, the floaters become more apparent.

RETINAL DETACHMENT. When the retina detaches from the back of the eye, it causes flashes of light and floaters, and a curtain is pulled down on one side of your visual field. This can happen in the later stages of diabetic retinopathy.

CATARACTS. This condition manifests as cloudiness within the eye's lens. It can cause blurred vision, poor night vision, glare sensitivity, and halos around lights.

GLAUCOMA. Excess eye pressure in the eyeball causes poor night vision, loss of peripheral vision (outer vision), blind spots, and eventual blindness if not detected and treated. There are two types, which I'll describe later in the chapter.

PRESBYOPIA. This is the medical term for aging eyes, a condition that generally occurs in the early 40s. The lens of the eye loses its flexibility and thus its ability to focus properly on objects that are close. I realize this condition sounds a lot like farsightedness, but these are two different conditions.

OPTIC NEURITIS. Inflammation of the optic nerve is a hallmark symptom of multiple sclerosis (MS). One statistic I read said that 15 to 20 percent of people who get optic neuritis go on to develop MS. If you have optic neuritis, the eyeball actually hurts when you move your eye from side to side. It usually affects just one eye (not both). Colors look washed out or faded, and you can experience complete vision loss in the affected eye for a period of time—as little as 10 minutes and up to several days.

OPHTHALMIC MIGRAINES. These are also called ocular migraines, but instead of that severe type of pain normally associated with migraines, there is

FLOATERS IN YOUR EYES

Floaters in the eye look like dots or strands in your vision. Though annoying, these floaters are just tiny pieces of protein that get trapped in the vitreous humor—the clear, jelly-like fluid that fills the space in your eyeball. They commonly show up as people age, strain, cough, or deal with chronic stress. Nonetheless, as I always remind you, please go to an ophthalmologist if you experience any changes in your eyes or your vision. As your vitreous humor thins with aging, inflammation, or disease, the floaters become more apparent. Poor diet plays a role too. Anecdotally speaking, people who are elderly, nearsighted, or infected with the fungus *Candida albicans* seem to have the most complaints.

Floaters are usually harmless and occur more frequently as we age because of degeneration to the retina or the vitreous humor. Floaters might gradually disappear over time. If you are bothered by floaters, I have two supplement suggestions—bilberry and hyaluronic acid. Both of these nutrients are important for anyone who wants to protect vision and improve general health.

Bilberry is an herb known to improve circulation, which helps release pieces of gunk that are stuck in your vitreous humor. My suggested dosage: 80–250 mg once or twice daily. Of course, remember to check with your doctor to see if this, or any other supplement, might interfere with any medications you're taking now. You'll find the full story on hyaluronic acid on page 125.

no head pain. It's all in the eyes. Scientists think it occurs because of a temporary spasm, only it's in the blood vessel behind your eye rather than in your leg. You might get a blind spot that starts to enlarge and move across your field of vision. You may see bright flashes of lights that flicker or what looks like a lightning bolt in the blind spot.

It's all very bizarre, but fortunately it lasts only 5 to 30 minutes before it resolves. Migraines of any sort, including this kind, are usually triggered by hormonal or neurologic changes. Experts feel that ophthalmic migraines are not cause for alarm and probably not harmful, but you should definitely get checked out by an ophthalmologist if you experience any changes in your eyes, including pain.

Ophthalmologists have years and years of training, not to mention some excellent diagnostic instruments, to evaluate what is going on. As for ophthalmic migraines, the visual changes occur because of some activity in the visual cortex in the brain (located in the back of the skull). They are not a problem of the eye. The supplements I recommend in this chapter have been shown to help nourish the visual cortex, as well as the eye.

PAMPER YOUR EYES

Eye fatigue is common, especially if you watch a lot of TV, work nonstop on the computer, or play video games a lot. Take it from me as a writer sitting in front of the computer for up to 18 hours a day—eyestrain is not fun! If you don't periodically rest your eyes, eye fatigue can cause blurred vision, heavy lids, redness, wateriness, and the frequent need to blink. Artificial tears and similar products can help, but they are most effective when used *before* your eyes get tired, blurry, and uncomfortable. This is because by the time your eyes get that way, they're already dried out and much harder to treat.

GETTING AT THE ROOT OF THE PROBLEM

Changes in vision, blurriness, blind spots, halos around lights, or dimness of vision should always be evaluated by a medical professional. Such changes may represent a specific disease of the eye, aging, an eye injury, or a condition such as diabetes that affects many organs in your body. If you have diabetes, it's doubly important to get routine eye examinations.

The National Eye Institute and the American Diabetes Association recommend that people with diabetes get a dilated eye exam annually. When I interviewed Gregory Johnson, MD, an ophthalmologist at Coastal Carolina Eye Clinic in Wilmington, North Carolina, he said that the number-one thing people can do to preserve their vision is to keep their body healthy. "What works for your body works for your eyes," he says. "For example, diabetics who maintain tight control of their blood sugar and blood pressure tend to maintain healthy eyes. Other important factors come into play, such as smoking. Don't do it. Also, make sure to exercise regularly and eat a healthy diet."

VISION LOSS AND DIABETES

There are many ways that vision loss occurs—including some that are very subtle and slow—and the key to protecting your vision is in fruits, not in the pharmacy. That's because fruits contain powerful antioxidants that protect the eyes and potentially reverse vision loss for some people. Numerous scientific studies have documented that antioxidants have this capability.

If you or your loved one struggles with the loss of eyesight, one the next page I've listed some helpful tips.

BEAUTIFUL NEWS FOR DRY EYES

You can squirt in all the lubricating eyedrops you want, but they will only bring temporary relief to your dry eyes. For longer-lasting relief you need to address the underlying cause of dryness. The solution to this problem is so affordable and easy. Go to your health food store or pharmacy and buy a couple of supplements—fish oil (or krill oil), which is rich in omega-3 fatty acids, and hyaluronic acid. These two supplements help lubricate and wet the eye like nothing else can.

And guess what else they can do? They can make you beautiful! Seriously, both of these dietary supplements have been associated with reducing fine lines and wrinkles. You will notice a lovely difference within 2 weeks. Take these supplements with a meal.

When purchasing fish oil (or krill oil), be sure to get the kind made from mercury-free fish. I recommend taking the standard dose of 500 to 1,000 milligrams one to three times daily.

For hyaluronic acid, I recommend taking 100 milligrams once or twice daily, but check with your physician to make sure this doesn't interfere with any medications you're taking.

SHADE YOUR EYES. Wear sunglasses with 100 percent ultraviolet (UV) protection. Sunglasses that are amber, or in the orange-brown color range, work best to prevent the most damaging UV rays from hitting the retina.

INVEST IN SOME PROTECTION. Shield your eyes from chemicals, dust, smoke, or debris. Safety glasses may not be stylish, but they guard your eyes when you are doing household chores or working in the garden.

AVOID EYESTRAIN. Take regular breaks when reading, watching TV, or using the computer. Consider using a lubricating eye solution, such as artificial tears, to relieve any dryness. If you experience frequent eyestrain, it's possible that you need glasses.

WASH YOUR HANDS FREQUENTLY. You are constantly touching your eyes unknowingly, and you need to protect them from germs.

STOP SMOKING. It only hastens your vision loss because of free-radical damage to delicate eye capillaries.

SLEEP PROPERLY. Without proper rest, you get puffy eyes or dark circles, but you also feel more eyestrain as capillaries struggle to deliver blood to your eye area.

KEEP YOUR EYES WELL LUBRICATED. Drops and gels are sold over the counter at pharmacies nationwide. Products include Systane, GenTeal, Refresh Tears, and Similasan homeopathic drops.

Also, believe it or not, essential fatty acids (like those found in fish oils) are fantastic oral supplements to take if you have dry eyes. While eyedrops work quickly to restore moisture to the eyes, it's important to fix the underlying cause rather than just treating the problem. Fish oils work from the inside out to lube you up and, in my opinion, address one potential underlying cause of dry eyes—essential fatty acid deficiency.

EAT MORE FRUITS AND VEGGIES. These are rich in eye-saving nutrients and antioxidants. I prefer organic produce because pesticides can be harmful to delicate eye tissue and cause free-radical damage.

LOOK INSIDE YOUR MEDICINE CABINET

Here is a list of medications that can adversely affect your eyesight:

- Anticholinergic medication
- Antihistamines (Claritin, Zyrtec, Allegra, Benadryl, Chlor-Trimeton, etc.)
- Cold medicine
- Digoxin
- Hydrochlorothiazide
- Indomethacin
- Lyrica
- Plaquenil
- Psychiatric medications (This list is long and includes many medications, such as tricyclic antidepressants, selective serotonin reuptake inhibitors, antidepressants, and certain norephinephrine reuptake inhibitors.)
- Thiazide diuretics (hydrochlorothiazide and Dyazide)
- Urinary incontinence medications (Ditropan and Detrol)

GLAUCOMA: COMMON IN DIABETES

Now let's go back and take a more detailed look at an eye disease that's especially common in people with diabetes. There are several types of glaucoma, the second leading cause of blindness in the United States (right behind macular degeneration). Glaucoma comes in two primary types, and it's important to know the difference.

OPEN-ANGLE GLAUCOMA. The predominant type is called open-angle glaucoma. It causes a slowly progressing, chronic type of vision loss. With open-

SUZY'S QUICK EYE COMFORT POTION

If you've overworked your eyes, there is a cool and comfy way to relieve them—and don't worry, you won't need to apply cucumbers to your eyes. Just make a soothing eye compress. Here's my recipe: First turn off your cell phone and BlackBerry and all other forms of communication that could distract you from a peaceful state of mind. Next, put a half-teaspoonful of witch hazel and 5 drops each of Roman chamomile and lavender essential oil into a cup of water. Chill for 10 minutes. Finally, apply the mixture to cotton pads or a soft washcloth and then lie down with the compress over your eyes. Now inhale the wonderful aroma and relax your tired eyes for 10 minutes.

angle glaucoma, the pressure of fluid builds up in the eye. Scientists term the eye fluid aqueous humor.

With glaucoma, the aqueous humor fluid does not drain well out of the eye.

Some researchers believe that open-angle glaucoma is the result of hyaluronic acid (HA) deficiency. Yes, it could be that simple. You can buy supplements of hyaluronic acid at the health food store. The substance is a component of connective tissue, and it is all over your body. HA can help firm your skin, reduce wrinkles, ease joint pain, and improve vision. It also lubricates the vitreous humor in the chamber of your eye and adds moisture to your eye.

I think HA may be helpful in treating both glaucoma and detached retinas. In fact, a recent article in a pharmacology/biotechnology journal noted that solutions of HA are used in many surgical procedures within the eye and on the surface of the eye to both prevent dryness and promote wound healing after the surgery. In 2009 scientists in Hirosaki, Japan, published a study in the journal *Ophthalmology* showing how applying a film of HA after eye surgery (in this case, the patients were rabbits) can prevent postoperative complications.

Hyaluronic acid has impressive health benefits for people with arthritis, hernias, TMJ (temperomandibular joint) syndrome, ligament tears, mitral valve prolapse, wrinkled skin, fibromyalgia, and other disorders of the skin and connective tissue. I honestly don't know why so few doctors tell their patients about this inexpensive, powerful supplement that has the potential to save eyesight and offer so many additional benefits.

Hyaluronic acid is a natural component of the body found in all tissues, but some of these supplements are derived from chicken cartilage. For that reason, if you are allergic to chicken or eggs I would suggest either avoiding HA completely or using it only if you're sure the product is not poultry derived. Contraindications to using HA include a prior allergic reaction to HA, an active infection or inflammation of the skin or the joints, or sensitivity to eggs or chicken. A typical dosage is 100 to 200 milligrams once or twice daily.

CLOSED-ANGLE GLAUCOMA. The other type of glaucoma is called closed-angle glaucoma. This type is acute and, fortunately, relatively uncommon. It constitutes a medical emergency and occurs when there are structural changes in the iris, which bows forward, as in an archery bow. With this type of glaucoma eye fluid does not drain out at all.

Closed-angle glaucoma causes excruciating pain. Vision can be irreversibly lost unless laser surgery is performed promptly, and even then vision may be lost. Staying with the kitchen sink analogy, in the case of closed-angle glaucoma, the disposal gets clogged with a tennis ball and doesn't work at all. The sink will overflow and flood your kitchen unless you get a plumber to come in and punch a hole in the tennis ball or get it out.

NEOVASCULAR GLAUCOMA. Another type of glaucoma is usually associated with diabetic retinopathy. This rare form is called neovascular glaucoma and occurs when the blood vessels surrounding the retina are damaged. The retina makes new blood vessels to accommodate, but they are abnormal and grow on the iris. (That's the pretty, colorful part of your eye.)

This abnormal growth impairs drainage, causing pressure to build. Laser surgery or drainage implants can help with this.

No matter what kind of diabetes condition you have, it's important to lower blood sugar. When we accomplish that, we ultimately protect the precious blood vessels and capillaries that lead to our eyes. This lowers our risk for all forms of glaucoma.

MEDICATIONS FOR GLAUCOMA

Medications have a role—they are prescribed to protect whatever function you currently have, slowing the progression of blindness. Unfortunately, they have limitations, so after you read this section, please also read the section on natural supplements and teas that can potentially help in the process of repairing underlying damage.

Here are some of the most popular prescription eyedrops and some of their common side effects:

Betaxolol (Betoptic S)

Carteolol (Teoptic)

Levobunolol (Betagan)

Optipranolol (Metipranolol)

Timolol (Timoptic, Istalol, or

Betimol)

These five popular medications are in the class known as beta-blockers and have long been considered the gold standard for glaucoma therapy. Despite newer, pricey alternatives, these agents are still excellent, effective, well-tolerated, and useful first-line medications.

These medications work by reducing the amount of fluid production in the eye. With less fluid, there is less pressure. One problem is that they can slow heart rate, so they are not useful to some people with heart disease or metabolic syndrome. Other side effects to beta-blocker eye drops are relatively rare but possible, so I'll mention them to err on the side of caution. These include hair loss, worsening of asthma (and possibly emphysema), and an inability to recognize hypoglycemia—when your blood sugar drops dangerously low.

ALPHAGAN P AND IOPIDINE. These medications are called alpha adrenergic agonists, and they slow down fluid production within the eye. They also help drain the eye. They are usually used twice daily for optimal effectiveness. There is some talk among scientists that Alphagan may help prevent degeneration of retinal nerve cells. In some people, these drops can make the eyes itch and turn them bloodshot. They are also capable of enlarging your pupils.

TRUSOPT, AZOPT, AND DIAMOX. These medications reduce pressure in the eye by halting the amount of eye fluid produced. Trusopt and Azopt are eyedrops, while Diamox is a pill sold generically as acetazolamide. These medications are classified as carbonic anhydrase inhibitors. Side effects include burning and itching, and strangely, a bitter taste in your mouth, even though the drops go into your eyes.

COSOPT, COMBIGAN, AND DUOTRAV. Combination drops are getting to be the rage. These brand-name prescription drugs are basically a combination of two different types of glaucoma medications that come out of one convenient dropper. This improves adherence and offers synergy with two medications in one formulation. Frequently, people with glaucoma require more than one medication, and combo drops are an awesome way to fill that need and save money. With a combo drop, you only have to buy one bottle, or pay one copay at the pharmacy.

XALATAN, LUMIGAN, RESCULA, AND TRAVATAN. These eyedrops are popular because they need to be used only once daily, and they cause very few systemic

WHAT ABOUT MARIJUANA FOR GLAUCOMA?

Some folks with glaucoma try everything and still, they are almost legally blind and living in a lot of pain. There is another option for those who suffer, but you have to be open-minded. If you live in a state such as California where marijuana is decriminalized—meaning that those who have prescriptions to take it cannot be arrested for possession—then you could speak to your physician about getting a prescription for pot. Seriously. Studies show that smoking marijuana has the ability to reduce intraocular pressure.

In 1992 the American Academy of Ophthalmology stated: "There is evidence that marijuana (or its components), taken orally or by inhalation, can lower intraocular pressure. However, there are no conclusive studies to date to indicate that marijuana (or its components) can safely and effectively lower intraocular pressure enough to prevent optic nerve damage."

So can pot really make the grass look greener on the other side? Probably, if you smoke enough of it, but I don't think this benefit is worth the side effects of drowsiness and hunger pangs. Still, it may possibly give you a respite from the pain of glaucoma.

Now if you prefer a more stimulating drug like caffeine, this is a good time to tell you that caffeinated coffee spikes intraocular pressure. That's right, coffeeholics have a great risk of developing glaucoma, while potheads may actually have a lower risk!

(full-body) side effects. They are in the prostaglandin class of medications and work by allowing eye fluid to drain more efficiently. With better outflow of aqueous humor, there is lower pressure in the eye.

Do note that with these drops the color of your eye might change, and that change is likely to be permanent. The color can darken, especially if your eyes appear to change colors normally, as hazel eyes frequently do. The brown will start to spread into the green color of your iris over the course of 6 months to a year. (With brown eyes, there would be no significant changes in color.)

And guys, you may indeed be very macho, but I'm alerting you: These eyedrops also have a pretty side effect. They might lengthen and curl your eyelashes (and yours too, ladies), just like mascara does. One of these medications (Lumigan, which is known chemically as bimatoprost) has been turned into a drug that is applied to your lashes in order to make them thicken and grow longer. It's called Latisse and is manufactured by Allergan, the same company that made millions of dollars from Botox for wrinkles.

(This company knows what women want, and they've done it yet again by

SURPRISING TWIST OF FATE FOR TWO POPULAR MEDICATIONS

A study published in the *New England Journal of Medicine* in 2009 came up with some surprising results. Researchers looked at the effects of two popular prescription medications—Cozaar and Vasotec—to determine their effect on kidney function in diabetics. (Medications often have more than one condition that they are prescribed for. The two primary indications for Cozaar and Vasotec include hypertension and kidney disease.) What the researchers found surprised them. While the study could not confirm that these drugs worked any better than a dummy pill in preventing kidney damage, they did appear to slow the progression of diabetic eye damage in more than 65 percent of patients with type 1 diabetes.

So if your physician prescribes these medications to you for either high blood pressure or kidney disease, it may give you the added benefit of protecting your eyes.

targeting women who have hypotrichosis, or thin, skimpy eyelashes. Latisse became the first eyelash-growing drug to be approved by the FDA in December 2008. It is available by prescription for approximately $120 a month.)

Finally, it's worth noting that with most eyedrops, stinging, burning, or itching can occur. It's unusual, but sometimes you hear of people developing muscle aches, cramps, or a flulike reaction.

NUTRIENTS THAT PROTECT YOUR VISION

Fortunately, if you have diabetes, you don't need to wait for problems to develop with your eyes. A number of nutrients can help protect your vision. And if problems do develop, these same nutrients can help protect your precious eyesight. Pay special attention to getting more of the following nutrients either from your diet or from supplements. The doses listed are standard doses for these nutrients.

LUTEIN

Lutein is a yellow-orange pigment called a carotenoid. It is responsible for the color in fruits and vegetables such as sweet potatoes, papaya, carrots, and even some green vegetables. It's also a powerful antioxidant, and several studies have discovered a direct relationship between lutein and better eye health.

SPECIALTY PRODUCTS FOR PROTECTING YOUR VISION

Health food stores and pharmacies offer a huge variety of supplements. I often find myself cruising down the aisles to see what new goodies companies have developed. Here are a few of the most popular products for protecting your vision.

Ocuvite Preservision. This is one of the most popular and easy-to-find supplements on the market. It contains lutein, omega-3 fatty acids, and vitamins C and E, as well as a few minerals. It's inexpensive, too. I like this combination of nutrients, especially for the price (under $20). But since I'm picky, I'll tell you that I'm unhappy with the soy in here, and also the peanut oil (which many people are allergic to), as well as the numerous artificial colorants in the formula.

Icaps. This multitasking formula contains lutein and zeaxanthin, along with a good dose of important eye-loving minerals such as zinc, copper, selenium, and manganese. On the upside, it also contains some antioxidants, such as vitamins A, C, and E. But on the downside, it contains some preservatives, anticaking agents, and other artificial ingredients.

Ultimate DHA Eye by Nordic Naturals. This product contains pure, mercury-free omega-3 fatty acids from fish oil extracts. Omega-3s relieve dry eyes and protect your retina. The unique formula also contains lutein and zeaxanthin, as well as pure natural vitamin E for stabilization. It is free of artificial preservatives and colorants.

Vision Formula with Lutein and Bilberry by Nature's Way. This product contains lutein, bilberry, vitamin A, biotin, citrus bioflavonoids, taurine, ginseng, grapeseed, and several other natural eye savers. It also contains cayenne pepper extract. The hot pepper fruit is thought to increase blood flow and reduce nerve pain (neuropathy), which is very common in diabetes.

Visual Eyes by Source Naturals. Each tablet contains bilberry, quercetin, lutein, zeaxanthin, grapeseed extract, vitamin A, and important minerals. The formula also includes *Ginkgo biloba*, which increases blood flow to the eyes (and everywhere else in your body). This formula is one of those all-in-one products that contains many nutrients to retain and regain vision. It does contain a few fillers and binders used in the tablet-making process.

Under the right circumstances, lutein even seems to be associated with the prevention of cataracts and macular degeneration. The Nurses' Health Study concluded that for some people, lutein intake reduces the need for cataract surgery. It's unfortunate that only plants can synthesize this wonderful nutrient—humans cannot—so we must take it into our body from outside sources, such as plant-based foods or dietary supplements.

HOW TO GET LUTEIN IN YOUR DIET. Eat five or more servings per day of dark, leafy green vegetables, especially kale, but also spinach, Swiss chard, mustard greens, red leaf lettuce, parsley, and broccoli. Other foods rich in lutein include tomatoes, corn, eggs, avocados, sweet potatoes, squash, mangoes, and papaya.

HOW TO SUPPLEMENT. Lutein is easy to find in health food stores nationwide in dosages ranging from 6 to 20 milligrams. A typical dosage is 20 milligrams taken daily with a meal. Lutein works better with its carotenoid sister zeaxanthin, so you will often find these two nutrients in a combination formula.

ZEAXANTHIN

Zeaxanthin (pronounced *zee-uh-ZAN-thin*) is another natural yellow-orange pigment, similar to lutein but even friendlier to the eye. In fact, of all the carotenoid nutrients, a number of studies have shown that the human eye prefers zeaxanthin and lutein. This nutrient quenches free radicals just as lutein does, thus preventing damage to the retina by protecting against cataracts and macular degeneration. Humans cannot make zeaxanthin, and therefore dietary intake or supplementation is needed.

HOW TO GET ZEAXANTHIN IN YOUR DIET. Raw spinach leaves, broccoli, corn, and persimmons have the greatest concentrations of this nutrient. Other foods to include are brussels sprouts, peas, cauliflower, kale, and egg yolks.

HOW TO SUPPLEMENT. Take about 4 milligrams of zeaxanthin daily with food, and ideally in combination with lutein. Many supplements are sold in combination this way.

BETA-CAROTENE

Beta-carotene is a carotenoid just like lutein and zeaxanthin. Beta-carotene gives carrots and pumpkins that familiar orange color. It's also the pigment that you see in beautiful autumn leaves. When the green chlorophyll dies, the orange-yellow beta-carotene can be seen in the leaves.

The difference between lutein, zeaxanthin, and beta-carotene is that beta-carotene can actually undergo a chemical reaction in the body and convert to a vitamin A derivative called retinol. Many scientific experts have mixed feelings about beta-carotene, especially after publication of a large clinical trial in the

March 2007 issue of *Archives of Ophthalmology*. This study followed 21,000 participants (physicians actually) and concluded that beta-carotene had no beneficial effect on vision after 12 years. The doctors were randomly assigned to take either 50 milligrams of beta-carotene every other day or a placebo pill.

I take issue with this study, which at the time made headlines stating that beta-carotene doesn't improve vision. How can they say that, when all they provided was a *synthetic* form of beta-carotene? And we're not even sure the participants took it. They filled out questionnaires saying they did.

Regardless, let's assume they took their synthetic beta-carotene supplement every day for 12 years. Does it shock you to hear that synthetic beta-carotene can increase mortality according to some studies? True story—not only does synthetic beta-carotene *not* protect your eyesight, but some studies show it can hasten your death, especially if you smoke. The *real* deal, pure natural beta-carotene, has repeatedly been shown in many studies over the years to protect your eyesight. And being a powerful antioxidant, I think it reduces your cancer risk.

This is a very important distinction for consumers who are hunting down the very best supplements they can find, so let me repeat it. Natural beta-carotene seems to be able to help you and improve vision, as do most eye-penetrating antioxidants. Synthetic forms of beta-carotene may not work, and in some people may be harmful.

Beta-carotene converts to vitamin A once inside the body. People with night blindness are almost always deficient in vitamin A. People short on vitamin A also experience a haze or glare even under normal lighting circumstances.

SPECIAL NOTE. Many medications are drug muggers of beta-carotene and steal this nutrient from your body. Drug muggers of beta-carotene include acid-blocking drugs for heartburn, antacids, cholestyramine resin (Questran), mineral oil, prescription fat blockers (Xenical and Alli), and Olestra (a fat substitute commonly found in potato chips).

HOW TO GET BETA-CAROTENE IN YOUR DIET. Eat more orange foods like sweet potatoes, carrots, butternut squash, red peppers, tomatoes, pumpkin, spinach, collards, cantaloupe, apricots, peaches, and broccoli. Lightly sautéeing or steaming veggies actually seems to make it easier to absorb the beta-carotene. To get vitamin A itself, you can include food sources such as meat, liver, kidney, butter, and eggs.

HOW TO SUPPLEMENT. I recommend about 5 to 15 milligrams per day. (That's 8,000 to 25,000 IU per day.) Pregnant women should take no more than 10,000

IU per day. Synthetic sources will say only "beta-carotene" on the label. I want you to take only natural forms (not synthetic), so look for phrases on product labels that say "natural beta-carotene," "from *D. salina*," "from an algae source," or "from a palm source." I also like Carrot Essence by Green Foods; this powder gets mixed with water.

ASTAXANTHIN

The antioxidant astaxanthin is another carotenoid and is found in very high concentrations in a red algae called *Haematococcus pluvialis*. Astaxanthin can be produced in a synthetic nonnatural form, and this product is often used commercially to color animal feed. But a natural form of astaxanthin is found in oceans all over the world and also in the very best dietary supplements.

Marine critters love to munch on natural astaxanthin-rich algae. Anything that eats the red algae turns red. Think lobster, salmon, and shrimp. Astaxanthin is food for flamingos, and this natural pigment is what puts the pink in pink flamingos.

Clinical studies done on natural astaxanthin supplements show that it improves blood flow to eye muscles, helping to improve accommodation and relieve eyestrain. It is an anti-inflammatory and can help neutralize free radicals. Studies do support its role in preventing macular degeneration. It is one of my favorite dietary supplements because it's a powerful immune enhancer, it lowers blood pressure, and it works to protect the heart.

HOW TO GET ASTAXANTHIN IN YOUR DIET. Dietary sources are insignificant unless you graze on algae.

HOW TO SUPPLEMENT. Just remember, you want it to say "natural astaxanthin" on the label. Take 4 to 6 milligrams once or twice daily. As always, check with your physician when it comes to these or any other nutritional supplements to make sure they don't interfere with any of the medications you're currently taking.

I take astaxanthin myself several times a week. I have enjoyed the following brands:

BioAstin 4mg by Nutrex-Hawaii. This brand is produced in Hawaii by Cyanotech, a world leader in dietary supplements derived from micro-algae. They harvest and process astaxanthin (and their spirulina) in tightly controlled and sterile open ponds. These are softgels.

AstraReal by AstaVita. I like the way this company produces its product, in controlled domes that provide a totally clean environment. Based in Sweden and also Hawaii, AstaVita is another world leader with a lot of science behind their incredibly stable product. These are small softgels.

BILBERRY

Bilberry is often called the European blueberry, whortleberry, or huckleberry. The American blueberry is a relative. Bilberry is actually blue in the center where the meat is, whereas blueberries are cream-colored in the center. Bilberries offer a dark pigment that colors these fruits bluish purple.

Bilberries contain a lot of vitamin C and some terrific chemicals called anthocyanosides, which are powerful antioxidants. These anthocyanosides give bilberry its pharmacologic activity. In other countries, especially Europe, bilberry is considered a gold standard in the treatment of many vision disorders, such as cataracts, macular degeneration, and glaucoma.

The European enthusiasm for bilberry actually got its start when some pilots ate bilberry jam and discovered that they could see better at night. These delicious berries can also lower blood sugar.

Bilberries can also reduce inflammatory chemicals, improve floaters, strengthen capillary walls, and protect the retina.

Bilberries were shown to quench free radicals in some studies done on lab animals. In one Russian study, published in the journal *Biochemistry* in 2004, researchers noted the many health-promoting benefits of berries rich in anthocyanin, which is found in bilberries and five other berries in the study—wild blueberries, cranberries, elderberries, raspberry seeds, and strawberries. Scientists in Finland have noted that substances made from berries have important applications for the food industry because of their natural antimicrobial, disease-killing properties.

HOW TO GET MORE BILBERRY IN YOUR DIET. You can find bilberry in juice or teas sold in many health food stores.

HOW TO SUPPLEMENT. Bilberry is available in extract form. I recommend that you take about 80 milligrams one or two times daily. Often this nutrient is combined with other antioxidants such as grapeseed or lutein. Even better!

The most potent formulas will state "25 percent anthocyanosides" on the label, meaning that the makers have extracted one of the beneficial active ingredients. Common sense may tell you that if you extract only one of the beneficial ingredients, you forfeit all the other goodies within, and yes, that's true. However, when you do that and "standardize" an herb using its most important isolate, it works almost like a drug because you have a very potent version of the active ingredient.

There is a lot of controversy regarding whether to standardize an herb. Sometimes I think it's valuable, sometimes I think you compromise some of the benefits. In the case of bilberry, I think it's fine.

GINKGO BILOBA

The herb *Ginkgo biloba* has shown promise for protecting the optic nerve in some people. A February 2003 study published in *Ophthalmology* concluded that people in a study taking *Ginkgo biloba* started to see a wider field of vision.

People with diabetes have circulation problems because of all those tiny little clots that clog up the blood vessels. In the eye, these clots form in and around the retina. Ginkgo thins the blood and allows more blood to flow. In one Taiwanese study, ginkgo was given to people with type 2 diabetes who had retinopathy. After a few months, blood clotting was reduced and blood flow to the retina was improved. With more blood flow, there is more oxygen to the optic nerve and to the retina, and that contributes to better eyesight.

HOW TO GET MORE *GINKGO BILOBA* IN YOUR DIET. Drink *Ginkgo biloba* tea, 1 cup once or twice daily.

HOW TO SUPPLEMENT. I recommend taking 40 milligrams of *Ginkgo biloba* daily with food. This is a natural blood thinner and its effect is considered beneficial. Do not combine it with aspirin, heparin, warfarin (Coumadin), or any other blood thinner unless under the advice and supervision of your doctor.

B VITAMINS

There is a connection between elevated inflammatory chemicals, such as homocysteine, in the body and age-related macular degeneration. One well-designed study, the Women's Antioxidant and Folic Acid Cardiovascular Study (WAFACS), published in 2008 in the *Journal of the American Medical Association*, showed that giving high-risk patients B vitamin supplements actually reduced their risk for age-related macular degeneration. Participants received either a dummy pill or a

B vitamin cocktail that contained 2.5 milligrams of folic acid, 50 milligrams of vitamin B_6, and 1,000 micrograms of vitamin B_{12} daily. After 7 years, women taking the B vitamin supplements had a 34 percent lower risk of macular degeneration and a 41 percent lower risk of "visually significant" macular degeneration.

HOW TO GET MORE B VITAMINS IN YOUR DIET. Eat green, leafy vegetables, such as kale, Swiss chard, turnip greens, parsley, and lettuce (not iceberg, though, as it has fewer significant nutrients compared to darker greens). Broccoli is a good choice, too.

HOW TO SUPPLEMENT. I recommend that you take a high-quality B-complex supplement that provides active nutrients, such as Thorne Research's Basic B-complex. You can find high-quality B supplements online and at some doctor's offices. You can also supplement with an organic green drink such as spirulina, Nanogreens, Ocean's Alive Marine Phytoplankton, or Greens Plus.

OMEGA-3 FATTY ACIDS

Studies show that omega-3 fatty acids can be especially helpful for people with dry eyes or Sjögren's syndrome, a chronic disease that causes drying of the eyes, salivary glands, and other mucous membranes. Taking omega-3 fatty acid supplements daily can improve the immune system, enhance blood flow and circulation, improve mood, and reduce inflammation. You will often find this ingredient in multitasking eye formulas.

HOW TO GET MORE ESSENTIAL FATTY ACIDS IN YOUR DIET. Eat more cold-water fish. Make sure it's wild caught, not farm raised, to ensure optimal levels of essential fatty acids and purity. Good choices include Arctic char, salmon, cod, herring, anchovies, mackerel, and yellowfin (also called ahi) tuna.

HOW TO SUPPLEMENT. Take an omega-3 fatty acid supplement that contains fish oil or krill oil. A typical dose is 500 to 1,000 milligrams two or three times daily with food. Krill oil holds an advantage over fish oils because it appears to cause less abdominal discomfort and "fish burp." Two of the better brands on the market are produced by Nordic Naturals (www.nordicnaturals.com) and Udo's Choice (www.udoschoice.com). These are sold online and at health food stores nationwide.

Improving Heart Disease

Most people are aware that routine exercise, a healthy diet, and refraining from smoking help reduce chances of cardiovascular problems. But what we call lifestyle changes are not enough for people with diabetes because they have poor bloodflow, high blood pressure, and many nutritional deficiencies. It's harder to stave off heart disease if you have diabetes, when blood sugar is high and inflammatory chemicals run amok. According to the Centers for Disease Control and Prevention (CDC), heart disease is the number one cause of death for all men and women in the United States.

The American Heart Association has some scary statistics taken from an ongoing, nearly 50-year-old study, called NHANES, which stands for the National Health and Nutrition Examination Survey. NHANES was created in the early 1960s by the National Center for Health Statistics and is run by the CDC.

NHANES consists of several studies designed to figure out the general health and nutritional status of adults and children in the United States. How do they do that? They choose about 5,000 people—of all backgrounds and ethnicities, both women and men, in various places across the country—and perform physical exams, as well as interview them about their health. The CDC people go to about 15 different locations each year. It results in some pretty amazing stuff. And I'm glad they're doing it, so I can present you with only a handful of their shocking statistics. Specifically, the most recent information from the study tells us:

- About 80 million American adults (one in three) have one or more types of cardiovascular disease; of these, 38.1 million are 60 years of age or older.
- 73.6 million Americans have high blood pressure (defined as 140/90 mm Hg or greater).
- 7.9 million Americans have had heart attacks, also known as myocardial infarction.
- In 2005, some 652,091 Americans died of heart disease (50.5 percent of them women), which was 27.1 percent of all U.S. deaths in that year. Worldwide, coronary heart disease killed more than 7.6 million people.

It surprised me to learn that cardiovascular disease—which includes heart attack and stroke—is the number-one killer of Americans, accounting for more deaths than all cancers. Without a shadow of a doubt, your heart is the most crucial part of your circulatory system. If it stops holding up its end of the bargain, life stops within minutes.

A person with diabetes who is stressed out and eating too many saturated fats, processed foods, and too little fiber, can expect to develop heart disease sooner rather than later. And if you smoke, it'll happen even sooner than that. If you are sedentary, then blood flow in your body becomes stagnant, which is why your doctor will tell you to get up and move around during long flights. In Chinese medicine this problem is known as qi (pronounced *chi*) stagnation. Acupuncturists and Asian folks reading my book will appreciate this analogy. Qi stagnation is just another way of saying that blood isn't flowing well.

Poor blood flow could very well translate into blood clots, thrombus (a blood clot in a vessel or in your heart), and tumors. You want your blood flowing, which is why exercise is so important for everyone, but especially for the people with heart disease. It's even more important for the cardiac patient who has diabetes. With diabetes, the body's repair systems don't work as well because all the circulating blood sugar messes things up.

The pharmaceutical industry offers people a quick fix-me-up with drugs that temporarily fix one part of the disease process. But these drugs are not a cure. They only offer time and, at most, prolong the life of an individual who needs a boost. Behind the pharmacy counter, we have strong blood thinners such as aspirin, Plavix, warfarin (Coumadin), and the newest member, Effient, approved in July 2009. We have medications for hypertension, such as diuretics (water pills), angiotensin-converting enzyme (ACE) inhibitors, calcium-channel blockers, and beta blockers others. We have statins to lower cholesterol. We have drugs to help regulate heart rhythm. But none of these drugs or procedures is without risk or side effects.

Well, I've got good news for you! There are some natural alternatives that could very well reduce your risk for developing complications of heart disease. But before we get to those, let's take a closer look at heart disease as it relates to diabetes.

SIGNS OF A FAILING HEART

Did you know that the cause of death for two out of three people with diabetes is heart disease or stroke? For people over the age of 20 (and I'm guessing that's most of the people reading my book), the highest risk factors for heart and circu-latory disease are having:

- High blood pressure (or taking medications for high blood pressure)
- High cholesterol
- Diabetes
- A weight that is considered obese (that is, having a body mass index [BMI] of 30 or higher). See page 23 to find out your own BMI.
- Cigarette smoking

That's five. Guess what the sixth is? Being sedentary or, as the CDC says, "engaging in no leisure-time physical activity." The last time this was measured it included 39.5 percent of us. That's shameful!

CIRCULATION 101

I call your blood vessels, arteries, and capillaries your body's pipeline. Maintain-ing a healthy pipeline is crucial to avoiding heart problems because when your blood vessels are flexible and wide open, blood can flow properly to all of your organs.

A perfectly healthy heart can pump about 9 pints of blood per minute when resting and about 50 pints while exercising strenuously. The heart is a dual-acting pump. The right side of your heart receives blood from your body and pumps it to your lungs so the blood can get some oxygen. The left side of the heart does just the opposite. It gets oxygenated blood from your lungs and pumps it out to the rest of your body.

With every beat (contraction), your heart squeezes out the blood that has collected and sends it to the rest of your body for energy and nutrition in the form of O_2. Yep, oxygen. The heart beats an average of 70 times per minute and 2.5 billion times during an average lifetime. Compare that to the heart of a blue-throated hummingbird, which beats up to 1,260 times per minute. Can you imagine?!

This may sound weird to you because most people associate muscles with biceps, quads, or abs, but your heart is really a muscle, and it's about the size of your fist. This muscle works 24/7 and pumps about 100,000 times a day. Imag-ine squeezing your glutes that many times a day—I'd have to be put in traction for weeks if I tried that! Why are we, especially we ladies, so concerned about getting a soft heinie when our heart muscle is the one keeping us alive?

HOW HEALTHY IS YOUR HEART?

Take this quiz to see if you have early signs of heart disease:

1. Do you ever experience the sensation of pressure or "squeezing" in your chest, neck, or at the top of your abdomen? (It can last anywhere from a few seconds to weeks, and the onset is unpredictable.)
2. Are you aware of irregular heartbeats, where the beat flutters or feels like a pause, and then it's followed by a very strong beat?
3. Do you sometimes feel lightheaded or dizzy?
4. Do you want to sleep during the day? (While common in dozens of other medical conditions, daytime fatigue is one hallmark symptom that your heart isn't circulating blood properly.)
5. Do you experience shortness of breath? (It can happen with very little exertion, or, in some cases, it can wake you up gasping for breath. These episodes are known as paroxysmal nocturnal dyspnea.)

If you answered yes to two or more of these questions, you could have the beginnings of heart disease. Obviously, you will want to see your doctor and possibly a cardiologist who specializes in heart disease to find out what treatments are right for you. In the meantime, let me walk you through the very basics of heart function so you can see why the supplements I recommend work so well.

We take for granted that our heart will always beat and that it will never go soft like our abs or buns. To drive this statement home and raise awareness with the public, I contacted the editor at *Vogue* magazine and asked her to put an actual heart on the cover of their magazine, instead of another airbrushed celebrity with Photoshopped thighs and a cellulite-free butt. They have yet to respond.

If you want to reduce your chances of heart attack or stroke, you have to reduce inflammation in your body by keeping your blood sugar down, which normalizes your insulin-to-glucose ratios and helps to keep your blood vessels clean and free of debris. Controlling blood glucose, blood pressure, and cholesterol are all important ways of reducing your risk of fatal heart disease and stroke. Now let's take a closer look at some of the most common problems that may be affecting you and your heart.

PROBLEMS OF THE HEART AND CIRCULATORY SYSTEM

I've created an overview of the common disorders of the heart to help you recognize any problems you might have and get needed medical attention. Don't just ignore these signs or symptoms, okay? They can turn into deadly complications. Please pay attention because cardiovascular disease is easier to prevent than to cure.

People with diabetes have a much higher risk of developing the conditions I've listed below. I have also listed some types of supplements you might consider taking. However, you must discuss all changes to your drug and supplement regimen with your physician, your diabetes educator, and your pharmacist. Discuss my recommendations with them.

We are dealing with your heart, after all, so please make sure you are under the care and supervision of your doctor and helped by your diabetes educator and pharmacist, and take your medications as prescribed until otherwise directed. In the meantime, here is a brief list of problems that occur within the circulatory system and some supplements that may help.

ANGINA PECTORIS. Sometimes angina pectoris is mistaken for indigestion. A symptom of coronary artery disease (CAD), angina pectoris is a condition that causes chest pain, heaviness, pressure, aching, burning, or squeezing sensations in the shoulders, arms, neck, throat, and back. All this occurs when the heart is suffocating from lack of bloodflow and oxygen, so it uses an alternative fuel to keep beating. The by-product of this fuel is a substance called lactic acid, which builds up in the heart muscle and creates pain. This is exactly the same reason your muscles are sore while you are working out. Angina may respond to arginine, ubiquinone, or nattokinase, supplements that I will discuss later on.

VENTRICULAR TACHYCARDIA (ALSO CALLED V-TACH). In this condition, the heart beats very fast, but it has a normal rhythm. Because it is beating so fast, the heart isn't able to adequately fill up its chambers with blood. Symptoms include dizziness, lightheadedness, shortness of breath, chest pain, or near fainting. The pulse is usually weak but rapid. Ventricular tachycardia is dangerous because if it lasts for more than a few seconds, it can progress to ventricular fibrillation and cause sudden death. Ventricular fibrillation is a leading cause of sudden cardiac death. Nonprescription decongestants, herbal remedies that contain ma huang or ephedra, diet pills, and energy supplements often contain stimulants

DRUG MUGGERS THAT STEAL POTASSIUM

These medications may lower your potassium levels, putting you at higher risk for a dangerous condition known as ketoacidosis. Read page 110 in Chapter 6 to learn how you can avoid this diabetic complication.

Albuterol (Ventolin, Proventil)

Acetazolamide (Diamox)

Alcohol

Amoxicillin, ampicillin, dicloxacillin, and other antibiotics

Aspirin

Butalbital/aspirin compound (Fiorinal)

Caffeine

Docusate/casanthranol (Peri-Colace)

Enalapril and hydrochlorothiazide (Vaseretic)

Furosemide (Lasix)

Hydrochlorothiazide

Hydrochlorothiazide and triamterene (Dyazide, Maxzide)

Levodopa/carbidopa (Sinemet)

Nifedipine (Procardia)

Steroids

Stimulant laxatives

Tacrolimus (Prograf)

Telmisartan and hydrochlorothiazide (Micardis HCT)

Verapamil (Calan, Verelan)

Valsartan (Diovan)

It's also possible that natural diuretics can cause a shift in potassium even though they are far weaker than medications. But do be aware that certain herbal diuretics may also affect your electrolytes if you are very susceptible. (Electrolytes are minerals that your body uses to keep fluids in balance. This balance can affect your heart rhythm, muscle contraction, and brain function.) Herbs that are cause for concern include uva ursi, dandelion, stinging nettle, cedar berry, licorice root, mullein leaf, and goldenseal.

that can trigger episodes of ventricular tachycardia. Prescribed medications used for high blood pressure can occasionally trigger episodes of V-tach.

The condition may respond favorably to ubiquinol (coenzyme Q10), hawthorn, and Cordyceps mushroom. Hypokalemia (low potassium) can trigger episodes, too, so see the box above for a list of prescribed drug muggers that steal potassium from your body.

PREMATURE ATRIAL CONTRACTIONS. These are extra beats, thought by most physicians to be harmless for most people, and do not require treatment if they are infrequent. I don't feel that way myself. If your heart is doing something out of the ordinary, I think that is a clue to improve heart health. Heart-loving supplements, such as D-ribose, L-carnitine, hawthorn, or ubiquinol (coenzyme Q10), are some of the substances that may be associated with normalizing your heart rhythm.

PREMATURE VENTRICULAR CONTRACTIONS. These are extremely common arrhythmias and can happen to anyone. When they happen, it feels like your heart has skipped a beat. They can be tied to stress, caffeine, nicotine, strenuous workouts, or sex. These are also thought to be harmless and do not require treatment if they are infrequent. That said, I think you should ask your doctor about the same heart-healthy supplements listed above for premature atrial contractions.

ATRIAL FIBRILLATION. This is another common irregular heart rhythm that causes the upper chambers of the heart—called the atria—to contract abnormally. It occurs because the electrical signals from the heart are firing in a different pattern than is normal. For some, it results in mild palpitations, and for others, it can cause life-threatening arrhythmias. Sometimes the heart beats dangerously fast, and sometimes it slows down dramatically. A general heart tonic such as hawthorn may be of value here, as well as taurine, D-ribose, arginine, Cordyceps, and L-carnitine.

ATRIAL FLUTTER. Similar to atrial fibrillation, but atrial flutters are usually more rhythmic and regular. They can occur after surgery and may progress to atrial fibrillation.

BRADYCARDIA. These are slow heart rhythms that occur because of problems with the heart's electrical conduction system. Examples include sinus node dysfunction and heart block. Sometimes bradycardia is associated with vagus nerve disorders, such as excessive parasympathetic stimulation, a condition that causes too much acetylcholine in the body. It is also associated with many other conditions, especially with hypothyroidism (low thyroid). A heart that beats too slowly may normalize over time, possibly with the assistance of supplements. Two good all-around supplements to try include essential fatty acids (from omega-3 fish oils) and a medicinal mushroom blend that contains several health extracts, such as MycoPhyto by Econugenics or 5 Mushroom Formula by JHS.

HEART-HEALTHY SUPPLEMENTS

With heart disease the number-one killer in the United States and abroad, it seems that more doctors would be telling you about the heart-healthy supplements that could potentially preserve your health and maybe even save your life. If you have heart disease or high cholesterol, it's high time you started thinking outside the pills that are typically dispensed via prescription.

Modern healthcare is obsessed with good-looking numbers, and I am banging my head wondering why more physicians aren't focused on natural alternatives that actually *repair* the damage. Repair it, don't mask it. That's not too much to ask for the good money you spend on doctor visits.

I bet if we lined up 20 health food store owners and 20 cardiologists, more of the health food store owners would know that the supplements I'm about to recommend can prevent heart damage. It's true that cardiovascular risk can be greatly reduced by modifying your diet, exercising routinely, and giving up toxins (like cigarettes). Adding dietary supplements has also been proven to support cardiovascular health in numerous studies, as you will see.

If you have had angina (chest pain) or have had a heart attack, then you will want to read this. Also, if you, or someone you love, has congestive heart failure or high blood pressure, these next few pages can save you (or your loved one's) life. I don't care if you have a 90 percent blockage to all your arteries, you'll still find hope here.

TERRY'S STORY OF TRIUMPH

Terry was sent home to die under hospice care back in September 1993 after having two massive heart attacks. According to his coronary arterial diagram done at the hospital, he had three arterial blockages at 100 percent, plus one at 90 percent, another at 99 percent, and yet another at 70 percent.

Terry's mitral valve, the heart valve that helps control blood flow, was so damaged that surgery to replace it was the only remedy proposed. But because of an only 40 percent chance of surviving the surgery, Terry opted not to have it done. The cardiologist and intensive care unit doctors gave him just a few days or weeks to live and sent him home under hospice care.

Terry gave away his pickup truck and most of his beloved personal belongings. His family members from all over Pennsylvania flew to Florida to say goodbye to him, and it was a very sad time for all of us. Terry is one of those men who would rather enjoy his life, eat what he wants, and watch sports. Like most men (and many women), exercising and eating healthy plant-based foods are not high on his list of things that constitute "enjoying life."

I totally understand this point of view. Look, I used to eat cheeseburgers, too, and cheddar-smothered french fries with ranch dressing. It's delish. But don't you think these meals should be served along with an open-heart surgeon?

Anyway, during the years that preceded this hospitalization, Terry ignored the warning signs of heart disease. He paid little attention to his body. He frequently ate triple bacon cheeseburgers (yes, triple) and clung to his first love, Lebanon bologna sandwiches. (He was actually born in Lebanon, Pennsylvania, where they make this stuff.)

At this apparently terminal stage of his life, it seemed like nothing *and no one* would be able to help him. We videotaped Terry telling his stories, and he did all the necessary things a man does when preparing to leave the Earth. That was in September 2007. As of the writing of this book, Terry is still here. He even underwent major abdominal surgery to remove his appendix and gallbladder in November 2009. They extracted a stone the size of a golf ball!

Between 2007 and now, there was a high point when Terry began climbing a flight of stairs four or five times a day for exercise. While he's not running any marathons, he is able to drive and do mild activities. Plus, much to my chagrin, he still sneaks meals that are known to clog up arteries. But generally speaking, he's doing well and enjoying life.

We never know when our time is up, but while we have time, we may as well make the best of it. Terry has gotten to enjoy a few more birthdays, the birth of two grandchildren, the graduation of his stepson, plus more years with his family.

I know that I'm not the sole reason for his improvement, as he has a loving wife who cares for him daily and cooks him healthy foods to offset the bacon cheeseburgers he consumes occasionally. But the supplements I have encouraged him to take have helped tremendously.

The take-home point here is that even a person who is given a death sentence may be able to enjoy a few good months or even years if he commits to taking the right combination of nutrients, herbs, and minerals. And, of course, an important part of this picture is maintaining good, solid medical care from a treating physician. During his recovery phase, Terry took a few of the supplements discussed in the coming pages. He continues to take them daily. They may or may not be right for you, so make sure you check with your personal team of physicians before taking any supplements for your heart.

HEART-HEALTHY SUPPLEMENTS

By now, I'll bet you're anxious to learn about all the nutritional supplements that medical science knows can be helpful for supporting heart health. Here's an overview of the best.

Arginine

Arginine, sometimes called L-arginine, is an amino acid, naturally produced throughout the body, even though there are high concentrations of it in your pituitary gland. It's first on my list because it has such widespread effects.

Arginine may be useful to people with diabetes in some very important ways because it is a jack-of-all trades. Arginine appears to be able to help one maintain healthy blood sugar levels and blood pressure while also boosting energy reserves and helping to sweep away artery-clogging gunk from the arteries. Furthermore, it appears to have cholesterol-lowing abilities, as well as kidney-supportive properties, because it helps remove waste products (such as ammonia) from the body.

If you're not impressed yet, let me tell you that studies on arginine show that it may also enhance wound healing. It works because arginine is a precursor to proline, which is ultimately converted to collagen for your skin. Arginine supports blood flow to the sexual organs, so it helps men with erectile dysfunction. This, and so much more! No small feat for one molecule.

In a groundbreaking study researchers in Barcelona, Spain, found that nuts show a lot of promise in supporting heart health because nuts are so rich in unsaturated fatty acids and other "good" fat. Researchers attributed these findings in part to the fact that nuts (especially walnuts) are so rich in L-arginine, as well as alpha linoleic acid, among other nutrients.

In 2009 researchers at the University of Virginia in Charlottesville found that arginine may help people with heart failure. They also found, as noted in my "Caution" paragraph on the next page, that arginine may be dangerous for people who have already had a heart attack. I don't personally agree, and I'll tell you why momentarily.

In the body, the amino acid L-arginine is a precursor to many molecules, one of which is nitric oxide. Nitric oxide helps blood vessels relax and pushes more blood to flow to your heart and all the other good parts, if you know what I mean. One study did, in fact, prove that arginine improved bloodflow to the heart.

On the basis of all this research, it's reasonable to conclude that arginine may ease symptoms of angina, coronary artery disease, intermittent claudication, and clogged arteries. Not all studies are positive, but the data I've read is firm enough for me to feel comfortable in recommending arginine to you.

Of course, as with any nutrient and medication, I want you to discuss the potential benefits of arginine with your doctor so he or she can make sure it's right for you.

HOW TO GET MORE ARGININE IN YOUR DIET. Vegetarians usually don't have any problem getting arginine into their diet. Rich food sources include brown rice, coconut, oatmeal, seeds, whole wheat bread, and raisins. Nuts are a very rich source of arginine, too. It is also found in poultry and red meat to some extent.

HOW TO SUPPLEMENT. Please refer to my caution note below before you go run out and buy this supplement. You'll want to take 500 to 1,000 milligrams of L-arginine one to four times daily. Start on the very low end of the range, say 500 milligrams once daily for a week, and if you do not see improvement, move to twice daily and so on.

I see products with very high dosages—even up to 6,000 milligrams per day total. If you want to do take this much, consult your physician and move up to that dosage very slowly. The reason dosages vary so much is because it depends on whether you are using it to reduce blood pressure, improve symptoms of heart failure, or lower cholesterol.

In clinical trials, arginine has been used safely with minor side effects for up to 3 months. Many brands are available, but since you are dealing with the heart, I'd be very choosy. I took this supplement myself to see how I would feel, and it appeared to improve my athletic performance. I was able to do longer periods of aerobics without feeling winded.

Some good brands that I've taken myself and recommended to others include Arginine TR, Perfusia SR, and Twinlab L-Arginine. See my Resources section on page 382 for more information about how to get those.

CAUTION. Possible side effects include blood thinning, stomach discomfort, bloating, diarrhea, and gout. A National Institutes of Health study testing the use of L-arginine after a heart attack was abruptly halted when six patients (who had had heart attacks) taking L-arginine died; none of the patients who did *not* receive L-arginine died. The researchers were worried that L-arginine aggravated the effects of a heart attack. All of this was discussed in an article in the *Journal of the American Medical Association.*

I take issue with the researchers findings because for one, the study participants may have died anyway. Two people died from *presumed sepsis,* meaning they were *very* sick to begin with and hospitalized. Why blame that on arginine? Two were found dead at home with no cause of death noted. One person died 3 weeks after stopping the arginine! And the silliest part of all is that the plasma L-arginine levels were *the same* in both the arginine group and the placebo (untreated) group!

So tell me, do you feel confident that arginine was the cause of death for these extremely sick people who had already suffered massive heart attacks? How can scientists sleep when they frighten people away from heart-healthy nutrients on the basis of weak findings that have no statistical significance in my book. Even the authors confess that the deaths are most like due to statistical chance but that's not what drug companies want you to think. They want you to run scared from natural supplements, into the arms of FDA approved drugs. Lots of them!

I am giving you these details because I do not want you to be frightened about arginine. Do, however, share these important details with our physician to see if it's right for you and if you have residual concerns, stick to low dosages that feel comfortable.

People with asthma need to be very careful with this supplement because it may worsen breathing problems. Taking high doses of the amino acid L-arginine can suppress levels of the related amino acid L-lysine, and in some sensitive individuals this imbalance increases outbreaks of arginine-driven infections, such as shingles, fever blisters, or other herpes-related infections.

An individual who has been diagnosed with any form of herpes or cancer should consult a healthcare provider for approval and dosage information. Arginine is often found in sex enhancement pills that are sold over the counter. I would not combine arginine (or sex supplements that contain arginine) with prescribed drugs such as Cialis, Levitra, or Viagra.

Coenzyme Q10

Coenzyme Q10 (CoQ10), a vitaminlike substance, is one of the most heart-healthy nutrients you can take. It should be considered just as important as arginine in this list. It is a powerful antioxidant, and it's in all your muscles, especially your heart.

The mitochondria of your cells are where energy is produced, and they contain the most CoQ10. Powering up your mitochondria—your cells' generators—can help you burn fat, improve cholesterol ratios, raise energy, and improve thyroid and pancreatic function. Think of CoQ10 as an energy molecule helping your heart pump blood in and out and helping every single cell to breathe. In fact, when you think "heart," think CoQ10 or its activated version, called ubiquinol.

Ubiquinone is converted within our body into ubiquinol, a potent antioxidant; but as we age, this conversion process becomes compromised. Ubiquinol, as a potent antioxidant, has been found to help minimize oxidative injury to DNA. Still, ubiquinone has other valuable properties, so it's best to try to get both in a supplement.

STATINS INCREASE BLOOD SUGAR

Your blood sugar may go up because of your cholesterol medication. If you take a statin, it can cause high blood sugar and you may be mistakenly diagnosed with diabetes. Please read more on page 103.

CoQ10 is really helpful for anyone, not just people with diabetes, who experiences leg cramps and muscle pain, often the result of the drug-mugging effect of statin cholesterol medicines such as Advicor, Pravachol, Zocor, Lipitor, and Mevacor. These drugs block production of cholesterol in the liver, but that's also where CoQ10 is made. So taking statin drugs can compromise your ability to make CoQ10, a heart-healthy nutrient, as can some diabetic medications. What an irony! A deficiency of CoQ10 may cause liver damage, muscle weakness, leg cramps, memory loss, fatigue, shortness of breath, cardiac arrhythmias, heart attack, stroke, or rhabdomyolysis (a potentially fatal condition in which skeletal muscle cells break down, even if you have perfect cholesterol).

Statins aren't the only mugger of CoQ10, however. Diabetic medications, such as metformin, Actos, and Avandia; estrogen hormones; antidepressants; and blood pressure medications all affect levels of CoQ10. Refer to "Drug Muggers of CoQ10" on page 152 for a more thorough list of drugs that deplete CoQ10. There is another, longer list that is updated periodically, posted at my Web site, www.DearPharmacist.com.

When you find out that every living cell makes a form of CoQ10, you realize the importance of this nutrient and its life-sustaining abilities. CoQ10 appears to help reduce cholesterol and improve symptoms of angina, as well as some types of abnormal heart rhythm.

In 2008, I interviewed the world's leading researcher on CoQ10, Peter Langsjoen, MD, and he had this to say regarding CoQ10: "The effects of ubiquinol on late-stage heart failure patients resulted in striking improvements beyond anything I've seen in 25 years of cardiology practice. It is my strong feeling that ubiquinol product is a major breakthrough."

In recent years, Kaneka, the world's largest manufacturer of CoQ10, has been able to produce and stabilize ubiquinol. Kaneka supplies centers that conduct clinical trials with their CoQ10, and most studies are positive, especially heart failure studies. One study by Dr. Langsjoen showed that ubiquinol offered "dramatically" improved absorption as compared to CoQ10. Moreover, this improved absorption was associated with both overall improvement for patients with heart failure, as well as improved functioning of the left ventricular portion of the heart.

HOW TO GET MORE COQ10 AND UBIQUINONE IN YOUR DIET. Dietary sources in descending order include sardines, mackerel, beef heart and liver, lamb, pork, and eggs. Some vegetables are dietary sources of CoQ10 include spinach and broccoli. Nuts and whole grains are also sources. Buy organic produce and wild-caught fish when possible.

HOW TO SUPPLEMENT. Product labels will state ubiquinone, CoQ10, or coenzyme Q10, all exactly the same nutrient. The more active form of CoQ10 will be labeled with "QH" or "ubiquinol" (notice the -ol on this word). These two names denote the active, more usable forms of the same nutrient.

So which should you take, ubiquinone (CoQ10) or ubiquinol (QH)? Since it's available, and it's stronger and probably easier for your body to incorporate into your cells, I recommend ubiquinol to everyone. If you are over 30 years of age, have heart disease, have reflux disease, take acid blockers, or take a drug mugger of CoQ10, then I also recommend ubiquinol.

However, plain CoQ10 is fine if you are in relatively good health or if price is an issue. I prefer that your supplements be softgel and free of soy or gluten.

I've done some legwork for you, and the bottom line is this: If you choose CoQ10, take 50 to 150 milligrams once or twice daily. Do check this amount with your doctor. Many brands are sold nationwide. Some good ones include Healthy Origins CoQ10, and Bluebonnet.

If you choose ubiquinol (QH), take 50 to 150 milligrams once or twice daily. Again, check this dose with your doctor. Only a handful of companies right now make this form, including Life Extension, Bluebonnet, Healthy Origins, Puritan's Pride, and Vitamin World. It's also sold under the brand name of QH-Absorb by Jarrow. These brands are sold widely at health food stores nationwide and online.

CAUTION. Work with your doctor to determine the best dosage for you, which varies widely—between 30 and 500 milligrams daily, sometimes more! I don't recommend high dosages because high amounts of CoQ10 (ubiquinol) can backfire and cause heart rhythm abnormalities, dizziness, or fainting (because blood pressure may drop too low).

The supplement is generally well tolerated; however, sometimes gastrointestinal upset or allergies occur. Quality differs greatly among brands. I prefer that you take bioidentical forms of CoQ10 (the kind that matches your own natural form) rather than synthetic, lab-created versions. The brands I've recommended above are considered bioidentical.

Ribose

Ribose, sometimes called D-ribose, is a naturally occurring sugar that the body uses to make adenosine triphosphate (ATP), your cells' energy molecule. Ribose is needed to make other energy molecules (such as nicotinamide adenine dinucle-otide [NADH], FADH [flavin adenine dinucleotide], and acetyl CoA) that your body needs to make your heart beat.

Ribose is found throughout your body and in many foods. It provides an essential component that acts as the backbone of your genetic code (DNA and RNA). Ribose is found in every living human cell, and what's so fascinating is that ribose is also a component of vitamin B_2 (riboflavin), which, incidentally, is thought to help people with migraines and teeth grinding. Ribose is frequently used by athletes who get muscle soreness because they have depleted their energy stores with high-intensity exercise.

Ribose seems to help people with heart failure by improving bloodflow, and with increased bloodflow more oxygen is carried to the heart. This means that ribose may ease feelings of shortness of breath, fatigue, and other symptoms of heart failure. It makes sense that ribose can improve heart failure (and athletic function) because the body's energy molecule ATP is depleted from the heart and skeletal muscles.

With more energy, the mitochondrial powerhouses work better. Ribose's effect on an individual with heart failure could be dramatic because it helps the heart pump better and improves breathing. This is one of the most important things that a person with diabetes could focus on; that is, improving the health of their cells' generators (mitochondria), so ribose becomes important for the whole body, not just the heart.

Ribose is also understandably an excellent supplement for those who suffer with muscle pain, soreness, and stiffness, as does anyone with fibromyalgia or chronic fatigue syndrome. I've recommended ribose to many readers of my syndicated column, with remarkable success. Some feedback came my way, saying that the supplement helped. Some noted that ribose helped "a little" (within 24 hours). Another said, "I felt complete relief after only 2 months," and that was after having moderate pain for many years. Again, it has to do with ribose's ability to improve ATP (energy) metabolism.

DRUG MUGGERS OF CoQ10

The following drugs can affect the level of CoQ10 (and therefore ubiquinol) in your body. If these drugs cause a deficiency of CoQ10, then over time, it could hasten the development of other side effects. Deficiencies of CoQ10 have been linked to liver damage, muscle aches and pain, memory loss, and increased risk for cardiac arrhythmias, congestive heart failure, and even cancer (since CoQ10 is an antioxidant).

The big shocker is that statin cholesterol drugs have a well-documented effect of depleting stores of CoQ10 because they work on the same pathway. This explains why statins may cause some of those challenging side effects.

Replenishing the CoQ10 can help many people feel better. Knowledge is power. Check this admittedly long list see if your medication depletes CoQ10. If so, you should ask your doctor about taking supplements of this nutrient.

Acebutolol (Sectral, Prent)

Acetohexamide (Diamox)

Acetophenazine (Tindal)

Alcohol

Amiloride and hydrochlorothiazide (Moduretic)

Amitriptyline (Elavil)

Amoxapine (Ascendin)

Atenolol (Tenormin)

Atenolol and chlorthalidone (Tenoretic)

Atorvastatin (Lipitor)

Benzthiazide (Exna)

Betaxolol (Betoptic eye drops, Kerlone)

Bisoprolol (Zebeta)

Candesartan and hydrochlorothiazide (Atacand HCT)

Carteolol (Ocupress eye drops)

Carvedilol (Coreg)

Chlorothiazide (Diuril)

Chlorpromazine (Thorazine)

Chlorpropamide (Diabinese)

Clomipramine (Anafranil)

Clonidine (Catapres)

Cyclothiazide (Anhydron)

Desipramine (Imipramine)

Doxepin (Sinequan)

Droperidol (Inapsine)

Enalapril and hydrochlorothiazide (Vaseretic)

Enoxacin (Penetrex)

Esmolol (Brevibloc)

Fenofibrate (Tricor)

Fluphenazine (Prolixin)

Fluvastatin (Lescol)

Gemfibrozil (Lopid)

Glimepiride (Amaryl)

Glipizide (Glucotrol, Glucotrol XL)

Glyburide (Micronase, DiaBeta, Euglucon)

Glyburide and metformin (Glucovance)

Haloperidol (Haldol)

Hydralazine (Apresoline)

Hydralazine and hydrochlorothiazide (Apresozide)

Hydralazine, hydrochlorothiazide, and reserpine (Ser-Ap-Es)

Hydrochlorothiazide (Hydrodiuril)

Hydrochlorothiazide and reserpine (Hydropres, Hydroserpine)

Hydrochlorothiazide and spironolactone (Aldactazide)

Hydrochlorothiazide and triamterene (Maxzide, Dyazide)

Hydroflumethiazide (Diucardin, Saluron)

Imipramine (Tofranil)

Indapamide (Lozol, Lozide, Apo-Indapamide)

Irbesartan and hydrochlorothiazide (Avalide)

Labetalol (Normodyne, Trandate)

Losartan and hydrochlorothiazide (Hyzaar)

Lovastatin (Mevacor, Apo-Lovastatin, Anlostin, Aztatin, Belvas)

Mesoridazine (Serentil)

Methdilazine (Bristaline, Dilosyn, Disyncram)

Methotrimeprazine (Apo-Methoprazine, Novo-Meprazine; Nozinan)

Methyclothiazide (Enduron, Aquatensen)

Methyldopa (Aldomet, Apo-Methyldopa)

Methyldopa and hydrochlorothiazide (Aldoril, Apo-Methazide)

Metolazone (Zaroxolyn, Mykrox)

Metoprolol (Lopressor, Toprol XL, Apo-Metoprolol, Betaloc, Durules, PMS-Metoprolol)

Moexipril and hydrochlorothiazide (Uniretic)

Nadolol (Corgard)

Nortriptyline (Pamelor)

Perphenazine (Trilafon)

Pindolol (Visken)

Polythiazide (Renese)

Pravastatin (Pravachol, Apo-Pravastatin)

Prazosin and polythiazide (Minozide)

Prochlorperazine (Compazine)

Promazine (Sparine)

Promethazine (Phenergan)

Propafenone (Trental)

Propranolol (Inderal)

Propranolol and hydrochlorothiazide (Inderide)

Protriptyline (Vivactil, Triptil)

Quinethazone (Hydromox)

Repaglinide (Prandin, GlucoNorm)

Simvastatin (Zocor, Apo-Simvastatin, Revastat, Simvacor, Lisac, Cardin)

Sotalol (Betapace, Alti-Sotalol)

Telmisartan and hydrochlorothiazide (Micardis-HCT, Micardis Plus)

Thiethylperazine (Torecan)

Thioridazine (Mellaril, Apo-Thioridazine)

Timolol (Timoptic, Apo-Timol)

Tolazamide (Tolinase)

Tolbutamide (Apo-Tolbutamide, Diabetose)

Trichlormethiazide (Metahydrin, Naqua)

Trifluoperazine (Stelazine)

Valsartan and hydrochlorothiazide (Diovan HCT)

An article published in the journal *Alternative Therapies in Health and Medicine* in 2009 concluded that "metabolic interventions" that preserve energy (think D-ribose) or those that help you produce more ATP energy molecules (think L-carnitine and CoQ10) are "the missing link" when it comes to treating congestive heart failure. That's a strong statement from a researcher!

HOW TO GET MORE RIBOSE IN YOUR DIET. Red meat (especially veal) contains some ribose, but it's really an insignificant source. There are no substantial dietary sources that I recommend. Here's one case where it's better to take a supplement.

HOW TO SUPPLEMENT. Ribose can be used to prevent muscle cramping and soreness and for increasing energy and stamina. Take 3 to 5 grams two or three times daily as directed. High-quality brands include Corvalen, Doctor's Best, Healthy Origins, and Life Extension.

CAUTION. This nutrient is found in every living plant and animal cell. Very large doses have been taken without ill effect, although I can't make any promises about how it will affect you personally. Check with your physician about whether this supplement is appropriate for you.

Ribose can lower blood sugar levels by improving the body's general health. For that reason, monitoring blood sugar is important to avoid hypoglycemia.

Hawthorn (*Crataegus oxyacantha*)

Hawthorn is an herb that grows all over the world and the bright red berries look similar to mistletoe. Hawthorn extract is the best all-around heart tonic I can think of because studies show that for some people, it can improve symptoms of heart failure, fatigue, chest pain (angina), and heartbeat irregularities. The berries, leaves, and flowers all contain cardio-active compounds.

Hawthorn works by increasing the amount of blood your heart pumps, and it lowers blood pressure over time. One human study did show that hawthorn was able to lower blood pressure in people with diabetes. I also think hawthorn is a great all-around cardiac protector because for some people it seems to be able to help normalize heart rhythm; in contrast, many other heart supplements just improve bloodflow/circulation. Hawthorn dilates the arteries that supply the heart muscle itself with blood, oxygen, and fuel. With continued use, people may experience a stronger, more efficient heartbeat.

One of the best aspects of hawthorn extract is its apparent ability to protect against free radicals that do so much damage in the arteries. That's right, it's a powerful free-radical scavenger, and by virtue of its ability to sweep away inflammatory chemicals it ultimately could reduce your risk for atherosclerosis. Researchers in France published a study in 2003 noting just that.

A diet rich in polyphenols, which hawthorn contains in abundance, apparently reduces the overall risk of heart disease. And guess what else? It activates an enzyme system that increases the activity of the PGC-1 alpha gene. That's a good thing because the more PGC-1 alpha activity you have, the easier it gets for you to burn fat and improve diabetes symptoms. So in essence hawthorn works in various important ways to take a load off your heart. The French researchers used hawthorn extract.

HOW TO GET MORE HAWTHORN IN YOUR DIET. There are no substantial dietary sources, although you can drink hawthorn tea once or twice daily. Hawthorn tea blends are sold nationwide at health food stores.

HOW TO SUPPLEMENT. A good choice is *Crataegus* extract standardized to 1.8 to 2.0 percent vitexin (that's an active ingredient in hawthorn). Take 250 to 450 milligrams one to three times daily or follow directions on the label. Best of all, take as directed by your physician.

CAUTION. With hawthorn, you get better effects if you take it for a longer period of time, like 3 months or more, rather than taking big doses all at once. People who are sensitive to the herb or who take excessive dosages may experience dizziness, drowsiness, a drop in blood pressure, tremor, nausea, or heart palpitations. In normal dosages, hawthorn is generally well tolerated.

Omega-3 Fatty Acids (Fish Oil)

Omega-3 compounds, particularly EPA (eicosapentaenoic acid) and DHA (docosahexaenoic acid), found in fish oil, plant themselves firmly into the membrane of your cells. And you have between 50 and 75 trillion cells in your body. That's a lot of planting!

Once in the cells, these omega-3 compounds affect the electrical signaling between your cells, as well as their structure and function. The effect on the human body is to cause your blood vessels to relax, so your blood pressure goes down; to squash inflammation, thereby reducing pain; and to inhibit blood clotting, thereby reducing your risk of stroke or heart attack.

This supplement could well be the number-one, simplest, most cost-effective fix for your heart, but of course, this is just my opinion. You need to ask your doctor.

The American Heart Association agrees that the intake of fish that contain essential fatty acids (EFAs) can reduce your risk of developing heart disease. Fatty fish contain two kinds of omega-3 fatty acids that love your heart—EPA and DHA. But the joy doesn't stop at your heart. Research is under way to determine whether EPA and DHA may also have positive effects on blood glucose in people with type 2 diabetes. Some early research does suggest that EPA and DHA may indeed be beneficial in such patients.

In 2002, the American Heart Association released a scientific statement called "Fish Consumption, Fish Oil, Omega-3 Fatty Acids, and Cardiovascular Disease," about the effects of omega-3 fatty acids on heart function. The statement noted that while the link between omega-3 fatty acids and reduction in risk for cardiovascular disease is still being studied, existing research shows that omega-3 fatty acids are associated with the following four positive health effects:

1. Decreased risk of arrhythmias, which can lead to sudden cardiac death
2. Decreased triglyceride levels
3. Decreased growth rate of atherosclerotic plaque
4. Lowered blood pressure (slightly)

The benefits of omega-3 fish oils don't stop with heart health, however. These oils have also been associated with easing depression, improving constipation, and even reducing wrinkles.

Many people get confused about the omega fatty acids because there are three types—omega-3s, omega-6s, and omega-9s. All three are important to the body; however, people who consume corn oil, soybean oil, cottonseed oil, fried foods, and many animal-based foods—unfortunately, all too big a part of the typical American diet—get more than enough omega-6 and -9 in their diet. It's the balance among all the omega fatty acids (3, 6, and 9) that is important.

Supplementing with just omega-3 fatty acids is right for some people, while others may need a combination. I can't tell from here who needs what, so you need to closely examine your diet and work with your doctor or a nutritionist to help you decide a right course of action. A blood test is available by Genova Diagnostics that assesses your levels of these fatty acids and can help anyone with inflammatory disorders. It's called an EMFA test, which stands for essential and metabolic fatty acids analysis, and your physician can call Genova to get it for you. (See the Resources section for the information on Genova.) I can tell you that if you eat a vegetarian, low-fat diet, you may need a combination. If you eat a lot of fried foods, animal proteins, and vegetable oils, you will probably need pure omega-3 supplements that supply EPA and DHA only. The labels clearly identify which omegas the products contain.

HOW TO GET MORE OMEGA-3S IN YOUR DIET. Eat wild-caught cold-water fish such as herring, mackerel, tuna, Arctic char, cod, and salmon. Farm-raised seafood does not contain the same amount of healthy omega-3s that wild caught does. If you're dining out, you should ask your server whether the fish on the menu is wild caught or farm raised.

Chia seeds and flaxseeds are two vegetarian sources that offer some EFA. Nuts, especially walnuts, Brazil nuts, hazelnuts, and almonds, contain some beneficial fatty acids that protect your heart. Many of my recipes in Chapter 17 are based on almond flour. And there is more about Chia seeds on page 163 of this chapter.

HOW TO SUPPLEMENT. The standard dose is about 500 to 1,000 milligrams one to three times daily with food. Taking it several times a day rather than all at once helps to minimize unpleasant side effects, such as abdominal discomfort. For people with high blood fats (cholesterol and triglycerides), the American Heart Association recommends a higher dosage, more like 2 to 4 grams of EPA and DHA daily, while remaining under a physician's supervision. Remember, fish oils have the positive effect of thinning blood, but this can also be problematic in sensitive individuals, so medical supervision is advised.

It's best to build up dosages rather than start all at once. Nordic Naturals makes a pure form of fish oils that doesn't taste fishy, and I have taken their product for many years with good results.

Doctors sometimes prescribe the drug Lovaza, which is a patented extract of fish oil called an omega acid ethyl ester that is especially good at reducing triglycerides. Some of the readers of my syndicated column have asked me if I like the drug version better than the natural version. As a pharmacist, you'd think I would, but I don't. I am staunch about your taking natural products, not those that are isolated or morphed into patentable (and profitable) versions.

CAUTION. Fish oils may thin the blood and cause digestive upset. Fish oil is best taken with food, meaning while you're eating or just afterward. Poor-quality products sometimes contain heavy-metal contamination, although this problem is getting better nowadays. If you experience "fish burp," you may need to switch brands because this could be due to inferior quality.

If switching brands does not stop the problem, fish burp could be a sign of poor digestive health. You may need to take digestive enzymes, probiotics, or other supplements to improve digestion. More often than not, fish burp is related to poor digestion, rather than inferior brands.

Taurine

Taurine is an amino acid, a building block for protein. The secret's out, however, that taurine also has antioxidant effects. That means it has the ability to mop up damaging free radicals that fire toxic bullets at your brain, heart, pancreas, liver, arteries, and everywhere else.

Taurine is another one of my secret weapons for people with diabetes who seek natural means to help themselves. Tests have detected low levels of taurine in many people with type 2 diabetes. And taurine may directly improve symptoms in people with type 2 diabetes. Research has shown that when depleted supplies of taurine are restored to study participants through nutritional supplements, symptoms improve.

In one study, Japanese researchers, for example, looked at 30 college students between the ages of 18 and 22 to see if taurine supplements could help them lose weight or improve their total cholesterol number and levels of fat in their bodies.

The students had a body mass index (BMI) of 25 or higher, which is technically right on the edge of being overweight, and no evidence of any kind of diabetes. During the 7-week study, neither the researchers nor the students knew which group of 15 students got the taurine (3 grams a day) and which group got the placebo. When the researchers completed the study, they found that the 15 people who received the taurine supplement had "significantly" reduced their weight and improved their cholesterol. Taurine, the researchers noted, "produces a beneficial effect on lipid metabolism and may have an important role in cardiovascular disease prevention in overweight or obese subjects." Not bad for an amino acid.

Another study, done in India and published in 2009 in *Current Protein and Peptide Science*, noted: "Nutritional intervention with taurine, phenylalanine, or branched chain amino acids can improve insulin sensitivity and postprandial glucose disposal." Translation: Taurine and other amino acids can help increase your body's sensitivity to insulin and can help get sugar out of your system after you eat.

Taurine acts kind of like insulin, helping to shuttle glucose into your cells where it belongs. That's just what insulin does. That little action makes taurine ideal for athletes as well as for those with high blood sugar.

Taurine is found everywhere in your body. It's really an interesting molecule. Here are some of the things it can do:

- It can help regulate your heartbeat.
- It can speed up the healing of wounds. (I'm thinking about your feet as well as cuts and sores.)
- It plays a role in regulating your blood pressure.
- It may protect the kidneys, which is fantastic news for those with diabetes.
- It may increase your liver's ability to detoxify harmful chemicals.
- It benefits the pancreas's beta cells, where insulin is made.
- It seems to lower blood sugar and helps people lose some weight.

HOW TO GET MORE TAURINE IN YOUR DIET. Protein-rich foods contain taurine. These include lean meat, poultry, fish, and eggs. Vegans could run low on taurine because they do not eat these foods.

HOW TO SUPPLEMENT. Dosages vary widely. Most product labels recommend 500 to 1,000 milligrams once daily. Some nutrition experts suggest 2,000 milligrams two or three times daily. Such higher dosages have been used in many research studies and are generally well tolerated; however, ask your doctor what is right for your individual needs. Taking taurine with a little vitamin B_6 (about 20 to 50 milligrams daily) may improve results.

CAUTION. Taurine is often found in energy drinks but it probably does not produce energy itself. In fact, it causes drowsiness once in a while. It may reduce blood pressure and blood sugar, so taking it in combination with your prescription medications may lead to an additive effect. It has a blood-thinning effect, too. That is generally considered beneficial, but caution is advised in people with bleeding disorders or those taking medications that also thin the blood. In those cases, dosing adjustments may be necessary. Taurine should be used cautiously or avoided if you have epilepsy. As always, please check with your physician when adding supplements to your regular medication regimen.

Nattokinase

In Japan, natto is a food. This salty, nutty cheese product derived from fermented soybeans is used in many Asian and European recipes, and it's usually mixed with spices or other cheeses and served with rice. Nattokinase is an enzyme extracted from natto.

Once purified and put into capsules and tablets, nattokinase as a supplement

CARDIAC TUNE-UP FROM TULSI TEA

The herb tulsi contains hundreds of different natural compounds, including essential oils, vitamins, minerals, and many cancer-fighting phytochemicals. In this one herb, you get one of the most powerful and healing substances in the world. Holy moley! Actually, I should say holy basil—the other name for tulsi, and the name that most dietary supplements of this herb goes by.

I love tulsi so much I want to marry it! Herb experts maintain that it revs up your immune system, reduces inflammation, and protects against harmful bacteria, viruses, and other germs. But here's the best part—it seems that tulsi helps your body adapt more easily to stress, making it one of the most powerful adaptogens ever known to man. Adaptogens reduce the burden placed on your body by stress, including the kind of stress caused by emotional trauma, chronic pain, pollution, and poor diet, not to mention dial-up Internet connections.

Herbal experts also maintain that tulsi can tune up your heart by lowering dangerous cholesterol and stress-induced high blood pressure. By lowering inflammation and sweeping away free radicals, tulsi protects the heart and blood vessels. It also has mild blood-thinning qualities, so perhaps it can reduce the likelihood of strokes.

I take my tulsi in the form of tea, which can be purchased at health food stores nationwide. You can also take a holy basil supplement. There are many brands, but because I'm picky, picky, the only one I'm willing to recommend to you today is New Chapter's brand called Supercritical Holy Basil. It's free of impurities such as chemical solvents and other contaminants.

New Chapter's brand is also free of soybean oil. The holy basil is mixed with organic olive oil instead.

becomes one of nature's most powerful natural blood thinners. Thinning the blood—which is often too thick in people with diabetes or metabolic syndrome—can really improve circulation and blood flow to vital organs.

Research shows that nattokinase may also be able to dissolve blood clots and prevent their formation in some cases. Researchers in Taiwan, for example, studied a group of 45 people and found no adverse effects from giving them two capsules of nattokinase (2,000 fibrinolytic units [FU] per capsule) a day for 2 months.

On the basis of their findings, the researchers concluded that because of its properties, including anticlotting abilities, nattokinase could be considered a nutriceutical to defend against cardiovascular disease. They published their findings in the journal *Nutrition Research* in March 2009.

Because nattokinase thins the blood, it may also help reduce blood pressure. Makes sense, right? If it can also help lower your risk for heart attack, stroke, phlebitis, pulmonary embolism, and deep-vein thrombosis, nattokinase should have a solid future in the nutriceutical industry, given the fact that annual healthcare spending in the United States has reached $2.3 trillion! That's trillion with a T.

Nattokinase has been found to work by dissolving fibrin (tiny fibers) that makes up the meshwork of the blood clot. If the meshwork is weakened, the blood clot dissolves. This is the same reasoning behind the use of streptokinase and urokinase, two medications usually given intravenously in the hospital after a heart attack or stroke.

Other experts think that nattokinase acts a little like plasmin—a natural enzyme in human blood that maintains the right viscosity. The debate about how it works could go on for years, but I think there are enough solid studies for me to comfortably recommend this dietary supplement to you. That said, please ask your cardiologist whether it's right for you.

Nattokinase may also be able to help people with angina (chest pain). Can it head off bypass surgery or angioplasty? I don't know, and I can't safely advise you about this, but I do know the risks involved with those procedures. It's certainly a good question, and I believe you should have a candid discussion with your cardiologist to seriously consider this supplement before going under the knife.

HOW TO GET MORE NATTOKINASE IN YOUR DIET. Natto is called cheese, but to be blunt, it's an acquired taste. My understanding is that it's rather slimy and somewhat aromatic. (Okay, fine, let's be honest. It's smelly!) Also, the health benefits are in the *raw*, fermented natto. To get the benefits you'd have to eat a lot, which Americans might find hard to stomach (and perhaps hard *on* the stomach). You can find recipes for natto online and give it a try, if you wish. But I am recommending an easy way out—just take a pure, high-quality extract of nattokinase instead. It's stronger, simpler, and far more palatable.

HOW TO SUPPLEMENT. Try Enzymedica's brand called Natto-K, which combines nattokinase and six other enzymes to really target clot formation. There is also Nutricology's brand NattoZyme or Source Naturals' Nattokinase. I found more good brands to recommend to you. One is Doctor's Best Nattokinase; the other is NSK-SD by Dr. David Williams. Both have had the natural vitamin K removed, which may be important to people on blood-thinning medications. Still, I want you to remain supervised while taking these supplements because they affect your heart and circulatory system.

Take about 2,000 FU one to four times daily or as directed by your physician. This could also be expressed as 100 milligrams one to four times daily. (The conversion is 2,000 FU equals 100 milligrams.) The higher the dosage, the stronger the blood-thinning effect, so please be mindful of that.

CAUTION. Combining nattokinase with warfarin, Plavix, Effient, or other prescribed blood thinners; aspirin; or any other herbs or medicines that thin the blood or prevent blood clotting may have a dangerous additive effect and lead to excessive blood thinning.

If you are allergic to soy, you should not use nattokinase. Also, people with very low levels of thyroid hormone may find that long-term nattokinase exacerbates their problem, as soy lowers thyroid hormone.

RESVERATROL

Resveratrol is the key ingredient that gives red wine its benefits. Research has found that this powerful antioxidant can improve cholesterol ratios, lower LDL (low-density lipoprotein, the bad cholesterol), and is otherwise good for you. My preference? I wish you would take it in supplement form or drink a tablespoon of purple grape juice. I'm not a big fan of people with diabetes drinking alcohol.

Studies have shown that we humans absorb resveratrol well. Problem is that we absorb it so well and so quickly that our bodies soak it in and eliminate it pretty fast. The real fascination with resveratrol began in the United States when scientists noticed its presence in red wine. They began to look into resveratrol as possibly being the reason behind the "French paradox." The French paradox is that despite a diet high in fatty foods, including butter and the ultimate fatty food, hard cheese, the French suffer from far less cardiovascular disease than do Americans.

Research has shown that resveratrol can inhibit the growth of cancer cells in yeast, worms, fruit flies, and fish, but the truth is we don't know for sure whether it can do all of this in humans. I happen to think it shows great promise. There is much more on resveratrol and how to buy supplements in Chapter 13.

HOW TO GET MORE RESVERATROL IN YOUR DIET. Consume more red or purple grapes or grape juice, organic peanuts, or peanut butter. If you don't have diabetes, red wine can be a good source, once in awhile.

HOW TO SUPPLEMENT. Take about 100 milligrams daily of the form derived from the Japanese knotwood shrub (*Polygonum cuspidatum*). Make sure the

> ## ANOTHER REASON TO LOVE VITAMIN C
>
> Matthias Rath, MD, founder of the Dr. Rath Research Institute and author of *Why Animals Don't Get Heart Disease and People Do* is reshaping the way modern medicine treats heart disease. His scientific discoveries in the areas of cardiovascular disease and cancer are impressive. In a nutshell, Dr. Rath has found that a little vitamin C goes a long way in protecting against heart attack and stroke. Vitamin C, which is abundant in citrus fruit, works indirectly to keep your arteries flexible, which, in turn, may reduce buildup of cholesterol and plaque, as well as reduce other risk factors of heart attack and stroke. There is an incredible wealth of information at his Web site, where you can learn more about the man and his mission: www.drrathresearch.org.

extract is standardized to at least 50 percent resveratrol, but preferably to 98 percent, if you can find it. You may find products called red wine extract, but this not the same thing as resveratrol.

CAUTION. Some people taking resveratrol report insomnia, dizziness, spikes in blood pressure, and stomach cramping. This occurs most frequently with inferior brands of supplements. Read more in Chapter 13 on how to get the best type of resveratrol supplement.

CHIA

Remember back in the 1970s those terra cotta figurines that sprouted green "hair"? C'mon, you can admit it. Everybody back then was part of the chia pet phenomenon (and you can still buy them!). It was tiny black chia seeds that sprouted to make the hair. But here's the cool thing. You can eat the seeds!

Chia seeds (*Salvia hispanica*) may be the richest *vegetarian* source of essential fatty acids (like omega-3s) in the world. As you know, EFAs are the good fats that protect our brain, liver, pancreas, heart, and what I call the pipeline—all our blood vessels and arteries.

Chia seeds were consumed by the Aztecs and Mayans and just might be the most nutrition-packed food (for the size) that I can think of. They are seriously tiny, the size of a flaxseed, but in many ways, easier to integrate into your diet. Why? Because you have to grind flaxseeds; you don't have to grind chia seeds. Also, they don't spoil quite as fast as flaxseeds do, so they have a longer lifespan in your kitchen.

These seeds are packed with power because 1 ounce of dried chia seeds contains almost 5,000 milligrams of omega-3 fatty acids and over 170 milligrams of calcium. Eating chia seeds may improve skin conditions, joint pain, and immune function. Here's the best part—and the reason I love chia seeds so much: They have the ability to absorb several times their own weight in water, so you feel full after eating them. This means chia seeds can curb hunger and help you lose weight if you need to. Fiber is fantastic for you, and so easy to get by sprinkling a few chia seeds on your food.

You can buy organic chia seeds at health food stores nationwide and online. Many readers of my column write in to ask me if the white chia seeds (often seen under the brand name Salba) are better than regular black chia seeds. You already know my stance on this if you read Chapter 1: no more white!

I think darker, more colorful foods are more nutritious, as a general rule. That said, there's nothing bad about Salba, but it's not what I recommend. The reason for that is because it's a patented white version of the natural chia seed, which is black, and the price tag for this heavily promoted version is much higher. Why mess with Mother Nature?

Real chia seeds may lack the hoopla that Salba receives, but it's the natural form that Mother Earth provides for us. And it's what I use in my own kitchen. I always want you to choose natural foods over patented, morphed ones.

WHEN TO GET HELP

I've been a syndicated columnist for over 12 years and I review readers' letters and questions carefully. One thing that is clear is that many readers tend to self-treat and play around with medications, dosages, and supplements without their doctor's knowledge. I'm never happy to hear that. I advise you to get your doctor's approval on any change to your treatment plan, including all the recommendations that I feature in this book. But in any case, I need to tell you that there are some signs you should *never* ignore or self-treat. The following signs and symptoms could mean impending heart attack or stroke, so pay attention:

- Sudden weakness or numbness of your face, arm, leg, or one side of your body
- Sudden confusion, difficulty talking, or trouble understanding
- Dizziness, loss of balance, or problems walking
- Trouble seeing out of one or both eyes or sudden double vision
- Sudden severe headache or chest pain

DRUGS THAT CAUSE ABNORMAL HEART RHYTHM

Some drugs can interfere with the heart's rhythm, causing palpitations. It can happen as a typical side effect for some popular classes of medications, such as antidepressants, blood pressure pills, medications for diabetes, statins, inhalers for asthma, and thyroid hormone. It can also be the result of dosages that are too high for you. If you experience palpitations, it's worth reviewing your medications with your doctor or pharmacist. Here are some common pharmaceuticals that can alter heart rate.

Antianxiety medications

Antibiotics

Antidepressants

Blood pressure pills

Breathing medications

Cough and cold remedies

Diuretics such as Lasix (furosemide) or hydrochlorothiazide (HCTZ)

Estrogen-containing drugs (birth control and hormone replacement therapy)

Pain-relieving narcotics

Potassium supplements

Pseudoephedrine (for sinus congestion)

Sleeping pills

Statin cholesterol medications (Lipitor, Mevacor, Prevacor, and others)

Thyroid medication

- Pain that radiates into the arm(s), chest, neck, or jaw
- Shortness of breath
- Breaking out in a cold sweat or feeling nauseated

Now I know that you may have some of these symptoms occasionally within the context of normal days, but your body has its own alert system. So if you have any of these symptoms and get a sense of foreboding or an awareness that something is very different, call 911 right away or have someone drive you to the hospital. You can help prevent permanent damage by getting to a hospital within an hour of a stroke.

There is also some research to suggest that if you take one regular-strength aspirin (325 milligrams) at the onset of a heart attack, you will reduce your risk of dying from it. It may even be wise to chew the plain aspirin (not enteric coated) for 30 seconds before swallowing. Apparently, this can speed up its clot-busting activity, putting it to work minutes faster than just swallowing it whole.

Aspirin and other nonsteroidal anti-inflammatory drugs (NSAIDs) have been known to trigger asthma attacks in people with asthma (or in those not yet diagnosed), so make sure you are not one of the sensitive folks.

With a stroke or heart attack, early intervention is very important. If your doctor thinks you have had a minor stroke, sometimes termed a TIA (for transient ischemic attack), you may undergo tests such as a neurologic examination to check your nervous system, special scans, blood tests, ultrasound examinations, or x-rays. You may also be given medication that thins your blood to help prevent blood clots from forming again.

Prescription blood-thinning medications include warfarin (Coumadin), Plavix, Lovenox, and heparin injections. Nattokinase is a natural supplement that you can ask your doctor about, which I mentioned on page 000 of this chapter. Am I telling you to switch to natural? Absolutely not! I am just telling you about options so that you and your team of healthcare practitioners can sit down together and decide what is right for you, including dosages of drugs and supplements, so that you start to feel better and ideally even reverse the damage.

EXERCISE: GET UP AND MOVE

Even though I'm a pharmacist and spend a lot of my time working with pharmaceuticals and natural supplements, I'd be remiss if I didn't also talk to you about one of the most important things you can do to protect your heart: exercise.

You can walk if that's all you're able to do, but it's important because exercising gets blood flowing. When you improve circulation, you also reduce stagnation and slow down your body's production of nasty inflammatory chemicals and free radicals. If you can't walk, move your hands, fingers, toes, ankles, arms, and legs while you're sitting. Even if you *can* walk, when you're sitting, move your body. Rotate your ankles, your wrists, or your neck. Shrug your shoulders, even if just a few times. I personally exercise 2 to 3 hours every week, and though I'm busy too, my priority is to maintain health so I do it!

Stretch while you're sitting, and stretch while you're standing. If other people are around when you stretch, tell them why you're stretching and moving, and encourage them to get moving. You may have read about Richard Simmons's campaign to go to schools across the country to get up and dance. He complains that budget cuts took physical education out of the curriculum, and kids are becoming more and more sedentary. He even talks about the effect on the healthcare system if the kids become overweight teenagers and then obese adults.

By moving, you are helping to make everything flow better in your body.

This is way better than just taking pills to artificially make things flow. I'm thinking here of prescribed anticoagulants and aspirin. Am I telling you to stop taking your medicine and just begin exercising? Of course not, but if you exercise regularly, you may be able to reduce dosage in time, with proper supervision.

Exercising the heart muscle is even more important than exercising your abs and glutes, but most people don't think of exercise as having an effect on their heart, only their waistline. Most adults have been told that engaging in exercise at least 30 minutes per day can reduce the risk of heart disease and increase insulin sensitivity. But most folks won't make that kind of commitment because of time constraints.

What if I told you that exercising just 7½ minutes per week could help you? Would you exercise then? It will go by in a flash, I promise. A study by exercise physiologist James Timmons, PhD, shows that it works, at least for young, healthy men between the ages of 20 and 40. Dr. Timmons' research looked at 16 men in their early 20s. He directed them to exercise in six short sessions—between four and six 30-second sprints. In this case, they were running, but they could get the same effect from running up a flight of stairs or going to a spinning class.

In the study, the men drank a sugary solution containing 75 grams of glucose, which equates to about one baked potato. Upon measuring blood sugar and insulin levels, the researchers found that after only 2 weeks, the duration of blood sugar elevation was decreased by 12 percent and the duration of insulin elevation decreased by 37 percent. Of course, this was a study on young, healthy males. You know that I recommend seeing your physician and getting clearance before you start any kind of exercise program. The point is to get up and MOVE—it's good for your heart and for your life.

ADD BEAUTY TO YOUR HEART

Finally, I want to mention that there's one more important thing you can do for your heart; and it's all in your mind.

I conducted my own experiment to see how thoughts and environment can affect heart rate. I conducted my one-person, non–placebo-controlled clinical trial in the loveliest forest in America. This study is not randomized, nor is it published in any journal.

While visiting northern California, I set out to a beautiful forest teeming with giant redwood trees, called the Armstrong Woods. What better place to set the mood for closing our heart chapter than in a place that makes your heart skip a beat because of its stunning beauty?

When I first arrived, I took my pulse using the stopwatch on my iPhone, and it was 84 beats per minute. Then I set a timer for 10 minutes and sat down near one of the giant redwoods and just breathed in and out, very slowly. I closed my eyes and focused on the light dancing off the canopy of trees. The energy of these giant beauties was almost palpable, with the sweet aroma of blooming rhododendrons, the sound of the birds and occasional footsteps of other people enjoying the forest on a nearby path. I just focused on the sheer loveliness of the moment, as I sat and breathed, in and out.

At the end of the 10 minutes I took my pulse again. This time it was 64 beats per minute, literally 20 beats less per minute. And all I did was sit still in nature, breathe, and think happy thoughts.

My personal foray into the redwood forest isn't the first study to prove that meditation (focused thoughts on the positive) can help reduce heart rate. Even though most of us don't have easy access to the woods, this inner peace is really just a state of mind. You can feel it at home, if you just set the mood.

Find a place in your home or garden and make it comfortable for yourself. This may mean that you light a candle or some incense, or you adjust the lighting. In the wintertime, perhaps you want to fill a hot water bottle or use a hot pack that brings instant warmth. You may feel relaxed sipping a warm cup of tea.

The point is, just sit still. Get comfy, close your eyes, and breathe. Think of people, places, or situations that make you smile. The goal is to smile and to breathe. And laugh if you can think of funny, happy times. Say something pleasant as an affirmation (for example, "I feel good today").

Forget about the pain, and the drugs, and the upcoming procedures and challenges in your life. Just think about how you are connected to all things in nature and become part of the field of nature. Try to hold your good thoughts and feelings of gratitude for as long as you can. It only takes 5 or 10 minutes to make a difference in your heart rate. I promise, this is the cheapest way to reduce heart rate, improve bloodflow, and have no side effects! Try it right now . . . my book can wait.

Kidneys Deserve Good Care

Many people, including those without diabetes, have the beginnings of kidney disease and don't even realize it. According to the National Kidney Foundation, approximately 26 million Americans actually have chronic kidney disease, also called glomerulonephritis.

The condition is more serious in people who have had diabetes for 15 years or longer, although this is not always the case. In someone with diabetes, the kidneys start to work less efficiently because the blood vessels in and around them become diseased. This happens, in part, because of free-radical damage, which is also the case in problems with the pancreas and heart. So antioxidants are very important to *anyone* with diabetes, but especially if you have kidney disease.

Kidney disease in diabetics is often called diabetic nephropathy (pro-nounced *nef-RAHP-athie*) and should not be confused with neuropathy, which is nerve damage. Catching on to the fact that your kidneys are in trouble is crucial because diabetic nephropathy is a prime cause for dialysis in the United States. A small percentage of people have a condition that will progress rapidly after initial lesions are found, and they could die within 3 years if not managed appropriately.

There are many ways to slow the progression of kidney disease in people with diabetes, and we'll get to all that good news shortly. First, we need to look at how this disease manifests itself.

Missing the signs of early kidney trouble is easy unless you know what to look for. Just take a look at the subtle ways in which kidney disease shows up and why it's so easy to overlook the condition. Here are some excerpts from letters that readers of my column send me:

"Suzy—I just feel extremely tired all the time. I'm totally drained, and I don't really do anything to cause this feeling . . ."

"Dear Pharmacist—My skin itches a lot. It's like I have a little rash somewhere all the time, and I have to constantly scratch it."

"Dear Suzy—My prostate function is fine, yet I have to get up at night to urinate a lot."

"Suzy—There is so much swelling in my ankles that my socks and shoes are uncomfortable. What do you think is going on?"

After reading those symptoms, you can understand why thousands of people are misdiagnosed and only told that they have high blood pressure, prostate trouble, atopic dermatitis, or some other medical condition that includes these symptoms. The importance of recognizing kidney disease cannot be overstated, because early detection allows you to intervene quickly and save your kidneys, and possibly your life.

SIGNS AND SYMPTOMS OF KIDNEY TROUBLE

Just how do your kidneys signal to you that they're in trouble? Unlike high blood pressure, kidney disease is not a silent disease. If your kidneys are malfunctioning, you'll start to notice changes. Some of these include:

CHANGES IN YOUR URINE. You may need to urinate less frequently, or you might feel the need to urinate but only a few drops come out, or you may experience pressure while urinating. Your urine may become foamy or darken because blood is leaking out into it. The color may be like a strongly brewed tea. If it's actually purple, that means you are in immediate danger. Seek help in the nearest ER.

EDEMA (SWELLING IN THE BODY DUE TO FLUID RETENTION). Your first sign of trouble could be swelling in one ankle. When the kidneys don't remove fluid properly, it pools in certain areas of your body. Your weight may temporarily increase as a result of the edema. This often occurs in a leg, or in both legs, the ankles, feet, or hands. Sometimes it shows up as a puffy face.

EXHAUSTION. Your kidneys help you produce red blood cells, which carry oxygen to all your cells and your brain. When the kidneys get tired, so do you. It occurs because the kidneys can't make the hormone erythropoietin. Without the big E, you have fewer red blood cells, so you get anemic. Once this problem is diagnosed, it's relatively easy to treat, but you have to pay attention to symptoms. If you don't know about this symptom, you may get misdiagnosed with chronic fatigue syndrome, fibromyalgia, or even depression. It happens all the time. In fact, you may be getting treated with antidepressants, mood stabilizers, or stimulant drugs (like Provigil or Nuvigil) when you are just anemic or displaying early signs of chronic kidney disease (CKD). Luckily you have my book to help you sort all this out and make 100 percent sure that you are being treated appropriately.

ITCHY SKIN. Your kidneys remove waste products from your bloodstream, so if they can't do their job for one reason or another, these waste products will begin to build up. This can cause some serious itching, the kind that makes you wish you had a cheese grater to rub on your skin. At this point many people are misdiagnosed and told they have some kind of allergy or dermatitis. They are given various antihistamines, steroid lotions, and a bucketful of other potions and body brushes that provide only temporary relief.

You may think you have the condition called multiple chemical sensitivities, and more than likely, you own all sorts of fragrance-free, dye-free, hypoallergenic cosmetics, cleansers, soaps, and detergents. I definitely think these kinds of products are a good idea, but they don't solve your discomfort if it originates in your kidneys. By the way, itching can be a sign of poor bile blow, jaundice, or pancreatitis.

I'm not suggesting that every person who itches has kidney problems, because that is not true. I am saying that some people who chronically itch might have CKD and not know it. So please, if you have chronic skin problems, you need to make sure your renal function is normal. And check out my anti-itch remedies on page 234.

FOUL TASTE AND BAD BREATH. When the kidneys stop filtering properly, a substance known as urea builds up in the blood. This condition is called uremia, and it can cause a funky metallic taste in your mouth. One of my patients described his food by saying, "it tastes like it's wrapped in a tin can." Bad breath occurs and appetite goes down because food doesn't taste so good anymore. This symptom could cause weight loss because you lose your appetite for food.

FLU SYMPTOMS. Uremia can cause you to feel nauseated and even throw up. You may also experience stomach upset and weight loss. Some people have trouble keeping down anything in their stomach, including nibbles of food or medication. Some people get the chills or feel cold all the time.

DIFFICULTY BREATHING. This symptom is quite frequent in CKD. The fluid that your body is no longer able to eliminate may accumulate in the lungs. To make matters worse, anemia is often present, and when you don't have enough oxygen-carrying red blood cells, your lungs are starved for oxygen. This causes shortness of breath or a sensation of not being able to get a deep breath very easily. Some people say they feel as if they are drowning, or they just have to stop and rest after very little exertion. This is one of the most alarming symptoms of kidney disease and may be misdiagnosed as a respiratory infection, asthma, or another lung disorder.

BRAIN FOG. It's that darned anemia again. When your kidneys can't help you make oxygen-carrying red blood cells, the brain starves for food. You lose the ability to concentrate and remember things. I'm not talking about Sudoku puzzles here. I mean losing the ability to do simple math or remember what you did last week or maintain a train of thought and complete a sentence—a sort of fuzzy cobweb brain fog. You may experience dizziness, too. Doctors may misdiagnose you with dementia or other neurologic disorders. It's all connected. People with memory problems and people with diabetes both have chronically high insulin because their body is resistant to insulin's effect.

FLANK PAIN. People who have fluid-filled cysts on their kidneys sometimes develop pain in the back or side, sometimes radiating down a leg. Since this kind of pain can be a symptom of many problems, it's easy to miss it as a symptom of CKD. Instead, arthritis, low-back pain, sciatica, or a disc problem might be diagnosed. People with mild versions of this symptom basically toss and turn all night trying to get comfortable.

You can see where I'm going here. If you're have diabetes and you experience any of the odd symptoms I've mentioned here, please seek help from a medical professional.

WHY DO WE NEED OUR KIDNEYS?

They come in a pair, and each kidney is about the size of your fist. There is one kidney on either side of your spine, slightly below the rib cage. The kidneys have a huge task on their hands because they must continuously filter your blood. Generally speaking, the kidneys filter approximately 200 quarts of blood during the day and strain out waste products that your body eliminates.

The process is absolutely remarkable. Millions of tiny blood vessels called capillaries act as filters (think of panning for gold), and the capillaries have microscopic holes in them that filter the blood. Tiny particles of waste squeeze through the holes and exit the body through the urine. The blood cells and useful protein molecules are too big to fit through the holes, and so they stay in the blood. That's what you want. With our gold example, the gold stays in the pan, and what you don't want filters out. Now, the gold nuggets get filtered out, too!

When kidney disease sets in, the capillaries don't function as well, the kidneys no longer filter properly, and blood or proteins squeeze out and get into your urine. Waste builds up in the blood, too.

The kidneys make all this happen through an amazing chemical exchange within the kidney cells, which are called nephrons. The kidneys work hand in hand with your bladder, ureter (the ducts that propel urine from the kidneys to the bladder), tiny blood vessels (called glomeruli), and tubules. Your magical kidneys are designed to work so that your body has exactly the right amount of sodium, potassium, phosphorus, and other substances you need to stay alive. They filter the blood, keeping essential minerals and nutrients, while dumping the rest.

It's hard to believe, but the average human kidney sifts out about 2 quarts of waste products and excess fluid every 24 hours. You didn't realize you had that much junk inside, did you?

Just like the pancreas, the kidneys happen to secrete a few important hormones of their own. They are:

ERYTHROPOIETIN. This hormone tells your bone marrow to make red blood cells, which carry oxygen. The oxygen nourishes every cell in your body and keeps them alive. It creates energy for you, too.

CALCITRIOL. You make calcitriol, the body's most active form of vitamin D_3, in your kidneys. This nutrient helps regulate calcium levels and protect the body from infection and immune disorders. Vitamin D helps improve insulin sensitivity, so having healthy kidneys to convert the vitamin D_3 into calcitriol is crucial. A medication called Rocaltrol (calcitriol) is frequently prescribed for patients with CKD.

RENIN. This enzyme is a protein that regulates blood pressure by stimulating the production of a hormone called angiotensin, which then causes your adrenal glands to make aldosterone. The aldosterone raises your blood pressure, which is fine because you don't want to faint, but if aldosterone levels increase too much, you can develop high blood pressure. Renin isn't the only thing that raises aldosterone (and blood pressure); anxiety does it, too.

Kidney function is obviously more complicated than all of this, but the take-home point is that you want your kidneys to be serene and content, for without them you would become a toxic wasteland and die within hours, or days at best. Dialysis, of course, changes things for the better, and many people live normal lives for many years with dialysis. More about that later.

(continued on page 176)

DISEASE INCIDENCE PREVENTION

BLOOD LEVELS OF VITAMIN D (NG/ML)	6	8	10	12	14	16	18	20	22	24	26	28	
Studies of Individuals													
Cancers, all combined													
Breast Cancer													
Ovarian Cancer													
Colon Cancer													
Non-Hodgkins Lymphoma													
Type 1 Diabetes													
Fractures, all combined													
Falls, women													
Multiple Sclerosis													
Heart Attack (Men)													
Natural Experiments													
Kidney Cancer													
Endometrial Cancer													
Rickets			50%						99%				

BLOOD REFERENCE RANGE

All percentages reference a common baseline of 25 ng/ml (nanograms per milliliter) as shown on the chart. Percentages reflect the disease prevention percentage at the beginning and ending of available data. For example: Breast cancer incidence is reduced by 30% when the Vitamin D blood level is 34 ng/ml versus the baseline of 25 ng/ml. This is an 83% reduction in incidence when the serum level is 50 ng/ml versus the baseline of 25 ng/ml. The Xs in the bars indicate "reasonable extrapolations" from the data but are beyond existing data.

LINKED TO VITAMIN D LEVELS

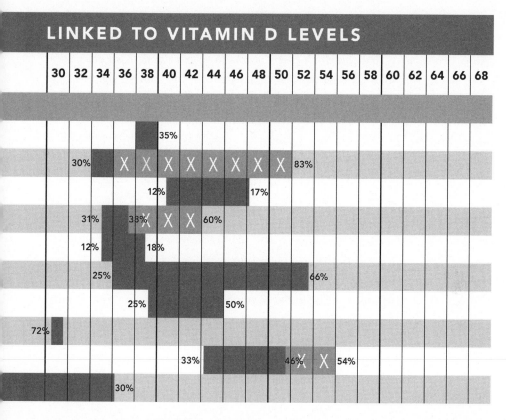

| 30 | 32 | 34 | 36 | 38 | 40 | 42 | 44 | 46 | 48 | 50 | 52 | 54 | 56 | 58 | 60 | 62 | 64 | 66 | 68 |

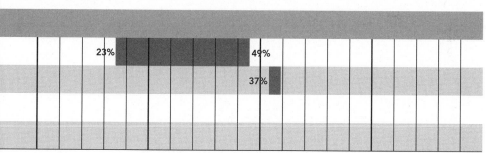

Data prepared by Garland CF, Baggerly CA
Copyright GrassrootsHealth, 10/16/08, www.grassrootshealth.org

KNOW THE SIGNS BEFORE IT'S TOO LATE

Many people with diabetes don't give their kidneys a second thought because there is no strong pain associated with declining renal function. When you have pins and needles in your fingers or toes, or numbness down your leg, you give that attention and attempt to relieve the pain. The kidneys, however, are usually quiet and unassuming, so unless you are visiting a nephrologist (a physician who specializes in kidney function), your kidneys may be ignored or misdiagnosed.

Knowledge is power. If you have diabetes, it's a good idea to see a nephrologist at least once a year to get the very best care from a doctor who really understands the complexity of your kidneys.

You can absolutely prevent kidney failure (and the need for dialysis) in many cases, if you catch small problems before they get bigger and get evaluated and treated by a nephrologist. The confusing part is that in some people, the filtering ability of the kidneys is actually higher than normal in the first few years of diabetes, so you and your doctor don't realize that your kidneys are starting to weaken. See now why it's important for you to get *all* the facts about CKD?

You need to pay attention to more than just numbers that appear on a blood or urine test. If you wait to find out that your filtering ability is low, a lot of damage has already been done. Here are some risk factors for CKD.

DIABETES. Chronically high blood sugar levels cause the kidneys to filter too much blood. When kidneys are faced with a continuous heavy burden, they tire out and begin leaking out small but much-needed proteins. This condition is called microalbuminuria.

HIGH BLOOD PRESSURE. Blood pressure that is too high damages blood vessels in the kidneys, and then they are unable to filter out toxins. An ideal blood pressure should be maintained at about 120/80 mm Hg.

HIGH CHOLESTEROL. This condition leads to the formation of plaque on the artery walls, which obstructs blood flow in the kidneys and leads to problems with your heart and with circulation and called hardening of the arteries.

HARDENING OF THE ARTERIES. When the vessels lose flexibility and become clogged up, they can no longer drain and filter properly. Think of your garden hose. You want it relatively soft and pliable, yet sturdy enough to shoot a strong stream of water out.

CHEMICAL TOXINS. In the scientific community these are called POPs, as in persistent organic pollutants. These poisons are termed persistent because they easily get carried through the food chain and through the water system. Once consumed or inhaled by a human, they are hard to unstick from the cells. POPs can tax and damage your kidneys and liver.

A study published in 2006 found a connection between blood serum levels of POPs and diabetes. People with a higher level of POPs, consisting of dioxins, DDT, PCBs, and chlordane, among others, were up to 38 times more likely to be insulin resistant than people who had lower levels. The study, however, did not demonstrate a cause-and-effect relationship.

CERTAIN TYPES OF ARTHRITIS OR AUTOIMMUNE DISORDERS, SUCH AS HASHIMOTO'S DISEASE OR LUPUS. When the body makes antibodies against its own tissue, the antibodies can lodge in the glomeruli and cause inflammation. People with autoimmune conditions sometimes require potent immune-modulating drugs, and the side effects of these medications also can damage the kidneys. So it could be the disease itself or the medications used to treat the disease causing a problem. Either way, kidney function should be closely monitored in these individuals.

WHAT DOES THE FUTURE HOLD?

I'm sure that by now you have one burning question: Am I condemned to have CKD just because I have diabetes?

No, not necessarily. CKD takes many years to develop, and some fortunate diabetics who take proper care of themselves never develop it. The good news is that the progression from early kidney disease to complete kidney failure usually takes years and can be eased—if not entirely avoided—by lifestyle changes, dietary changes, supplements, and medications.

CKD occurs in part because of free-radical damage. As you have already learned in earlier chapters, you can mitigate the amount of hits your body takes from free-radical damage and therefore control the level of damage to your kidneys, nerves, heart, and pancreas. So having a diagnosis of diabetes does not necessarily mean that you are headed for kidney trouble.

Here are some of the kidney-related conditions that can manifest down the road and that you need to be on the alert for.

MICROALBUMINURIA. The kidneys function normally during this stage, but small amounts of a tiny blood protein called albumin leak into the urine. It is detected through a urine sample.

PROTEINURIA, ALSO KNOWN AS MACROALBUMINURIA. In this condition, larger amounts of the protein albumin begin to show up in the urine as the filtering ability of the kidneys begins to decline. A urinalysis will show this. You can sometimes see it because your urine gets bubbly or foamy after eating fish, chicken, meat, or whey-protein supplements. What you can't see well here, you can actually feel. The body is retaining wastes that begin to overload your system, and you may start to itch, feel fatigued, lose your appetite, experience weakness, or have difficulty concentrating.

HIGH BLOOD PRESSURE. This condition develops because the body is retaining more fluid. Because the kidneys are not filtering and eliminating properly, pressure builds up in the blood vessels and you may get frequent headaches.

CREATININE IN THE BLOOD. The substance known as creatinine is produced from the breakdown of creatine phosphate, which is used to power your muscles. The kidneys normally filter the creatinine out, so if your doctor alerts you to a high level of creatinine, it means that for one reason or another your kidneys aren't functioning up to par. As a general rule, men tend to have higher levels of creatinine because they have more muscle than women, and also because they tend to eat more meat. In turn, vegetarians have been shown to have lower baseline creatinine levels. A doctor may estimate your GFR from your blood level of creatinine. Any measurement below 30 is a sign of trouble, and if you haven't already seen a nephrologist, you must go if your level dips below 30. The earlier you seek help, the better. If you don't get help and your GFR gets all the way down to 15, that's when you need to have dialysis or get your name on a kidney transplant list. But promise me you won't let that happen.

WHAT ABOUT DIET?

Dietary changes are important for people with compromised kidney function because certain foods can speed up the damage.

PROTEIN. Studies have shown that eating lots of protein-rich foods such as eggs, milk, meat, and cheese can tax your kidneys. They have a hard time filtering out the protein from the waste material. Too much protein burdens weak kidneys, so limit protein-rich foods such as these to a few times a week.

Protein is not the only concern for people with CKD, though. Fat is problematic too. That's because fat adds to the high levels of cholesterol found in the blood of most people with diabetes and those with CKD. When cholesterol builds up in the blood vessels, it taxes the heart and increases risk of heart attack and stroke.

SALT. Believe it or not, even the small amount of salt you use at the table to

WHAT IS DIALYSIS?

Dialysis is a procedure that does the job of failing kidneys. It's a phenomenal thing, too! Even though there are different types of dialysis, the basic goal is the same—to filter your body of unnecessary wastes so you don't become toxic. It helps your body filter out waste so the waste products don't build up in your blood, which makes you feel sick. Dialysis can be done for cases of acute kidney failure, or for people with chronic kidney disease. There are two primary types of dialysis: one that filters your blood, called hemodialysis, and the other type that filters wastes through the abdominal cavity, called peritoneal dialysis. These procedures can offer a person with chronic kidney disease many years of enjoyable life, so it is wonderful to have this technology.

season your food makes a big difference. There is a lot more about salt and the best types to use in Chapter 16. You probably didn't realize that salt could be problematic, did you? That's because salt is considered just a condiment, and it's served in millions of restaurants.

Regular iodized table salt is not the healthiest salt for you. Table salt has been stripped of the minerals that naturally occurring sea salt has. These are the very minerals that your body needs to regulate blood sugar, including magnesium, potassium, chromium, selenium, zinc, iron, and copper. In any case, both regular salt and sea salt (apart from the minerals) are actually composed of two elements, sodium and chlorine.

It's the sodium that's a big problem for people with kidney disease. It can actually be a problem for anyone. For people with CKD, the sodium in your salt causes you to hold on to water, and that means that your kidneys have more fluid to filter out.

You should be aware that only a small amount of the sodium in our diets (about 11 percent) comes from adding a pinch of salt to our soup and a dash to our eggs. The vast majority of sodium in our diet comes from processed foods.

There are a number of salty, high-sodium foods that you should avoid. These include frozen dinners, processed meats, and snack items, such as chips and pretzels. Be especially careful with prepared soups, whether canned or in a carton. And check the label on those ramen soups—the sodium count is astronomical. However, these are not the only foods to watch out for; there are many more.

If you want to salt your foods, please use natural sea salt, which provides your body with essential minerals, not just sodium. I use two brands in my home, Real Salt (www.realsalt.com), which I use while cooking if needed, and Fusion, a gourmet finishing salt that I sprinkle on top of food.

I love good salts, and if you want to indulge in the best, see my Resources on page 378 for the names of some companies that produce pure and delicious salts. Some of them are even flavored with ginger or rosemary.

One more thing about salt: Salt substitutes should be avoided, too. Most of them consist of potassium, and weak kidneys don't remove potassium very well. When it builds up in the bloodstream, excessive potassium causes abnormal heart rhythm, tingling of the hands and feet, and muscle weakness. Potassium is found naturally in fruits, vegetables, beans, and nuts. Of course, all these foods are fine to eat. You don't need to avoid them.

SODA. Finally, I want to mention that there is a seriously good reason to stay away from soda. New information from researchers at Loyola University Health System says that women who drink at least two cans of soda pop a day are nearly twice as likely to develop early signs of kidney disease as those who don't drink that many sodas. This result was based on findings from a urine test that women participating in the study took 24 hours after drinking two sodas. The women who drank the beverages were almost twice as likely to have albuminuria, excessive protein in their urine.

What in soda is the problem? It is probably a combination of several things. For one thing, soda contains phosphorus, and the kidneys are not happy when they have to deal with excess phosphorus. Soda also contains sugar's more sinful sister, a highly refined sweetener called high-fructose corn syrup (HFCS). And here's the kicker: HFCS is sometimes contaminated with mercury, a dangerous poison that sparks free-radical damage to your cells, including those in the kidney cells. You think I'm joking? Not. A 2009 study published in *Environmental Health* found that nine of 20 samples of HFCS were contaminated with mercury. So please trade in the soft drinks for good old H_2O (water) or herbal tea.

So what should you be eating? I recommend a low-fat, low-protein diet rich in fresh, organic fruits and vegetables along with healthy nuts and seeds. This is pretty much the same dietary plan I've outlined for you in many other chapters. The reason is that foods such as these offer your body genuine nourishment, rather than artificial additives, chemicals, trans fats, and cancer-causing ingredients.

Becoming conscious of the foods that you put into your body will translate

> **BRING THAT A1C DOWN**
> If you can reduce your hemoglobin A1c from 7 percent to just 6.4 percent, this reduces your risk of kidney disease by up to 25 percent. Read Chapter 13 for natural supplements that help reduce blood glucose and A1c.

into better health for your kidneys, because after all, they have to filter what goes into your body. Kidney disease can't be cured, but it can be managed. Eating better is number one on my list for getting well.

MEDICATIONS TO HELP YOUR KIDNEYS

Today we are lucky enough to have some powerful medications that slow the progression of kidney disease. People with kidney disease have to be vigilant about controlling blood pressure, so achieving a target range of 120/80, for example, can offer dramatic benefits. This is one of the reasons that doctors usually prescribe blood pressure pills for people with kidney disease.

There are lots of medications your doctor can order for you, and sometimes multiple medications are needed to do the job. The most popular medications used in the treatment of kidney disease fall into the following basic categories.

ANGIOTENSIN-CONVERTING ENZYME (ACE) INHIBITORS. These medications work by slowing down (inhibiting) the activity of the enzyme ACE, which in turn reduces production of a substance known as angiotensin II. This action keeps the blood vessels large so blood can flow more easily through your kidneys, which have the job of filtering your blood.

ACE inhibitors take a load off the work of your kidneys. Some of them can protect the kidneys' glomeruli and lower the amount of protein that spills into the urine. (As noted earlier in this chapter, the glomeruli are structures within the kidney that are composed of tiny capillary blood vessels. Their job is to filter the blood of wastes.) This delays deterioration. ACE inhibitors are also very good at reducing blood pressure.

Side effects include dry cough, headache, elevated potassium levels, drowsiness, weakness, or taste abnormalities (for example, a very salty or metallic taste, no matter what you eat).

Some examples of ACE inhibitors include:

Captopril (Capoten)   Lisinopril (Zestril, Prinivil)

Enalapril (Vasotec)   Ramipril (Altace)

ANGIOTENSIN II RECEPTOR BLOCKERS. These drugs are even more specific in their action than ACE inhibitors, so they produce fewer side effects, while also lowering the risk for heart problems. They work by keeping angiotensin from squeezing off your blood vessels.

Some examples include:

Candesartan (Atacand)   Losartan (Cozaar)

Irbesartan (Avapro)   Valsartan (Diovan)

These medications are sometimes combined with diuretics. One example of this type is Hyzaar, which is a combination of losartan and hydrochloro-thiazide.

ERYTHROPOIETIN (ALSO CALLED E-POIETIN OR EPO). EPO is actually a hormone that circulates in the blood. It was discovered about a century ago, on the heels of bloodletting experiments on rabbits. Your kidneys naturally produce EPO when they're healthy. EPO stimulates the production of red blood cells (erythrocytes) because it is sort of like a sensor. If you are low in iron or ferritin (the stored form of iron) then your anemia should trigger the production of EPO from your kidneys so that you can make more red blood cells and overcome the anemia. If your kidneys are unhealthy, this system fails and you may need blood transfusions.

Today EPO formulations are available as drugs, and each varies slightly. Some contain a little albumin, and some are alpha versions or beta versions, but they are all produced using recombinant DNA technology. This means they are relatively pure and free of allergy-causing substances.

Because EPO increases red blood cells, it also increases a person's hematocrit—which is simply a measurement of the percentage of red blood cells. You want red blood cell counts and hematocrit to be within normal ranges. But hematocrit levels tend to fall in people with CKD or other diseases that induce anemia.

Erythropoietin (alpha version) is sold under the brand names of Epogen and Procrit in the United States and as Eprex in other parts of the world. These inject-able medications are sometimes combined with iron supplements. In 2007, the cost of each injection was approximately $2,000. Yes, that's right. It may or may not be covered by your insurance plan. You should work with your doctor's office to find out if it's covered under your plan, and if so, how much and how often you can get these injections and still have your insurance plan cover the high cost.

Of course, pharmaceuticals are not the only substances that can help your kidneys. As you've probably guessed by this point in my book, I have a lot of helpful supplements and additional dietary strategies to recommend.

SUPPLEMENTS THAT CAN HELP

If you have kidney disease, nutrition experts who specialize in kidney disease maintain that you need different amounts of vitamins and minerals than someone with healthy kidneys. There are many reasons for the changing needs. For one, you have more toxins building up in your bloodstream, which means you need more detoxifying nutrients.

Also, individuals with CKD often take drug muggers—medications that happen to steal important vitamins and minerals.

Low appetite or dietary changes can also alter your nutritional needs. For example, a low-protein diet will cause you to run lower on certain vitamins such as B_{12}, or amino acids such as L-carnitine. Becoming deficient in those nutrients can wreak havoc throughout your body. So knowing what you need to replenish and what you need to protect your kidneys is key to getting better.

You can ask your doctor about several supplements that support kidney function. I've put them in the order that I think is most important for you; however, each individual is different. Before you take any of these supplements, I want you to get your doctor's blessings.

L-Carnitine

The amino acid L-carnitine is often just called carnitine. It helps your body turn fat into energy. Our bodies make carnitine naturally, but a little extra may be in order if you have CKD and have to eat a low-protein diet. Carnitine can help to shuttle artery-clogging fat out of your blood vessels and give you an energy boost.

The reason I give the number-one spot on my kidney-supporting supplement list to carnitine is because it has other wonderful attributes as well. For instance, studies show L-carnitine has heart-healthy benefits. Also, some small studies suggest that the version known as acetyl-L-carnitine (the acetylated version) may help with nerve regeneration, thereby reducing the pain of diabetic neuropathy.

And that's not all. The main reason I've recommended carnitine is that it helps control levels of a free-radical chemical called tumor necrosis factor alpha that (in excess) is tied to insulin resistance. In addition, your kidneys help produce it. When your kidneys malfunction, supplemental carnitine becomes necessary. It also helps men with erectile dysfunction. See why I've put carnitine at the top of this list?

DIETARY SOURCES OF CARNITINE. Red meat (particularly lamb), dairy products, and wheat are some primary sources of carnitine. But since you should not be eating too much protein or wheat gluten, better sources of carnitine for you would be fish, poultry, asparagus, avocados, and cashew butter. (Restricting wheat gluten is a good idea for anyone, not just diabetics with kidney disease.)

HOW TO SUPPLEMENT. Look for supplements called carnitine or L-carnitine. You can also buy acetyl-L-carnitine instead. Avoid D-carnitine because it is not natural and could interfere with your body's ability to use L-carnitine. It also could spark side effects.

My general suggested dosage is 500 to 1,000 milligrams two to four times daily. Do ask your doctor, however, because the dosage is based on your renal function, diet, and overall status.

CAUTION. This amino acid is usually very well tolerated. However, people who are sensitive to it or those who take high doses of carnitine may experience diarrhea or digestive upset. Certain antiseizure medications (often prescribed for people with neuropathy) are drug muggers of carnitine, meaning the drug lowers levels of carnitine and speeds up complications for a person with CKD. One such drug is valproic acid (Depakote). So if you take that medication, you definitely want to ask your doctor whether you should supplement with carnitine to replenish what the drug mugger stole.

Horsetail (*Equisetum arvense*)

The herb horsetail, sometimes known as shave grass or bottle brush, has been used for centuries to help treat kidney problems, strengthen bones, and heal ulcers or wounds. The stems of the plant provide the body with silica, which helps form collagen, a protein found in ligaments, cartilage, and connective tissue.

DRUGS THAT MAY LEAD TO KIDNEY DAMAGE

While medications that help kidney disease can save lives, you should be aware that many commonly prescribed medications can damage kidneys as a side effect. If you have kidney disease and are taking any of the following medications, you should discuss this with your doctor.

Aspirin

Excedrin

Meloxicam (Mobic)

Nonsteroidal anti-inflammatory drugs (NSAIDS), such as ibuprofen, naproxen, and diclofenac

Certain drug interactions can lead to kidney failure, too. Among the dangerous combinations are:

Advil and Prograf

Aldoril and calcium

Anaprox and Prograf

Cardizem and cyclosporine

Cardizem and Sandimmune

Dristan Sinus and tacrolimus

Dyazide and calcium

Dyazide and NSAIDs

Ibuprofen and tacrolimus

Methotrexate and ciprofloxacin

Statin cholesterol-reducing drugs and erythromycin-based antibiotics

Tricor and simvastatin (Zocor)

Silica by itself is a fantastic supplement, and horsetail herb provides a source for it. Silica is often used for osteoporosis and to increase nail and hair strength. Silica is necessary for pancreatic health too.

As for kidney function, horsetail can act as a diuretic, helping you to filter the blood and eliminate some of the fluid overload. You might say it lends your kidneys a hand.

DIETARY SOURCES OF SILICA. Whole grains (before they've been stripped and refined to make basic all-purpose flour) contain silica. However, I think the best way to get silica is to take a silica supplement such as horsetail herb or the one made by Cellfood. Follow label directions.

HOW TO SUPPLEMENT. You can buy horsetail in various ways, including tinctures (1:5 ratio), teas, and oral supplements.

My general suggested dosage is to drink the tea once daily in the morning or twice daily if your doctor permits.

Oral supplements are fine too. General dosage range is about 300 milligrams, two or three times daily, standardized to contain 10 to 15 percent silica.

CAUTION. People with kidney disorders need to be careful about dosing. As with all the other supplements in this chapter (and in the whole book), you need to ask your doctor whether this one is right for you, especially because the herb has a diuretic effect on the body. Diuretics can enhance side effects of many other medications and lead to drug-related problems. This effect poses a problem for people who take the heart drug digoxin, blood thinners, and seizure medications. Horsetail herb is a drug mugger of vitamin B_1 (thiamine), which means that long-term use of the supplement may cause a nutrient deficiency of B_1. That could make your peripheral neuropathy worse, so if you take horsetail regularly, you want to also supplement with some thiamine. Take about 25 milligrams daily or take a high-potency B-complex supplement, which contains B_1 and other important B vitamins. Read more about the importance of thiamine in the next entry.

Thiamine

Thiamine, also known as vitamin B_1, is easy to find in health food stores, and it's cheap. The body uses thiamine to help keep the nerves and brain healthy. A deficiency can cause depression, irritability, nerve pain, muscle atrophy, and muscle weakness. Later stages of thiamine deficiency (called beri beri) can cause an enlarged heart, rapid heartbeat (tachycardia) and neurologic problems.

Diabetic specialists may wonder why I'm mentioning this nutrient in the kidney chapter, because it's not usually considered a kidney-loving vitamin. But "cutting edge" is my middle name. The main reason little old B_1 has made it to my list is that this nutrient was recently found to have dramatic effects on the body's ability to excrete albumin and reverse early-stage kidney disease in some people with type 2 diabetes. The study was published in *Diabetologia*.

In one study scientists found that oral supplements of thiamine were able to reverse the early-stage symptom of microalbuminuria by 41 percent in the people studied. The researchers used high doses of thiamine (300 milligrams per day total)—higher than I would personally recommend—but the effects are noteworthy. Also, many people with diabetes have a deficiency of thiamine, which could underlie cardiac and neurological complications that occur as untreated diabetes persists.

Thiamine has also been shown to have some beneficial effects on the pancreas. So I'm going to give this B vitamin an A-plus for all its protective benefits.

DIETARY SOURCES OF THIAMINE. These include whole grains, fortified cereals, meat, and yeast. This is one of those rare times that I'd prefer you just supplement rather than eating large quantities of these types of foods.

HOW TO SUPPLEMENT. Look for thiamine pyrophosphate, the active form of this vitamin. I also want you to ask your doctor about taking a B-complex supplement too, right along with thiamine. The reason is that people with CKD are often low in all the B vitamins, not just thiamine. In addition, thiamine works harder for you when its other family members are present. These include folic acid, vitamin B_{12}, vitamin B_6, and riboflavin.

My suggested general dosage is 25 to 50 milligrams of thiamine once daily, unless your doctor agrees to supervise your taking the higher doses found to be effective in that study mentioned above—100 milligrams three times daily. In either case, you should also take a B-complex supplement, one capsule daily.

CAUTION. Whenever you take high doses of one B vitamin, you often need to have a B complex on board because a high dosage of one B vitamin could cause a relative deficiency of other B vitamins. Generally speaking, the B vitamins work better together.

Vitamin D

When you think of a vitamin, you probably think of a nutrient in your food or a supplement that you need to take by mouth. Vitamin D is, indeed, a nutrient that can be taken as a supplement. But its metabolic end point, its active form, is really produced within the body, and it's called calcitriol. Calcitrol is a hormone. The body takes external sources of D and converts them into the hormone in your kidneys.

Chronic kidney disease causes the body's level of calcitrol to decrease as the kidneys weaken. So people with CKD need to pay special attention to getting enough calcium and vitamin D.

There is a strong connection between vitamin D and diabetes. Vitamin D is often low in people with type 2 diabetes, so maintaining healthy levels of this nutrient is important. Why? Studies have shown that vitamin D can help lower blood sugar. Vitamin D also protects the nerves and is thought to benefit people with multiple sclerosis, an autoimmune disorder that destroys the sheaths of the nerves. Are you with me? I'm thinking of vitamin D to help you with insulin resistance, nerve damage, immune function, and bone strength. Not too shabby for one nutrient, eh?

The sun is a beautiful, life-giving star, the star closest to Earth and at the center of our solar system. This amazing star promotes natural vitamin D production in our skin. Some people can get enough vitamin D by basking in the sun for 15 minutes on each side (belly and back). But never sunbathe between the hours of 11 a.m. and 4 p.m., when damaging ultraviolet rays are strongest.

There are many reasons you may want to opt for a vitamin D supplement rather than relying on the sun for this important nutrient. As people age, their ability to convert vitamin D to its active form decreases. You may need to avoid sunlight because of the free-radical damage it causes to your skin. And, for sure, if you've ever had skin cancer, your doctor will probably tell you to avoid sun exposure.

Even though I think the sun is healthy for us, I usually just recommend a high-quality dietary supplement because it works quickly and raises D levels better than sunshine in the elderly population. Ask your doctor whether you can supplement with oral capsules of cholecalciferol (D_3), about 2,000 IU every morning. High-quality brands of vitamin D_3 are sold at health food stores nationwide. Supplements are a better option for people who have a history of skin cancer or those who are homebound or shy of the sun. There is much more on vitamin D in Chapter 12.

Pau d'Arco

If you're dealing with anemia as part of kidney disease, you should know that it is possible to help your body thrive by giving it nutrients that improve your ability to make red blood cells. That's important because red blood cells carry oxygen all over the body.

Pau d'arco bark, also known as taheebo or lapacho, is an herb from the Amazon rainforest that has been used for centuries to treat all sorts of immune problems. Data isn't clear, but pau d'arco bark appears to support red blood cells. It is sold in the United States at health food stores nationwide in a variety of forms—extract, capsules, tablets, liquids, and tea.

Herbal experts maintain that pau d'arco thins the blood and is a blood purifier and blood builder that aids the liver and endocrine glands.

One of the naturally occurring substances in pau d'arco is hydroquinone, which also happens to be a substance used to fade age spots. You find this substance in some over-the-counter creams and prescription versions too. Pau d'arco has many other powerful compounds in it, including benzenoids and flavonoids.

Even though pau d'arco does not require a prescription and is sold at health food stores, please ask your doctor whether it's appropriate for you. Drinking pau d'arco tea daily for 30 to 60 days is usually enough to spark the production of new red blood cells. Or you can take supplements and follow your product's dosage recommendations on the package.

CAUTION. Pau d'arco is usually well tolerated by people. Side effects of pau d'arco can include dizziness, nausea, vomiting, diarrhea, and thinning of the blood. It is a blood thinner, which is wonderful, but this also means it could have an additive effect with aspirin, heparin, warfarin (Coumadin), Plavix, Lovenox, and other blood-thinning agents, which could be dangerous. Be sure to check with your doctor about any interactions.

Astragalus

Astragalus is a plant native to Asia whose name in Chinese means "yellow leader." Its root (the part used medicinally) is considered one of the most essential herbs in traditional Chinese medicine. This herb is also known as *Astragalus membranaceous*, huang qi, bei qi, hwanggi, and milk vetch.

In traditional Chinese medicine, astragalus is used primarily to boost immune function and to treat people who suffer from night sweats or diarrhea. It is also found in energy tonics.

Astragalus may help you fend off colds—some studies have indicated that it has mild antiviral properties. It has been found to increase the effectiveness of antiviral medications such as Zovirax (acyclovir) and Symmetrel (amantadine).

In traditional Chinese culture, astragalus is used for various heart conditions. I mention it in the kidney chapter because it is also a diuretic, which can help to lower blood pressure and cause blood vessels to relax.

If you have high blood pressure or problems with water retention, you might want to consider using this herb.

As a general rule, don't be afraid to tell your doctor what supplements you take. For one thing, it's your body, for another, your doctor *needs to know* in order to ensure that the supplements don't interfere in any way with other prescription medications you're taking.

CAUTION. Astragalus is not for you if you have type 1 diabetes or if you have other autoimmune diseases (such as psoriasis, rheumatoid arthritis, Crohn's disease, multiple sclerosis, and lupus), unless your doctor recommends you take it. If you have had transplant surgery, you shouldn't use astralagus because this immune-enhancer will counteract the effectiveness of immune-suppressing drugs such as:

CellCept (mycophenolate)

Imuran (azathioprine)

Prograf (tacrolimus)

Rapamune (sirolimus)

Sandimmune (cyclosporine)

Steroid (methylprednisone or prednisone)

SUPPLEMENTS TO ASK YOUR DOCTOR ABOUT

Your kidneys need potassium and phosphorus to help regulate fluid balance. When your kidneys are weak, they have a hard time removing the potassium and phosphorus from your blood. These electrolytes can be easily monitored by your doctor, but since they are sold as over-the-counter supplements I need to go into a little more detail here, in particular about the phosphorus. As phosphorus builds up in the blood, your bones spit out calcium to balance the phosphorus. As a result, your bones begin to weaken and break more easily from lack of calcium.

This is a catch-22 because as your bones become more brittle, your doctor may suggest a bone-building supplement to prevent (or address) osteoporosis. But bone-building supplements usually contain minerals, among them phosphorus. So it may mean the start of a vicious cycle for which I don't have the answer. The discussion of whether you need more or less phosphorus—or potassium or any mineral for that matter—needs to take place with your nephrologist, a professional who devotes his or her life to solving challenging puzzles like this.

It's also a good idea to keep foods rich in phosphorus to a minimum. Such foods include soft drinks, cow's milk, yogurt, ice cream and most dairy products, split peas, lentils, peanut butter, and kidney beans.

ANTIOXIDANTS ARE APPROPRIATE

Because free-radical damage contributes to declining renal function, it makes sense that taking antioxidant supplements can protect your kidneys and slow down the progression of disease. This has been shown in the scientific literature. With that in mind, I think that people with CKD would be smart to consider taking proven and strong antioxidants under their physician's guidance.

The best antioxidants penetrate the delicate tissues of the brain, heart, liver, pancreas, *and* kidneys. This is why I think the following antioxidants are sensible choices if you have kidney disease, but of course discuss my recommendations with your physician to see whether they are right for you.

ASTAXANTHIN. This is a marine-derived type of carotenoid found in the highest concentrations in algae. *Haematococcus pluvialis* is home to one of the world's most powerful biological antioxidants. Today, purified astaxanthin is bottled and sold as a dietary supplement. We know that it can help protect against heart disease, but a study published in 2004 in the journal *Biofactors* showed that astaxanthin had protective abilities against diabetic nephropathy in mice as well. Does that mean it can perform this function in humans? Scientists do not yet have an answer to that question, but this supplement is undeniably a good antioxidant and worth taking. My suggested dosage is 4 to 6 milligrams daily.

RESVERATROL. This substance is found in the skin of red grapes, as well as in both cocoa and peanuts. I often recommend supplementation with resveratrol because I think it offers numerous benefits to the human body. It is one nutrient that appears capable of generating more mitochondria for us. Mitochondria are the powerhouses that your cells use to generate energy. The more of them you have, the less fat you have stuck inside your cells and your body as a whole.

A study published in the August 2008 issue of the journal *Clinical Interventions in Aging* concluded that a healthy diet and lifestyle have been found to stave off the typical age-related diseases—such as heart disease, obesity, and diabetes. In that same article, the researchers noted that "the future bodes well for the use of resveratrol."

If you have kidney disease, please check with your physician before you use resveratrol. A study published in the journal *Free Radical Biology & Medicine* in 2009 showed that treatment with resveratrol consistently limited damage from free radicals in mice. But the study also showed that long-term treatment with resveratrol could be toxic to the mice's kidneys. Of course we're not mice, but just make sure you clear the use of this with your doctor. And just to be on the safe side, take it every other month. That way you are not undergoing long-term treatment.

And to be even safer, make sure that your nephrologist agrees that resveratrol treatment is right for you. I think it's fantastic because it amps up activity of your longevity genes and improves insulin sensitivity via the PGC-1 alpha pathway discussed in Chapter 3.

If you clear it with your physician, I think resveratrol is one of the best possible antioxidants that one can take in diabetes, especially if complicated with CKD.

Should you get your resveratrol by drinking red wine? Not in my opinion. The risk that consuming alcohol poses for pancreatitis and liver failure outweighs the benefits.

My suggested dosage: Try taking about 100 milligrams of *Polygonum cuspidate* standardized to contain at least 50 percent resveratrol (preferably closer to 98 percent).

VITAMIN E. Natural forms of vitamin E work in several ways to protect the kidney. Vitamin E is a strong antioxidant that has been shown to sweep away free radicals. It also reduces cholesterol and helps protect against atherosclerosis. A study published in the journal *Hypertension* showed that vitamin E reduced high blood pressure for some of the people involved in the study. My suggested dosage: Try about 400 to 800 IU natural vitamin E, mixed tocopherols and tocotrienols.

I want you to get natural vitamin E because this is easiest for your body to absorb, put to work, and ultimately eliminate. You want mixed tocopherols and tocotrienols. Mixed simply means that you are getting the full range of vitamin E—all eight of the family members. Surprised? Vitamin E is the term given to the eight compounds that make up this nutrient. That is how it appears in nature. If you take one of the nutrients (as in alpha tocopherol and that's how most vitamin supplements are sold) then you are cheating yourself out of the seven other incredible compounds that make up the family.

HERBAL TEAS THAT REALLY WORK

I am aware that if you have diabetes you probably fear getting kidney stones. Perhaps you even have them right now. Herbal teas contain little if any tannins and tannins are thought to promote the formation of kidney stones. Tannins are found in regular black tea, green tea, and white tea.

Herbal teas are a great way to promote good health without fear of stone formation and without medication. Herbal teas do not contain medications, however, they have medicinal value, meaning they may do things like help you lower blood sugar or benefit your kidney and heart. (I'll mention those actions below in the discussion of individual teas.)

Also, high-quality pure herbal teas do not contain artificial ingredients, colorants, preservatives, or sweeteners for that matter, one more plus. The following herbal teas taste great.

Chamomile

You may not have heard of manzanilla, but you've probably heard of this herb by its more common name, chamomile. Chamomile was also known as the "plant's physician" because some people observed that if it was planted beside any dying plant, the dying plant would recover within a week's time and continue growing normally.

Chamomile is one of my favorite after dinner teas for digestion and relaxation. The word chamomile comes from the Greek word *kamai*, which means "ground apple." If you smell chamomile, you'll notice its blossoms smell like freshly cut apples. Delish! The taste of chamomile is fruity, slightly sweet, and very mild.

This botanical has been used for centuries and is best known for its ability to settle down the mind and body and induce relaxation. It may also relax muscles and nervous tension, as well as settle the stomach and improve immune function. But it gets better.

One study conducted (on rats) by researchers from Aberystwyth University in Wales and the University of Toyama in Japan was published in the *Journal of Agricultural and Food Chemistry*. Rats were fed a chamomile-mimicking extract every day for 3 weeks. The animals showed a 25 percent reduction in blood sugar. Researchers think that people might be able to gain similar benefits.

Special note: Chamomile is caffeine-free and is best taken at night because it may induce sleep.

Rooibos

You will sometimes find rooibos in health food stores sold as African Red Bush tea because this botanical is native to South Africa. Some people think it has a sweet enough flavor that they don't feel the need to add stevia or honey to it. I drink this almost every day, and it's true. It's sweet enough for me to enjoy all on its own.

Rooibos contains many healing polyphenols along with minerals that are associated with protecting the pancreas. It is rich in zinc, calcium, magnesium, manganese, iron, potassium, and copper.

One shining star substance in rooibos is alpha hydroxy acid, which is found

WONDERFUL WATERCRESS

Watercress is a green herb, similar to parsley, that belongs in the cabbage family. It's a wonderful addition to your salad. It's one of the most nutritious greens you can eat because it gives you fiber, iron, B vitamins, and carotenes. Watercress happens to contain almost three times as much calcium as phosphorus, which is important for people with kidney disease. See chapter 19 for the recipe for my mouth-watering watercress soup.

in many beauty products, so rooibos has the added ability to beautify and protect your skin. This is important, and if you doubt me, please read Chapter 10 on foot and wound care. You want to keep your skin as healthy as possible.

Another shining-star ingredient in rooibos is quercetin, which is known for its ability to increase the strength of capillaries. This is of major benefit to people with diabetes because when you improve capillary strength, you improve heart function, reduce blood pressure, and get the blood flowing to your eyes, to your kidneys, and all the way down to your feet.

Improving the health of your capillaries means that rooibos could scrub away some of that cholesterol buildup, too. So it could very well reduce your risk for heart attack, stroke, and other microvascular complications that occur with poor circulation.

In addition to quercetin, rooibos contains rutin. These two ingredients are associated with reducing the release of histamines in the body, so this is a good tea for people with chronic allergies. Rooibos also has a lot of antioxidant activity and thus is an excellent and tasty way to sweep away nasty free radicals from your body. Science teaches us that when you reduce free-radical damage to the body, you are protecting your DNA (genetic code), and this in turn minimizes risk for cancer.

Special note: Rooibos tea may increase your energy levels, so enjoy this one in the morning and early afternoon. It also naturally boosts levels of iron, magnesium, and potassium, and this may improve energy levels over time.

Bitter Melon

You can buy bitter melon tea at health food stores. It contains extracts from the fruit of the bitter melon, which gets its name because the plant turns bitter so

---

SNUFF THE BUTTS

If you have diabetes and kidney disease, smoking puts you on a faster track for complications such as stroke and heart attack. So do yourself a favor and stamp out cigarettes! Gee, where have you heard that before?

---

quickly. High-quality herbal teas are created within a day of harvesting the fruit, which keeps all the nutritionally packed ingredients from degrading.

Just so you know, bitter melon extracts are also sold as supplements to help lower blood sugar, and those are more potent than the tea. The brand that I've tried is made by Charantea. They make their tea from 100 percent dried, whole bitter melon fruits and I buy it online it their Web site.

Drink bitter melon tea after you eat lunch to get some of its blood sugar–lowering properties. Just when your body starts to digest the food after eating, the bitter melon tea helps stabilize your blood sugar. Studies show that bitter melon helps increase insulin secretion, which allows both muscle and fat in the body to absorb glucose and keep it out of your kidneys.

PART 4
STAYING WELL BELOW THE WAIST

CHAPTER 10

Natural Approaches to Relieve Neuropathy

Most people with diabetes, or prediabetes, aren't motivated to retrain their palate and eat better, or to exercise and take supplements, until they start to experience nerve pain (neuropathy). Let me tell you, if there is one thing that motivates a person to lower their blood glucose and set about trying to reverse diabetes, it is the onset of nerve damage in the body.

In fact, most people who have painful neuropathies don't even realize that they may also have diabetes. Some people find out they have the disease when they visit a doctor to find out what's causing the pain.

The pain of neuropathy often gets off to a slow start. A tingle may start in one of your toes, and it won't register as any big deal at first. As neuropathy progresses, however, and works its way up your calves and your legs, it becomes more painful. As one of the readers of my column said, it gets "more interesting in a rotten way."

To give you a better picture of this painful syndrome, here are some of the most common symptoms:

Balance problems

Burning pain

Erectile dysfunction in men

Faintness or dizziness when standing up (loss of blood pressure regulation)

Gait (walking) problems, such as stumbling or poor coordination

Loss of bladder control, urgency to urinate, or painful urination

Muscle pain or weakness

Nausea, vomiting, diarrhea, or constipation

Numbness

Sensation of pins and needles

Shooting pain

Stabbing or ice-pick pain

Tingling

Trigeminal neuralgia (facial pain)

Vaginal dryness in women

THE PROBLEM WITH SUGAR

Your blood sugar (blood glucose) is not a poison. It's a nutrient that the body needs for survival. But too much of any good thing—including nutrients—*can be* poisonous. When blood sugar is high, and remains high for prolonged periods of time, it causes nerve damage.

There are several reasons that nerve damage takes place. In part, the high blood sugar damages blood vessels that carry oxygen and nutrients to the nerves. You may have heard it described as a microvascular complication, which means it affects the ability of the teeniest, tiniest blood vessels of the body to deliver oxygen. Cells cannot survive without oxygen. So you might say the neurons (the cells that make up the nerves) starve to death and begin dying in the face of chronic high blood glucose. Not to be morbid about this, but it's just as if the cells were being strangled.

Also, there can be inflammation in the nerves, or an autoimmune attack on the nerves. Genetics play a role, and as I've explained in various chapters, those nasty free-radical molecules attack the nerve cells. People who smoke or drink alcohol have more free-radical damage than those who don't.

Some people begin to lose their myelin sheath, a coating that protects the nerve cells. When this happens, numbness and random nerve firing begin, which can feel like "pins and needles." People with the autoimmune disorder multiple sclerosis know exactly what I'm talking about, as do people who have celiac disease (allergy to gluten). With demyelination—loss of the myelin sheath—the pain can progress pretty rapidly. There is some evidence that an inexpensive B vitamin can help protect your myelin. I'll get to that soon enough.

What we do know is that there is an increase in the polyol pathway activity on neuron cells and on protein kinase C. In English, it just means *OUCH*. For the purposes of this chapter, it doesn't really matter how we describe it. What I'd like to do is offer you the very best ways to stop the pain. I have ideas to help shuttle more oxygen to your cells, reduce systemic inflammation—that is, inflammation throughout your entire body, inside and out—protect the myelin coating around your delicate nerves, quench toxic free radicals, and control protein kinase C. It's not terribly difficult to do all these things. It's just that most doctors trained in Western (also known as allopathic) medicine are trained to medicate you to reduce the symptoms rather than to correct the cause.

Medications may well be necessary for you. But whether or not you require prescription medication, I will still recommend some wonderful and extremely helpful supplements. First let's take a closer look at some of the forms that diabetic neuropathy can take.

THE MANY FACES OF DIABETIC NEUROPATHY

People experience neuropathy in many different ways. There are four different types of nerve damage: peripheral, autonomic, proximal, and focal. The sooner you can identify the kind of neuropathy you're experiencing, the sooner you can begin the path to healing. Here is a brief description of these four types of neuropathic pain.

PERIPHERAL NEUROPATHY. The word *peripheral* means around the outer edge, away from the central part, and refers to nerve damage that is in the toes, feet, legs, fingers, hands, and arms.

AUTONOMIC NEUROPATHY. Autonomic neuropathy affects the nerves that are part of the autonomic nervous system (ANS) in the body. The ANS is responsible for all the functions in our bodies that we don't consciously control, such as breathing, digestion, sexual arousal, and, of course, our own heartbeat. Nerves that extend from the ANS are connected to the heart, stomach, lungs, sexual organs, eyes, and bladder.

Cranial nerve 10, also called the vagus nerve and the wanderer nerve, gets in on the action. It wanders in and around some important organs. If you have autonomic neuropathy, you may not have the strange sensations, such as pain or numbness, that characterize peripheral neuropathy, but you could experience an abnormal heart rhythm, blood pressure swings, difficulty breathing, bladder problems, and increased or decreased sweating.

In the gut, you may have to deal with irritable bowel syndrome, diarrhea, constipation, and diabetic gastroparesis. This last one—gastroparesis—is the medical term for the stomach taking too long to empty its contents. It happens when nerves to the stomach are damaged or stop working.

The vagus nerve controls the movement of food through the digestive tract. If the vagus nerve is damaged, the muscles of the stomach and intestines do not work normally, and the movement of food is slowed or stopped with autonomic neuropathy. Men have to contend with erectile dysfunction, and women may develop vaginal dryness or inability to reach orgasm.

PROXIMAL NEUROPATHY. Proximal neuropathy is the nerve damage that affects the muscles of your thigh, including the front, back, and sides; your hip;

or your bottom. It results in pain or weakness and can cause you to literally fall down without any warning, once the affected muscles are severely weakened.

Some people experience balance problems or fall when they stand up, twist, or turn sideways. It disturbs me to think about how many people are misdiagnosed with osteoporosis and are prescribed bone-building drugs when they may be suffering from diabetes and proximal neuropathies, which can cause them to fall and break a hip.

A few simple blood tests described in Chapter 6 could determine whether you have diabetes, at which point you could begin to repair the nerves rather than simply take bone-building drugs that address neither the pain nor the underlying cause of hip fracture.

FOCAL NEUROPATHY. Focal neuropathy typically involves a single nerve and comes on suddenly. It's most common in older adults, and while it can cause intense pain, it usually disappears within a few weeks or months.

Sometimes focal neuropathy occurs when a nerve is compressed. Carpal tunnel syndrome is the most common type of compression neuropathy in people with diabetes. With focal neuropathy, the nerves that surround the eye are most often affected, creating pain in or behind the eye, as well as double vision or difficulty focusing.

Eye pain can be one-sided, and there may even be facial paralysis. The pain can come on suddenly, making focal neuropathies quite unpredictable and scary. Although many people experience focal neuropathy of the eye, it is possible that a cluster of nerves can cause pain in your lower back, chest, stomach area, or feet.

Signs of focal neuropathy include:

- Difficulty focusing your eyes, double vision, or aching behind one eye
- Paralysis on one side of your face (Bell's palsy)
- Pain in your shin or foot.

I hope that after reading all these possible symptoms, you're motivated to take nutritional supplements, lose weight (if that applies), exercise, and eat more raw, fresh foods.

GETTING NEUROPATHY UNDER CONTROL

Neuropathy is one of the most maddening and painful complications of diabetes. There are certain factors you cannot change, such as your age. The older you are, the more likely you are to develop nerve pain. You can't help that, but there are other things that you *do* have the power to change, and with courage, effort, and persistence, you can dramatically reduce your risk of developing painful neuropathies. For example, whether or not it feels that way all the time, you do have the power to control your:

Blood glucose	Weight
Blood pressure	Choice to exercise
Lipoprotein(a) (a measurement of bad cholesterol)	Intake of supplements shown to protect nerve cells

While lowering blood glucose levels will eventually help reduce your pain and may help to prevent the kind of severe damage that will be irreversible, this takes time. And I know that any amount of time is too much time if you are in a great deal of pain. There are several terrific natural ways to help yourself. I'm going to share some of the best ways to reduce pain, numbness, and neuropathic pain. Let's start with the hottest tip of all.

CHILE PEPPER CAN EASE THE BURN

I'll bet you think I'm kidding, but I'm not. Now please don't take a swig of Tabasco! That's not how it works.

There's a compound that puts the "hot" in hot pepper sauce, and it can honestly relieve nerve pain (and joint pain) for some people. It doesn't happen overnight. It may take a few weeks or even a month, and you have to stick with it, not just use it once in a while.

You can buy products with this ingredient—capsaicin (pronounced *cap-SAY-sin*)—at any pharmacy. These topical creams and patches work by numbing your nerve endings so you don't feel the pain. This works great for arthritis in the fingers, elbows, and knees—even better than those cooling menthol creams, which basically only distract you from the pain by giving you a cold sensation. With capsaicin-containing creams, you actually do something to block the pain.

I've helped so many people over the years with this hot little secret, even people with the most horrible nerve pain known to humankind. It's called trigeminal neuralgia (TN), and it's basically a neuropathy in the fifth cranial nerve. This is the nerve that allows you to feel sensations on your face, like when your grandbaby caresses your cheek.

With TN, it feels like someone has plugged the nerves that supply one side of your face into an electrical outlet. One individual described it as "a lightning strike on my face." Surgery doesn't usually help, and medications have limited use, which is why TN has been dubbed the suicide disease. It can be a complication of multiple sclerosis as well as diabetes. With that in mind, I think a gluten-free diet would be sensible, as gluten attacks nerves in certain people. You can read more about gluten sensitivity in Chapter 4.

In January 2007, I published a syndicated newspaper column on ways to help TN, and I included the benefits of hot chile pepper cream. You can read that article (and hundreds of other ones) at my Web site, www.DearPharmacist.com. A few weeks after I wrote the column on this type of neuropathy, I got an e-mail from a woman named Marilyn:

> *You have incredibly changed my life. In 2006, I had two surgeries designed to relieve the pain of trigeminal neuralgia. By September 06, my neurosurgeon told me that there was no treatment or relief for the type of pain I was experiencing. He was wrong! Since using the capsaicin you recommended in your column, hours of pain have been reduced to minutes. I am now living an almost normal life. I owe you an enormous debt of gratitude. Thank you, Thank you, Thank you!*
>
> *Marilyn in Gainesville, Florida*

Isn't that just amazing? I was moved to tears after reading that note because there is so little help for people with facial neuropathies. And here was Marilyn, after two surgeries doing so much better with a $10 cream I had recommended. I later got to meet her at a book signing in Florida, where I got the best hug and a jar of her delicious homemade strawberry preserves.

It's not just Marilyn—many people benefit from capsaicin. Articles and studies support the use of capsaicin for neuropathy. For example, the peer-reviewed journal *Current Opinion in Supportive and Palliative Care* published an article in its June 2009 issue called "Advances in the Management of Diabetic Peripheral Neuropathy" that mentions capsaicin as a therapeutic treatment

According to a 2009 article in the *Southern Medical Journal*, using capsaicin cream is one of the few ways of reducing the pain in diabetic neuropathy, and the only proven topical (applied to the skin) treatment. Capsaicin works because it numbs nerve endings by reducing a pain-causing chemical called substance P. It's very simple. If you have less of this "P," you have less pain to deal with.

Apply capsaicin cream to the area of your skin where it hurts, but never near the eyes or genitals and *never* during a painful neuropathy attack. When the hot sensation is gone, reapply it, usually every 3 to 6 hours. This should numb nerve endings within a week or two.

The cream causes a warm sensation, sometimes a burning sensation, but the burning sensation is transient and goes away after you have used the cream regularly for a week or two, if you remain compliant. The trick—and listen carefully now—is to apply the cream when you are NOT feeling much pain, preferably none at all. If you don't adhere to this rule and apply it to burning/tingling skin, then you will make your condition worse.

Repeated applications give you even more relief, as long as you massage the cream into your muscle (or joints) really well. If you are applying it to your hands, leave it on for 30 minutes (wear gloves while you leave it on), and be careful not to touch your eyes or any mucous membrane in your body, including your nostrils, mouth, genitals, or any open sores or wounds. Then wash with soap and water at least twice to remove all residue. Use a little nail brush to clean underneath your fingernails.

Trust me on this one, you do not want to go to the bathroom or touch your eyes or nostrils with capsaicin residue on your fingers. Again, normal sensations include burning or stinging, but it diminishes with continued use. And with continued use, the painful neuropathic sensations should subside. Two popular brand names sold nationwide at pharmacies are Capzasin and Zostrix. If you search the Web for capsaicin, you'll find all sorts of information about pepper creams and their use in reducing neuropathic pain.

SUPPLEMENTS TO SOOTHE THE PAIN

There are also many oral supplements that may prove helpful.

Alpha Lipoic Acid

Alpha lipoic acid (ALA) is a powerful antioxidant that can slip into all of your cells and neutralize those unstable dangerous free radicals. If that isn't good enough, ALA can breathe new life into other antioxidants in your body, such as vitamins C and E, coenzyme Q10, and intracellular glutathione. The net effect of all this is to build a stronger body, one that will take fewer hits from nasty free radicals that are trying to destroy your pancreas and nerve cells. Its effect on nerve health is well established, and it works by promoting healthy circulation in the tiniest capillaries (microcirculation).

Researchers have found that ALA has improved neuropathic symptoms—including reducing pain—in some 10 studies. Back in 2003, scientists from Moscow published an article in the journal *Diabetes Care*, based on an ongoing large study called the SYDNEY trial (named for "The sensory SYmptoms of Diabetic polyNEuropathY are improved with alpha-lipoic acid"). While the Russian scientists used intravenous ALA in that 2003 study, 3 years later, scientists in Germany undertook the SYDNEY 2 study and found the same wonderful effect by using ALA in oral supplements. They concluded that a dosage of 600 milligrams daily offered the most benefits with the lowest risk.

If I were going to take only one supplement for neuropathic pain and, for that matter, diabetes, it would be ALA. I believe it's the most important nutrient for a person with neuropathy because it helps reduce the nerve pain while also reducing blood sugar. How cool is that?! It's like a "buy one, get one free" kind of supplement, and who here doesn't love a bargain?

ALA is a cofactor, meaning it assists in chemical reactions, in this case chemical reactions that generate energy and oxygen. Having more oxygen flood your nerve cells is like having insurance to prevent premature cell death. Remember, you want to keep your nerve cells alive and thriving for as long as possible, and they crave oxygen. ALA gives them nourishment, and, in mild enough cases, it can completely relieve the pain.

While you may notice some effect in a few days, most people require several weeks before they notice a difference. It all really depends on how severe the damage is and how long you have been in pain. The more severe the damage and the longer you have been in pain, the longer it takes to feel any benefit.

MY SUGGESTED DOSAGE. 200 milligrams two or three times daily along with food, to enhance absorption.

Another related supplement called R-lipoic acid is available now. This form may be even more effective than ALA. It is just another isomer, which in this case is like a chemical mirror image, and it's natural and more potent.

My suggested dosage of R-lipoic acid is only about 100 milligrams two to four times daily because it's a little stronger than ALA.

You can boost the effect of ALA (or R-lipoic acid) by taking it with a high-quality fish oil supplement that contains an essential fatty acid called DHA.

My suggested dose for DHA is 1,000 to 2,000 milligrams daily. (See more information regarding fish oil in the heart chapter, page 137).

Curcumin

Curcumin is one of the active ingredients found in the spice turmeric and is responsible for its bright gold color. Curcumin is derived from the plant *Curcuma longa*, commonly used in India for both its health-promoting qualities and to preserve food and give color to fabrics (as those of us who have spilled Indian food on our clothes don't need reminding)!

Not only has curcumin been scientifically shown to reduce blood sugar, but it also has pain-relieving activity. It works in part by reducing a pain-causing chemical called TNF alpha (tumor necrosis factor alpha). In addition, there's this chemical in the body called nitric oxide, and we know that an overproduction of nitric oxide is implicated in certain pain pathways. Guess what? Curcumin chases away some of that nitric oxide, which helps cool the burn you feel in your nerves. It really helps to reduce the pain.

In fact, scientists in the Department of Experimental Therapeutics at the MD Anderson Cancer Center in Houston, Texas, are so impressed with curcumin's inflammation-fighting and pain-relieving properties that they call it the spice for life. They published an article about it in the peer-reviewed journal *Advances in Experimental and Medical Biology*. The scientists of MD Anderson are doing research on discovering or formulating a "super curcumin," and they published an article about that research in the journal *Biochemical Pharmacology*.

You can spice your food with turmeric, but you'd have to eat quite a bit to get any therapeutic response. I certainly recommend using turmeric in recipes, but you will need to take a supplement to get the best effect. Be patient. The beneficial effects for neuropathy may take 3 to 6 weeks for you to notice, especially if you've had the pain a long time. For some lucky people, relief may be experienced within a week or two.

MY SUGGESTED DOSAGE. Take 300 to 500 milligrams two or three times daily since curcumin activity in the body is short-lived. Dosing more frequently gives you more benefit than taking a big dose all at once. It works even better if taken with ALA. You will notice that some proprietary blends contain biopterin, a substance derived from black pepper (*Piper nigrum*). If your curcumin product contains it, it will be printed on the ingredient label. This is fine. In fact, I believe it's even better than taking curcumin alone, as biopterin enhances your body's ability to absorb curcumin. However, you will find that opinions differ as to whether plain curcumin supplements work as well as those combined with biopterin. Now, if you're asking me (which it looks like you are), I much prefer the combination of curcumin and black pepper.

Methylcobalamin or Vitamin B_{12} (Methyl B_{12})

I believe one of the most overlooked ways to help people with terrible nerve pain is the simple B vitamin called methylcobalamin. For some reason, most doctors don't think about this. Instead, it seems they'd rather prescribe a battery of prescription drugs, including nortriptyline. For the record, a study performed at the University of Medical Sciences in Iran showed that vitamin B_{12} outperformed nortriptyline in terms of reducing the symptoms of painful diabetic neuropathy. Scientists who ran the study on 100 people concluded, in an article published in 2009 in the *International Journal of Food Sciences and Nutrition,* "Vitamin B_{12} is more effective than nortriptyline for the treatment of symptomatic painful diabetic neuropathy." In fact, they found it tw times more likely to relieve pain than the drug.

Having a deficiency of vitamin B_{12} can cause you to lose the protective covering around your nerve cells. It's not that you really run out of B_{12}. It's more that you run out of beneficial micro-organisms in your gut, as well as another natural substance called intrinsic factor, which is a protein your gut needs to have in order to absorb vitamin B_{12}. That causes you to stop making and using B_{12} properly.

Some people develop numbness and neuropathic pain because they lack a certain B vitamin. Sometimes it's B_6, but most of the time it's B_{12}. When your body starves for B_{12}, you lose the myelin sheath that protects your nerve cells. It's as if they get stripped of their skin, and they get touchy.

As the deficiency of B_{12} continues, your nerves literally crumble and start to short-circuit, causing all sorts of neuropathies and bizarre sensations. One of my patients told me that he felt as if a pot of hot water were dumped on him, and he was also getting sores on his tongue and losing memory. I immediately recommended some methyl B_{12}, and he came back about 2 months later to say he was completely cured. Completely! The best part of this story is that he was able to get off two strong medications—an opiate painkiller (Percocet) and an antiseizure drug (Neurontin) that was causing undesirable side effects, such as blurred vision and balance problems while walking.

Here are some of the symptoms you may experience from a B_{12} deficiency:

Depression	Memory loss
Easy bruising	Pins-and-needles sensation in
Enlarged liver	your hands and feet, like ant
Hallucinations and dementia	bites all over
Headaches	Tinnitus (ringing in the ears)
Inflamed tongue and mouth sores	Vibration or buzzing in the legs

The most stupefying (and disgraceful) thing to me is that many popular diabetic medications can cause you to run low on B_{12}. And when you become deficient in B_{12}, your neuropathy will worsen, plus you suddenly develop those new medical conditions listed above. Then you get on the medication merry-go-round as your doctor tries to treat each new disease—dementia, depression, liver damage, and so forth. See how crazy it can get? And you know what I'm talking about, because I'll bet you have been on that medication merry-go-round. And all because a B_{12} deficiency is overlooked. So I'll repeat it:

Your diabetic medications can cause neuropathy even while they lower your blood sugar.

Here are just a few of the prescribed diabetic drugs known to be drug muggers of B_{12}, and therefore suspected to cause or contribute to nerve pain:

Glimepiride (Amaryl)	Glyburide/metformin (Glucovance)
Glipizide (Glucotrol)	Metformin (Glucophage)
Glyburide (Diabeta, Glynase,	Pioglitazone (Actos)
Micronase)	Rosiglitazone (Avandia)

You'll find a more thorough list of medications that rob you of vitamin B_{12} in "Drug Muggers of Vitamin B_{12}" on page 210.

Should you stop taking medications that rob you of vitamin B_{12}?

That decision is up to you and your doctor. I would be happy if you told me that you were supplementing with the vitamin that the drug mugger stole. When you replenish methyl B_{12}, the fire and pain in your body should cool off. It's so simple, and so overlooked.

Because vitamin B_{12} is available in hundreds of preparations, make sure that you take the best form, methylcobalamin, also called methyl B_{12}. Simply put, it's the active form that makes its way into the brain and nervous system, so it helps specifically with nerve pain.

Don't make the mistake of buying cyanocobalamin, which is not natural vitamin B_{12}. Cyanocobalamin is a semisynthetic version of the real deal. It's extremely hard for your body to use and integrate the synthetic compound into your nerve cells. Regrettably, it's very popular and is sold nationwide.

Cyanocobalamin is also the primary form used in over-the-counter supplements, such as multiple vitamins and injections sold at the pharmacy. It's unfortunate, but true, that this form is not going to help you nearly as well as the methyl B_{12}.

Go to the health food store or a natural grocery store and get methylcobalamin, preferably with intrinsic factor. As I mentioned earlier, the intrinsic factor makes the methylcobalamin work better. But it's not a deal breaker if you can't find it. This kind of product is hard to find. Methylcobalamin is the biologically active form of vitamin B_{12}, so it will be absorbed much better than cyanocobalamin, with or without the intrinsic factor.

In some people with anemia, or severe neuropathies, you can give them all the B_{12} you want, but if they don't have healthy gut flora and lack this intrinsic factor, there will be no response. Taking probiotics may help.

It's basically trial and error. If the methylcobalamin works great and pain is reduced within a few months, then wonderful. But if it doesn't, you'll have to bring out the big guns, that is, methylcobalamin that is combined with intrinsic factor. If you have trouble finding it, look for B_{12} with Intrinsic Factor sold online at www.stages-of-life.com, or Metagenic brand's Intrinsi B_{12}/Folate, which is sold only through healthcare practitioners' offices. Sublingual B_{12} is convenient and may offer you faster absorption. Try Natural Factor's Sublingual B_{12} lozenges. Another good one is Allergy Research's B_{12} (Methylcobalamin) Sublingual Liquid, sold at health food stores and online.

People who opt for injections of B_{12} almost always are prescribed cyanocobalamin because that is the product available at pharmacies. Regular pharmacies do not have methylcobalamin. To get the methylcobalamin form of B_{12}, you'll have to ask your doctor—okay, you may actually have to nag!—who will have to phone the local compound pharmacy and ask them to make it. It's really not that difficult, and if you are in pain, you should *insist* upon having the appropriate form of B_{12} that is proven to help remyelinate (reconstruct your nerve fibers) and therefore relieve nerve pain.

DRUG MUGGERS OF VITAMIN B$_{12}$

The following drugs can affect the level of vitamin B$_{12}$ in your body and therefore cause or contribute to painful neuropathies.

Acid blockers
  Ranitidine (Zantac)
  Cimetidine (Tagamet)
  Nizatidine (Axid)
  Famotidine (Pepcid and Pepcid Complete)
  Omeprazole (Prilosec OTC)
  Esomeprazole (Nexium)
  Lansoprazole (Prevacid)
  Pantoprazole (Protonix)
  Rabeprazole (Aciphex)

Alcohol
Antibiotics—Just a few examples here; there are many:
  Amoxicillin (Amoxil)
  Azithromycin (Z-pak)

Cefaclor (Ceclor), cefdinir (Omnicef), cephalexin (Keflex)
Ciprofloxacin (Cipro), levofloxacin (Levaquin)
Clarithromycin (Biaxin), erythromycin (E.E.S.)
Doxycycline (Doryx), minocycline (Minocin)
Tetracycline (Sumycin)
Trimethoprim-sulfamethoxazole (Septra, Bactrim)

Cholestyramine resin (Questran)
Colchicine
Colestipol (Colestid)
Dicloxacillin (Dynapen)

MY SUGGESTED DOSAGE. 500 to 1,000 micrograms daily for 2 weeks taken along with a B complex so that you have all the Bs on board. You need the B complex because B$_{12}$ needs its sisters to increase utilization and prevent a relative deficiency in the other Bs. As long as we are discussing B vitamins, I need to tell you that thiamine (vitamin B$_1$) can also be taken along with B$_{12}$ and is especially helpful to people who have a history of alcoholism.

Acetyl L-Carnitine

This amino acid undergoes a chemical reaction in the brain to turn into acetylcholine, whose job, among many others, is to facilitate memory. Can you imagine? Supplementing with acetyl L-carnitine, which is sold over the counter at health food stores, could help you remember things better. Even medications for Alzheimer's disease fail at sparking new production of acetylcholine.

Estrogen-containing drugs
(hormone replacement therapy
and birth control)
*Conjugated estrogens (Premarin,
Prempro)*
*Estradiol (Estrace, Climara, Estra-
derm, Estring, Activella, Femring,
Combipatch. EstroGel, Menostar,
and many others)*
*Ethinyl estradiol (found in many
birth control pills)*

Fibrate cholesterol medicine
Fenofibrate (TriCor)
Ezetimibe (Zetia)
Gemfibrozil (Lopid)
Clofibrate (Atromid S)
Levodopa/carbidopa (Sinemet)
Methotrexate (Rheumatrex, Trexall)
Methyldopa (Aldomet)
Norethindrone (Aygestin)

Phenobarbital
Phenytoin (Dilantin) (When
supplementing for B_{12} depletion
caused by this particular
anticonvulsant medication, space
the supplement at least 2 hours
away from the drug. In other
words, don't take the medication
and the supplement together.)
Potassium supplements and drugs
(Micro-K, Slow K)
Primidone (Mysoline)
Psychiatric drugs such as
chlorpromazine (Thorazine),
thioridazine (Mellaril),
fluphenazine (Prolixin),
haloperidol (Haldol)
Stavudine (Zerit)
Trimethoprim-sulfamethoxazole
(Septra or Bactrim)
Zidovudine (AZT, Retrovir)

Acetyl L-carnitine has also been shown to have powerful effects in reliev-ing painful neuropathies associated with diabetes. It works so well that drug companies want in on the action. Well of course! So phase II testing is under way in the United States right now, although it's been sold by prescription in Italy since 1994. I'm so happy to tell you that this powerful compound with potential to protect your nerves (and memory) is still sold over the coun-ter in the United States as of this writing. You can find it at most health food stores.

MY SUGGESTED DOSAGE. 250 milligrams three times daily. Give it a few months before you expect results.

David Perlmutter, M.D., practices in Naples, Florida, as a board-certified neurologist, and he sees a lot of people with neuropathic pain. He explained to me how well acetyl L-carnitine works when combined with other substances that

IF YOU MUST INDULGE . . .

Do you enjoy an occasional glass of wine? (I wish you wouldn't, but that's a whole other topic.) Just be aware that drinking a glass of wine can steal a nerve-protective nutrient called thiamine from your body. The B vitamin thiamine protects your nervous system and reduces burning sensations, as well as painful and tender feelings from your head down to your toes. If you indulge in alcohol, take thiamine, about 100 milligrams daily, ideally in the morning because it has weak diuretic-like effects. In fact, even if you don't drink alcohol, take thiamine to help reduce neuropathy.

fix the damaged and inflamed nerve tissue that causes peripheral neuropathy. In his product NeuroActive's Brain Sustain, he has combined several key nutrients that not only improve memory and reduce the risk for Alzheimer's disease (now being called type 3 diabetes by some) but also heal those touchy, painful nerves. NeuroActive's Brain Sustain combines acetyl L-carnitine with various nutrients, among them, the antioxidant coenzyme Q10, *Ginkgo biloba* for improved bloodflow, and phosphatidylserine, a compound that naturally repairs damaged cell membranes.

You might say the product cools the fire of hot, touchy nerves, but it takes a few weeks to months before it kicks in. It may be able to help those with diabetic or gluten-induced neuropathies. Suggested dose is two capsules twice daily with food. Available at www.inutritionals.com.

Minerals

If you are going to improve your health and reduce your symptoms of diabetes, you must have the right minerals. In fact, the deficiency of minerals within our soils has contributed to the nutrient-void foods we consume now.

Minerals are hugely important to a person with diabetes. There is a more thorough discussion of minerals in Chapter 14. As it relates to neuropathy, you need adequate amounts of calcium, magnesium, zinc, selenium, vanadium, chromium, and copper. These are all poorly absorbed from the gut unless you take them as an organic salt, more commonly called the chelated form.

It's unfortunate that most nutriceutical manufacturers don't go the extra mile for you. They provide their minerals as inorganic salts (for example, magnesium oxide or calcium carbonate), and so it is extremely difficult—if not impossible—to absorb those minerals into your bloodstream and shuttle them over to your nerve cells, or bone cells, or wherever they are needed to help you.

MY SUGGESTED DOSAGE. To begin with, look for chelated minerals, which means they will be less likely to upset your stomach and more likely to penetrate hungry nerve tissue. Minerals as they occur in nature are also better for your body, as opposed to synthetic irritating salts. Synthetic brands are the ones sold in most pharmacies, so when shopping for minerals, go to your local health food store or shop online.

Only a few easy-to-absorb types of minerals are available. Among the best sources are Solgar's VM-75, sold at health food stores, and Stages of Life's Magic Minerals, sold online. You can also get a good supply of minerals from a spirulina supplement or naturally by eating oysters, seafood, and seaweed. And this is a good excuse for eating more sushi. (Gosh, now you've got me craving a tuna roll.)

DO YOU HAVE HIGH CHOLESTEROL?

If you have high cholesterol in this country, chances are your doctor has pre-scribed a statin drug for you. Millions of prescriptions have been written for these blockbuster drugs, which include:

Atorvastatin (Lipitor)   Rosuvastatin (Crestor)
Lovastatin (Mevacor)   Simvastatin (Zocor)
Lovastatin and niacin (Advicor)   Simvastatin and niacin (Simcor)
Pravastatin (Pravachol)

Why are we talking about cholesterol in the neuropathy chapter? Because these popular drugs can actually cause numbness, tingling, burning, and pain. Statin-induced neuropathy has been well documented since at least 2002. And here's the worst part: People with diabetes who take statin drugs are approxi-mately 16 times more susceptible to neuropathy than non–statin users, according to an article published in the journal *Neurology* in 2002.

I believe that one reason behind the statin-induced pain is the depletion of coenzyme Q10 (CoQ10), a powerful antioxidant that protects your nerve cells from damage. It's known that statins are drug muggers of CoQ10, and when you run low on that nutrient, your nervous system pays a price. So does your heart. (Details are in Chapter 8).

When you run out of CoQ10, that's a huge problem for your body because without CoQ10 you lose an important defense mechanism against toxic poisons and free radicals. Statins also deplete a few other fat soluble nutrients you need for good health. The solution? Take CoQ10 along with some natural vitamin E (about 400 IU). Some studies have shown that CoQ10 and vitamin E work well together because of the synergy. CoQ10 recycles vitamin E in the body. Many formulas are sold with the two of them in a single formula. You'll need some additional beta-carotene (for the A) and vitamin D.

MY SUGGESTED DOSAGE. Take 100 milligrams of CoQ10 two or three times daily. Even better, take the active form of CoQ10 called ubiquinol. It has a stronger effect. My suggested dosage for that is 50 to 100 milligrams once or twice daily. You may notice effects as early as a week after taking it—or perhaps even earlier.

THE OVARY CONNECTION

Polycystic ovarian syndrome (PCOS) is connected to neuropathy. In the face of high blood sugar, insulin production goes up. Insulin is a hormone that also affects sex hormones, namely androgens, which are high in women with PCOS. So women with high levels of insulin could have higher levels of androgens, which means acne, weight gain, ovulation problems, and this not-so-sexy catch-22—extra facial hair while it thins out on your head.

PCOS also means a higher risk for diabetes and microvascular complications, such as painful neuropathies. The take-home point is that if you have PCOS, treat yourself as if you had diabetes. Please remember that if you have PCOS and take metformin, you need to pay attention to your levels of vitamin B_{12}, a nutrient that I covered at length earlier in this chapter. Metformin can make it more difficult for your gut to absorb vitamin B_{12} because it mugs the intrinsic factor, a protein that I also discussed earlier. So metformin is a drug mugger of vitamin B_{12}, and this can lead to deficiency. When you run out of B_{12} (and other B vitamins), your levels of the inflammatory substance homocysteine go up, and that opens up Pandora's box.

Elevated homocysteine is a bad thing because it could put you at a higher risk for chronic fatigue, fibromyalgia, memory problems, stroke, heart attack, or other unpleasant or dangerous conditions. Please have your doctor measure levels of homocysteine (an inflammatory marker) with a simple blood test. And do talk to your doctor about your homocysteine levels, especially if you take metformin or other drug muggers of B_{12}. (See page 210 for other drugs that rob you of B_{12}).

MEDICINE THAT CAN HELP

This chapter is all about natural solutions for neuropathy, but as a pharmacist I'd be remiss if I didn't pay some attention to medications as well.

Some medications work by preventing your brain from registering pain. They don't work in everyone, but the people these drugs do work for will experience less pain. It's like a fake-out. If you do take one of these medications, please just realize that you should also be taking something to address the underlying damage (like the supplements I detailed earlier in this chapter). None of these drugs reverse the damage in your nervous system. The damage continues at full speed, but you just don't feel the pain. If you ever stop the drug, the pain will come back like wildfire. That said, here are your best pharmaceutical options.

Antidepressants:

Elavil (amitriptyline)   Prozac (fluoxetine)

Imipramine (nortriptyline)   Cymbalta (duloxetine)

Antiseizure:

Dilantin (phenytoin)   Neurontin (gabapentin)

Tegretol (carbamazepine)   Lyrica (pregabalin)

Trileptal (oxcarbazine)   Vimpat (lacosamide)

Lots of people love Lyrica. This medication is getting to be quite popular. Lyrica was first approved in December 2004 to treat epilepsy, diabetic neuropathy pain, and pain from shingles. But doctors weren't supposed to prescribe it to treat the pain of fibromyalgia until the FDA approved it for that indication in 2007.

By 2008, Lyrica had generated $675 million in sales for its maker, Pfizer. Believe it or not, the drug is actually an anticonvulsant, and one of its side effects is sedation. This is a good combination for people who have a seizure disorder or neuropathic pain and insomnia to boot! It manages all three conditions.

My own patients seem to have a love-hate relationship with this drug. They either love it and think it is heaven-sent, or they hate it and develop all sorts of side effects. My experience is that it helps most people and so far, the majority of people taking Lyrica tolerate it well and derive more benefits than side effects.

Having said that, be aware that Lyrica is a relatively new drug, so as the years go by, we will have more data on its safety profile. Let me put it this way: If I had to take a drug for chronic neuropathic pain (that was unresponsive to

---

GET INTO THOSE MEDICINE BOTTLES

If those child-resistant caps on your medicine bottles are giving you grief, ask your pharmacist for easy-open caps that just pop off. There are laws designed to protect children and minimize household poisonings, which is why child-resistant caps are used in the first place. But if numbness and pain affect your hands, then I assure you, this problem is quick and simple to remedy. Just sign a little waiver at your pharmacy, and they will put a note in the computer to remind the pharmacist to use easy-open caps every time you refill your prescription. After you sign it, your request is immediately honored and each time you have your prescriptions filled, you should get a nonsafety cap that doesn't hurt to open. It's that easy!

---

natural supplements, methyl B_{12}, and a gluten-free diet), then I would try Lyrica, primarily because it reduces substance P, a chemical that causes pain.

I also appreciate that this drug is derived from a natural substance called GABA, one of our natural brain neurotransmitters. It's sold as an OTC supplement, too. GABA is short for gamma-aminobutyric acid, and at nighttime, our brain becomes flooded with natural GABA, which makes us fall asleep. The pharmacist in me wants you to start Lyrica at the lowest effective dosage, usually 50 to 75 milligrams taken at bedtime. Your doctor will probably have you increase your dosage every few days, or each week, until you reach the right dosage for your pain level. That dosage varies according to several factors your doctor can discuss with you. If the dose is increased slowly enough (titrated properly), you should not experience too many side effects. But do be aware that your vision may get fuzzy on this drug. Blurred vision is a frequently reported side effect, along with easy bruising, dizziness, drowsiness, stomach pain, increased appetite, or joint and muscle pain. Taking natural GABA is another option, but discuss that with your doctor.

WHAT ELSE CAN YOU TRY?

Here are several more ideas to help you deal with the pain of neuropathy.

GET MOVING. Try walking or another regular exercise to help maintain muscle mass. Yoga is great.

APPLY SOME PRESSURE. Elastic stockings may help relieve pain for some.

SOAK IT. There's a lot to be said for a warm bath, especially with Epsom salts.

TRY A TENS UNIT. It's kind of like fighting fire with fire. For localized pain, TENS (transcutaneous electrical nerve stimulation) sends tiny electrical impulses into a localized area. I know that you are thinking, "She's out of her mind—I have enough tingling and pain as it is!" But this treatment can honestly *interrupt* pain sensations for some people. It doesn't cure it, but it might give you a temporary deep breath because of the distraction, and it's sometimes recommended for this very type of pain.

Ask your doctor if TENS is appropriate for you, and if so, get a prescription. Many insurance companies cover the cost—anywhere from $40 to $400 depending on the brand. These units are sold at medical supply shops and distributors, and online.

Be careful buying online. I would sleep easier at night knowing that a medical professional—a physical therapist, chiropractor, or medical doctor—taught you how to use this little machine. After all, don't you want personal instruction? To use the unit, tiny electrodes must be attached to your skin.

CONSIDER MASSAGE THERAPY. A relaxing session reduces your body's output of cortisol, a pain-causing chemical.

LEARN BIOFEEDBACK. In this form of treatment you begin by wearing sensors on your head and body that read the tension of your muscles or other bodily functions, such as digestion, body temperature, or heart rate. It sounds like science fiction, but it's mind over matter, literally.

You train yourself to feel less diabetic neuropathy pain by staying relaxed and keeping your muscle tension low. Biofeedback may also reduce frequency and pain from migraines, and help with seizure disorders, heart disease, hypertension, bladder problems, and Raynaud's disease (cold hands and feet).

STAYING ON TOP OF THE PAIN

Finally, there's one natural, over-the-counter topical treatment I want to mention that you can try for pennies on the dollar compared to pricey drugs. It's called Neuragen. Generally speaking, the great advantage of topical treatments is that they target the specific area where the pain originates, such as the feet, with very little or no effect on other parts of the body. This avoids the most common side effects associated with medications you swallow, which can sometimes put too much of a burden on the liver and kidneys. Those organs have to do the work of filtering what goes into the body.

With topical formulations, so little is absorbed into the circulation, very little extra load is placed on the liver and kidney—the organs responsible for detoxifying substances in the body—and there is very little chance of unwanted interactions with other drugs or foods. Many people have found that topical treatments for neuropathic pain relief are the best choice among medications.

Neuragen contains a homeopathic blend of ingredients to reduce pain on contact. Two ingredients are hypericum (which you may know by its other name, St. John's wort) and *Aconitum napellus*, a flower extract that used to be used as a toxin on spears. This soothing blend also contains geranium, bergamot, and eucalyptus oils and was specifically designed for the relief of neuropathic pain.

In clinical trials to date on over 160 individuals, Neuragen, when applied topically, has been shown to be effective for postherpetic neuralgia (a painful complication of shingles), diabetic peripheral neuropathy, and all-cause neuropathies. The latter are any condition resulting in neuropathic pain, including the two mentioned above as well as chemo-induced neuropathy, HIV neuropathy, reflex sympathetic dystrophy, trigeminal neuralgia, trauma-induced neuropathy, and other idiopathic (unknown cause) neuropathies.

Users of Neuragen, regardless of the cause of the neuropathic pain, report pain relief, typically within 5 minutes, that lasts for 2 to 8 hours after only a few drops are applied topically. Remarkably, up to 80 percent of people get some pain relief, and nearly half get a 50 percent reduction or greater. Many have found that Neuragen is more effective than any other medicine they have tried. There is more information about this product on the Internet. Visit www.neuragen.com.

Walking Away from Diabetes: Foot and Wound Care

CHAPTER 11

About 20 years ago, I worked as a nursing home consultant for long-term care facilities around Florida. My work in nursing homes included reviewing drug protocols and lab tests to make sure that all medications were necessary and in proper doses.

I was deeply affected by the patients who had lost limbs because of amputation. Some of them were confined to a wheelchair and never ventured beyond the interior halls of their nursing homes. Others were confined to their bed because of multiple amputations.

I'll never forget one poor woman named Dottie who had no arms and no legs. Her arms were amputated at the shoulders, and her legs gone from the mid-thigh. Her torso just lay in her bed from morning til night. She never smiled. What would she have to smile about with no quality of life, and no ability to scratch an itch, brush her teeth, or even roll over? She would occasionally nod when I entered her room, but mostly, she'd stare blankly out her window, as if to say, "Please let me get out of here," and I doubt she meant out of her room. As if this wasn't bad enough, the fact that she could not turn herself in her bed caused her to develop painful bedsores all over her back.

Dottie's state was beyond pitiful to me. I felt so helpless as a consultant pharmacist. There was little I could recommend except medications to keep her comfortable. It left a deep impact on me as a young woman, along with a deeply rooted sense that *there has to be a way to help people before all hope is gone.* I filed that in my brain's to-do list.

There was nothing I could do for Dottie. She had long-standing diabetes and had been in this condition for 14 years. No arms, no legs! I know today that her fate was completely preventable. Did you know that every 30 seconds, somewhere in the world, someone loses a lower limb as a result of diabetes?

There were many amputees in the nursing homes that I worked in, almost all the result of diabetes. Did you know that having a toe, foot, or lower leg surgically removed is 10 times more likely in people with diabetes?

Many patients in these nursing homes would sit and cry, as they were often experiencing pain and were frightened, hungry, or in need of human companionship. But one thing was for sure, the amputees were by far the saddest people that I had ever met in my life.

Visions of them haunted me outside of work, and I shared their stories with my husband, Sam, who is a chiropractic physician. At the time, he was dedicated to his growing practice and helping to relieve the pain of many people. Sam understood my desire to help others in a meaningful (and nondrug) manner and devised a way to help people with their health *before* major challenges occurred. And so the idea of my nationally syndicated newspaper column, "Dear Pharmacist," sprang to life, with its first printing in 1999 in Florida.

I also offer my column to the public for free. Just sign up at my Web site: www.DearPharmacist.com. But the point here is that this chapter hits very close to home for me. It conjures up so many memories of the faces of patients (who became friends) that I used to know, those who had lost their hope for an independent life. I wish I could go back in time and teach them what I know today, about holistic options to maintain blood sugar and about ways to protect their feet against injury and infection. Amputation is a devastating complication of diabetes, so I want to teach you the best ways to take care of yourself and about the warning signs so you don't lose those precious limbs.

FOOT-PROTECTING FACTS

People with diabetes often experience nerve damage and loss of feeling in their feet. This is why they may not feel a tiny cut or sore until it becomes a blister or until it gets infected. If you have diabetic neuropathy (nerve damage due to diabetes), and you've ever had a diabetic foot ulcer, then your odds for developing more ulcers and dangerous foot complications are much greater, even if you are doing everything right and following the recommendations below.

Anyone who has diabetes can develop a foot ulcer. For whatever reasons, members of certain ethnic minorities are at higher risk for having some part of their foot or leg amputated. Native Americans are at highest risk, followed by African Americans (second), and Hispanics (third). Sadly, but not surprisingly, studies show that having complications of kidney disease triples the risk of having some part of the toe or leg amputated. People of Asian lineage were most likely to have a toe amputated than a foot or entire limb.

Additionally, older men and people who use insulin are at a higher risk of developing a foot ulcer. Regardless of whether you've found yourself in any of these categories, I've developed a list of the most important things you can do to protect your feet and reduce the likelihood of developing a diabetic foot ulcer or facing amputation. Some of these items may surprise you.

CONTROL BLOOD SUGAR. I took a personal survey with some of my patients at the community pharmacy one day and asked them what they thought was the most important thing they could do to avoid diabetic foot problems and amputation. They responded with all sorts of good answers, such as "wear shoes," "check for sores," "keep feet clean and dry," but no one, not one person in 17, replied "reduce blood sugar." But I think this is the *best* way to ensure that you don't get symptoms of peripheral neuropathy that prevent you from noticing dangerous foot problems that could lead to amputation.

All the research I can get my hands on points to keeping your hemoglobin A1c to below 6.5 or 7 percent as one of the factors you can control to prevent complications from diabetes that could lead to amputation. (Your A1c is a standard blood test that tells you how your blood sugar has been doing over the prior 3 months.)

Regulating your blood sugar also helps minimize the risk of kidney failure and vision loss. So from your head down to your toes, you have many reasons to do everything you can to keep blood sugar under control—avoid processed food, refined sugars, and oils, and take healthy supplements that work to help you

WATCH OUT FOR GANGRENE

Gangrene—the word for "dead tissue"—occurs when blood supply and nourishment is cut off from a part of the body. That part of the body dies even though it is still attached to you, hence the need for amputation. For many diabetics, gangrene occurs in the toe. Don't miss the first signs of gangrene; ignoring these can lead to amputation, so please pay attention.

It's shocking, but statistics show that worldwide, some 1 million amputations are performed every year, and about 85 percent of those are preventable. If you spot the beginnings of a problem, the sooner you get medical attention, the less likely it is you will have to endure amputation. You need to see a physician immediately if you develop *any* of these symptoms:

Brown or black discoloration of the skin	Numbness
Cold sensation	Shriveling up of skin
Fever	Swelling
Foul smell, pus, or oozing (signs of infection)	

regain total health. Picture poor Dottie, and keep that image of her in your head when you feel tempted to indulge in something you know you should not be eating. Am I coming on too strong? Good.

LOOK AT YOUR FEET EVERY DAY. You want to make sure that there are no sores, cuts, splinters, or ingrown toenails. Looking at your feet each day is important because neuropathy (nerve damage) may not allow you to fully feel the sensation of problems occurring with your feet. But your eyes won't lie.

It's important to check both of your feet, tops and bottoms and in between your toes, because you want to head off problems before infections and blisters occur. Keep your feet away from hot flames. Well, duh, that sounds so obvious, doesn't it? But I know plenty of people who put their feet by the cozy warm fireplace during the wintertime. If you don't feel sensation quite as well as you used to, they can get burned. It has happened.

When temperatures dip, people with diabetes have to deal with frostbite, whereas in the warmer regions, diabetics may find that their legs and feet get sunburned quickly. So, you see there are lots of reasons to give yourself a visual checkup daily.

You can carefully place a little handheld mirror on the floor and position your foot so you can view it better. If you have some problems with your vision, or trouble bending over to see your feet, you can ask a relative or friend to help you.

I tried to view the bottom of my feet just now and realized that I practically had to assume a yoga cobbler's-pose to see them clearly. With arthritis and poor flexibility, or advanced age, this could easily become one excuse that prevents you from daily visual inspections; my next suggestion takes away all of your excuses. Buy a telescoping mirror—one that is extendable. The good ones have 2× magnification, so you can really see the bottom of your feet more clearly.

MedPort is one company that produces this product to assist diabetics. The handle on it extends from 6 inches to 24 inches. The mirror portion is about 4 by 4 inches.

Check your feet every day to make sure there are no signs of infection or, heaven forbid, gangrene developing. This is the single most inexpensive and easy way to head off trouble, so do it! No excuses. Telescoping mirrors are available at some home medical supply stores, compounding pharmacies, and online at various Web sites, including www.lifesolutionplus.com.

TELL YOUR DOCTOR ABOUT FOOT PROBLEMS. *Any* changes to your feet, toes, legs, or hands could signal the beginning of neuropathy. Many people miss the early signs of foot infection, which could include itching, redness, swelling,

ARGININE HEALS WOUNDS

The amino acid arginine is fully discussed in Chapter 8. It's helpful because it punches up bloodflow throughout the body by revving up production of nitric oxide (NO). The NO pathway is one of the most influential in your body. Increasing NO in the body means you can help build more mitochondrial powerhouses in your cells and, therefore, unload fat and sugar from the tissues. Arginine, in appropriate dosages, can be extremely helpful for someone with diabetes and heart disease because it has a positive effect on the NO pathway and it activates PGC-1 alpha.

You may not realize how helpful arginine is when it comes to healing wounds. That extra bloodflow provides a steady supply of nutrient-rich blood and oxygen to a wound, which is helpful for healing. Arginine is a precursor to proline, a substance that ultimately gets converted to collagen, which creates beautiful skin. Arginine affects hormones that promote wound healing, and it is a precursor to polyamines, your cells' own building blocks that are critical in healing wounds. Arginine also seems to improve immune function, so this could reduce your risk of infection and complications to your wound.

and tingling. If you ignore any changes in sensation—such as pins and needles or numbness—then a foot problem could eventually progress to something worse, like amputation. See why it's so important to speak up?

KEEP 'EM SQUEAKY CLEAN. Hygiene is important, so give both of your feet a quick washing every day, even if you do not shower daily. You want to gently soak the feet for a few minutes using warm soapy water, not hot water. Test the temperature with your hands before you put your feet in, because nerve-damaged feet will not be able to tell whether the temperature is scalding. If your hands don't feel sensation very well either, then buy a set of infant spoons, the kind that change color when exposed to heat. Then you will know for sure whether the temperature is right for you. And if you like rubber duckies or other floatable fun thermometers, visit your local bath and linen shop.

Avoid soaking your feet too long in water, since waterlogged sores have a harder time healing. Plus, soaking your feet too long makes them dry out, and this increases your risk for cracking and sores. Pat your feet dry right away, and remember to dry between your toes. You don't want moisture in between the toes because this could cause athlete's foot, a type of fungal growth. Use a soft towel and don't rub them too hard. Just pat them dry.

SOFTEN CRACKED HEELS. Your skin can become dry when blood glucose

> ## SIMPLE SOLUTION FOR CRACKED HEELS
>
> Home remedies are inexpensive and often work as well as expensive moisturizing creams. A great way to soften cracked heels, which helps prevent foot infections, is to soak your feet in a warm-water foot bath with about 5 to 10 drops of eucalyptus essential oil. Soak for 5 to 10 minutes, then pat them dry. Next apply pure coconut oil, straight from the jar, to your dry, cracked heels, and dry the area. Coconut oil is a solid at room temperature but with the slightest warmth—like rubbing it in your hands or microwaving it for 5 seconds—it will turn into a liquid.

levels are high. Dry, cracked heels are common in people with diabetes, and you should apply some lotion daily to keep your feet soft and moist, not wet or sticky.

You can use inexpensive, nongreasy moisturizers such as Aquaphor or Eucerin. Other specialty products have soothing ingredients. One product that I like contains the amino acid L-arginine. In Chapter 8 you learned that arginine widens arteries and capillaries, increasing bloodflow. This formula is called DiabetiDerm Heel & Toe Cream. Another product, Diapedic Foot Cream (sold at www.amlab.com), contains vitamin C, bergamot, and eucalyptus oil among other soothing ingredients.

Another interesting one is Kerasal's Moisturizing Foot Ointment. It contains a form of aspirin (salicylic acid), which exfoliates your skin, along with an intensive moisturizer called urea. This is sold at many pharmacies and discount stores. The makers offer free samples on their Web site (www.kerasal.com). You can also use a soft pumice stone after showering to help soften corns and calluses.

WEAR SHOES. Walking around barefoot is not an option. Always wear shoes or slippers, even if you are just strolling out to get the mail or to the pool, or walking on the beach. I think it's very important that you wear sneakers or closed shoes rather than open-toe sandals or flip-flops. Also, you should wear socks, because not wearing them could lead to blisters from too much rubbing against your shoe, and blisters can lead to infections. Today's styles offer a wide variety of shoes that look good and protect your feet. See "Get Free Shoes" on the opposite page for information about getting free shoes if you are diabetic.

If your shoes don't fit you well, even the slightest friction can cause a blister, sore, or corn that may become infected and possibly lead to amputation. Unfor-

GET FREE SHOES

Third-party insurers are concerned about keeping diabetic feet from going bad, so more and more insurance companies—including Medicare, some state Medicaid programs, and other insurers—are now paying for one pair of special, customized shoes for diabetics per year. And the shoes don't look like your grandma's ugly old clogs. Shoe lovers can take pride in the fact that many stylish shoes are part of the deal. A footwear specialist can fit you properly too, so some of these shoes can even be customized.

Preventing foot problems is the most important thing you can do to avoid complications from diabetes (in addition to lowering your sugar levels), because small problems often lead to more serious foot problems.

Your foot doctor will carefully size and fit your foot to a shoe that will exactly fit your feet. Look at your insurance card and call the phone number on it. A representative can tell you if you qualify for free shoes.

tunately, foot blisters, sores, and corns are all too common in people with diabetes. So when I ask you to invest in good shoes, my intention is to protect your precious toes, feet, and legs.

BREAK IN NEW SHOES GRADUALLY. When you buy new shoes, break them in slowly by wearing them for short periods instead of wearing them until your feet hurt or you get a blister. Check the insides of your shoes for damage on a regular basis. Rough edges can be abrasive on your delicate skin.

If you are prone to heel pain, you are better off wearing a half size up rather than a half size too small. Also, consider shoe inserts sold at pharmacies nationwide. They add comfort and a squishiness to your step that might make walking more enjoyable. Podiatrists and some chiropractors know how to fit you for professional orthotics.

MOVE AROUND. If you're able to, please take up yoga, tai chi, swimming, walking, or ballroom dance. These types of minimal-impact exercises help increase circulation and get the blood flowing to your feet. The more circulation down there, the more oxygen and nutrients that reach your feet, which helps reduce your risk for wounds. Besides all that, mild exercise helps you manage weight and improves heart function.

TAKE YOUR FEET TO THE DOCTOR. Get corns, calluses, bunions, and hammertoes fixed. See a good podiatrist to help you take better care of your feet and address these types of issues. Podiatrists are trained to find the beginnings of diabetic foot ulcers, where other doctors may overlook the initial warning symptoms. Don't use over-the-counter remedies or medicines for corns and calluses unless your podiatrist tells you to, because some people experience more problems from the medicine. Don't try to cut or trim your corns or calluses, either. Taking care of your feet *prevents* problems, which, as you know, is much easier than trying to fix problems.

DO FOOT MASSAGE OR REFLEXOLOGY. Because diabetes causes your blood flow to slow down, your feet don't get as many nutrients or as much oxygen as normal, healthy feet do. So if you do get a sore or wound on your foot, it can take a long time for it to heal. Add in some neuropathy, and you have the makings of a lot of discomfort and problems in the diabetic foot.

The long-term solution to improving circulation throughout the body is to do aerobic exercise, meaning any exercise that causes your heart to beat faster than normal and increases your breathing. This gets more and more oxygen moving through your body via your blood. The short-term way to improve circulation in your feet is by rubbing them. It moves the blood around, and it feels great. You can do it yourself or trade the joy with a loved one.

You can also have a foot massage done professionally by a massage therapist. I believe that a foot massage or a qualified reflexology treatment could be an extremely important part of the diabetic care program. It's natural and holistic, and it feels good.

USE CAUTION WITH PEDICURES. Many people have asked me whether I recommend pedicures for diabetic feet. There is a lot of debate in the community because some salons do not cleanse their tools properly between clients, and they may nick or cut you by accident if they are not paying attention. If you are certain that your salon uses professionally licensed and experienced technicians (who are gentle!), then yes, I think a pedicure is nice.

Ask to see the salon's certification and make sure it's current. A good pedicurist could be the first person to spot a suspicious area on the bottom of the foot of someone with diabetes, as it's hard to see the bottom of your feet. (But you will be using the telescoping mirror I mentioned earlier, so I'm not going to worry.)

Make sure the salon's pedicure tools are properly sanitized and disinfected, or bring your own clean tools to the salon. Fine salons do not mind this, and in fact encourage it. Pedicures are relaxing, and it gets blood circulating to your lower legs and feet. That feeds them with what they are starving for—blood with lots of oxygen in it.

KEEP THEM COOL. Keep your feel properly ventilated so moisture doesn't build up and lead to bacterial or fungal infection. You can do this by wearing ventilated shoes or by airing your feet during restful periods of the day.

BE CAREFUL WHEN TRIMMING TOENAILS. Cut them straight across and smoothly. If necessary, file them with a gentle nail file. Resist the urge to cut into the corners of your toenails, because this could create a cut or sore that leads to infection (and possibly eventual amputation). If your toenails are ingrown, or if they are thick and yellow, it would be best if your podiatrist cuts them.

HOW TO CARE FOR A WOUND

Despite your very best efforts to protect your feet from injury, from time to time you may very well have to deal with cuts and small wounds. What is the best way to treat these?

For very small or basic wounds, wash them with normal saline, which is just a form of sodium chloride (table salt) in water that matches the saltiness of our normal bodily fluids. You find normal saline in many contact lens or nasal irrigation solutions and, of course, in the first-aid department at any pharmacy. Packages say Normal Saline on them. Then apply a topical antimicrobial cream or ointment, such as Neosporin ointment, triple antibiotic ointment, or bacitracin ointment. This will help to speed healing and prevent infection.

Apply the cream or ointment two or three times daily. You don't want to keep the wound constantly moist, though, or a scab will have a harder time forming. If a wound is clean, it will heal faster under the scab, so don't pick at it. But if it's dirty, you are more likely to develop an infection. You can apply a cotton gauze bandage or Band-Aid bandage. If what began as a minor cut or sore turns ugly or does not start to heal within a couple of days, see your physician.

What about foot ulcers? Foot ulcers absolutely require professional care, so let's delve deeper.

First and foremost: See a podiatrist or your primary care physician if you have any cut or wound on your foot that is not healing. There are some critical factors involved in the appropriate treatment of a diabetic foot ulcer, so don't delay. Make an appointment and go, even if you are not sure whether there is a problem. If you're not sure, when it comes to a diabetic foot, there's a problem!

Let your doctor determine whether the foot ulcer is infected. Noninfected foot ulcers can usually be treated without surgery. Even small ulcers on the foot need to be treated vigilantly. As your doctor will tell you, the goal is to prevent infection,

> ## SEEK TREATMENT FOR SKIN AILMENTS
> Healthy skin patches itself up rather quickly. If you notice a cut, sore, wound, or blister that does not begin to heal after a couple of days of treatment, please consult your doctor or pharmacist.

so it must be kept clean; debridement may be necessary. Debridement means freeing the area of dead skin and tissue. It is not comfortable, but it must be done.

Your doctor may want you to begin a course of antibiotics, and may apply medications or other dressings to the ulcer. Pressure must be taken off the ulcerated area; this is called off-loading and is accomplished with a crutch, walker, brace, special footgear, or wheelchair.

NUTRIENTS TO KEEP YOUR SKIN HEALTHY

When it comes to keeping your feet healthy, one of the most important preventives is actually what you put in your mouth. A number of nutrients and herbs can help protect your skin.

Vitamin C

Did you know that you need vitamin C to make collagen, a substance that helps you build strong bones and have beautiful skin?

Foods rich in vitamin C include citrus fruits, camu camu berries, and green vegetables.

HOW TO SUPPLEMENT WITH VITAMIN C. Look for natural vitamin C brands. Two good brands that I've tried include BlueBonnet's Buffered Vitamin C Plus Citrus Bioflavonoids and Solgar's Citrus Bioflavonoid Complex. There are others, but these brands are sugar-free, gluten-free, and kosher, and they contain a powerful blend of bioflavonoids derived from fresh fruit. Both are sold at most health food stores. In my home, I supplement with the herb Camu Camu. I use either Royal Camu by Whole World Botanicals or Camu Camu by Bright Earth Foods. These are powders and you mix them with water.

DRUG MUGGERS OF VITAMIN C. Drugs that may deplete vitamin C in your body (and therefore contribute to slower wound healing) include aspirin; estrogen-

---

SKIN-SAVING TEA

Here's a quick and inexpensive way to drink tea that saves your skin. You will need regular red rooibos tea, also known as African Red Bush tea. You will also need hibiscus herbal tea (yes, hibiscus as in the flower). Hibiscus is also known as the sabdariffa flower, and purified teas are sold at health food stores, fine tea shops, and online. Neither of these teas contains caffeine, so don't worry about a jolt to your system. Mix them together and steep.

Red rooibos tea is traditionally known for its ability to improve blood-flow, something you need for healthy skin all over. The hibiscus is very rich in vitamin C and healing flavonoids. It is useful in powering up your immune system, and the bright red tea may very well lower your blood pressure, too.

Why do I think hibiscus combined with rooibos is so good? Because after you drink this delicious tea, you can pull the hibiscus tea bag out and apply the (cooled-down) tea bag directly to your skin. It is known to soothe dry, irritated skin and could help your cracked heels.

---

containing drugs; diuretics, such as furosemide and hydrochlorothiazide; and most anti-inflammatory drugs, such as ibuprofen, naproxen, and diclofenac. Cigarettes are also muggers of vitamin C.

CAUTION. You are getting too much vitamin C if you start to develop stomach upset, gas, or bloating. Taking 200 to 600 milligrams per day is usually okay, but some people take 3,000 to 6,000 per day. That's the point where you're getting too much.

Beta-Carotene

A precursor to vitamin A, beta-carotene is often associated with eye health, but it is also a powerful skin protectant. It's found in many antiaging creams because it reduces fine lines and helps cleanse the skin of damaging free radicals. Some experts maintain that it boosts fertility and improves the body's ability to stave off infections.

Foods rich in beta-carotene include fruits and vegetables that are orange or orangey red, such as carrots, yams, apricots, winter squash, pumpkin, cantaloupe, and mangoes. Dark green leafy vegetables, such as broccoli, kale, collard greens, spinach, and leaf lettuce are also good sources. There are more mentioned earlier in Chapter 7.

HOW TO SUPPLEMENT WITH BETA-CAROTENE. Take about 5 to 15 milligrams (8,000 to 25,000 IU) per day. Pregnant women should limit their dosage to 10,000 IU per day.

CAUTION. It's true that excessive amounts of vitamin A in supplement form can be toxic, but beta-carotene is safer, and easier for your body to metabolize. Buy only natural forms of beta-carotene, which will be identified on the label. Look for phrases that say "from *D. salina*," "from an algae source," "natural beta-carotene," or "from a palm source."

Vitamin E

An antioxidant, vitamin E is well known for its antiaging effects on the skin. You will find vitamin E in thousands of moisturizers, eye creams, and skin care products. It is thought to minimize scarring, reduce the risk for skin cancer, and also regulate vitamin A, another skin-protecting nutrient.

Good food sources of vitamin E include walnuts, almonds, seeds, wheat germ oil, leafy greens, and egg yolks.

HOW TO SUPPLEMENT WITH VITAMIN E. Always buy natural vitamin E because it is easier to absorb, and it works better in your body. It's designated as d-alpha tocopherol. The synthetic forms, which don't work as well, are designated dL-alpha tocopherol. The best brands actually say *natural* on them and combine the entire family of vitamin E, which consists of four different tocopherols and four different tocotrienols. If you want this type of vitamin E, look for "mixed" tocopherols or "full spectrum" on the label. Good products include Full Spectrum E with Tocotrienols by Swanson, or New Chapter E Food Complex, which contains vitamin E along with anti-inflammatory ginger, turmeric, and blueberry extract and several other powerful antioxidants. This is good for your feet and for your whole body!

DRUG MUGGERS OF VITAMIN E. Fat blockers such as Alli and Xenical, and kidney bean starch blockers and also statin cholesterol drugs.

CAUTION. Taking synthetic forms of vitamin E is unhealthy because they tax your liver to convert the nutrient into something more usable. Generally speaking, when you take a vitamin or mineral, you want it to be as close to your own body as possible. Synthetic vitamins are not how nature makes them, and your body has trouble converting them to an active, usable form. You want to get natural vitamin E only, preferably mixed or full spectrum. Taking excessive amounts of vitamin E can cause a relative depletion in other fat-soluble nutrients, such as coenzyme Q10, vitamin D, and vitamin A. So don't overdo it.

Selenium

The mineral selenium is also an antioxidant. It works well on its own, but it works even greater with its best buddy, vitamin E. Some research shows that people who are selenium deficient and who take selenium in supplement form may reduce their risk for developing lung, colon, rectal, and prostate cancer. One such study by researchers at the Roswell Park Cancer Institute in Buffalo, New York, was published in the journal *Nutrition and Cancer*. The Nutritional Prevention of Cancer study of 1,312 people at high risk for skin cancer found that those given 200 micrograms of selenium were at a lower risk of cancer of these organs.

Another study, this one with 424 participants, reported an overall 25 percent decrease in the occurrence of all cancers with 200 micrograms of selenium supplementation.

Selenium can rev up thyroid production in the human body, and so it helps people who have hypothyroidism—Hashimoto's or Graves' disease. As you know, a poorly functional thyroid gland (low thyroid hormone) is one contributing factor in the development of diabetes. Low thyroid also means slower wound healing.

Selenium is a strong free-radical scavenger, so it protects the skin from these damaging bullets aimed at destroying it. Selenium ramps up production of glutathione, one of your most powerful free-radical scavengers. So with selenium, you get double your money, in terms of protection against harmful toxins.

Foods rich in selenium include Brazil nuts. They are an incredibly dense natural source of selenium because 1 ounce gives you about 540 micrograms. Other food sources include seafood, meat, turkey, rice, and oatmeal.

HOW TO SUPPLEMENT WITH SELENIUM. The best form is selenocysteine or selenomethionate. Take about 50 to 200 micrograms per day.

DRUG MUGGERS OF SELENIUM. Steroids; estrogen-containing drugs, such as hormone replacement therapy and birth control pills; sulfa antibiotics; and some sulfa-based diabetic medications, such as sulfonylureas.

CAUTION. Excessive amounts of selenium may cause heart palpitations gastrointestinal upset, hair loss, garlic breath, white blotchy nails, and fatigue.

Zinc

The antioxidant mineral zinc is best known for its ability to improve male sexual health by protecting the prostate gland. But zinc is incredibly important to the skin as well because you need it to make collagen, a substance that helps heal wounds. A deficiency in zinc could spell a lot of trouble in the form of delayed wound healing and acne breakouts. Oral zinc supplements might help you improve overall skin tone and heal bedsores, skin ulcers, surgical incisions, burns, and other minor skin irritations. The best part is that zinc will help drive the production of thyroid hormone, just as selenium does, and so it could also improve your fat-burning capabilities and energy reserves.

Food sources rich in zinc include seafood, particularly oysters and shellfish; beef; and nuts. It is also found in dairy products, pumpkin seeds, and various green vegetables.

HOW TO SUPPLEMENT WITH ZINC. Try zinc lozenges, one daily. They are flavored to mask the somewhat metallic taste of zinc, and good brands do not contain sugar or HFCS.

DRUG MUGGERS OF ZINC. Acid-blocking drugs used for ulcers and reflux, antacids, blood pressure pills that belong to the angiotensin-converting enzyme inhibitor class (captopril, lisinopril, enalapril), statins, and diuretics (water pills).

CAUTION. It's best to take zinc on a full stomach. Some people experience symptoms of nausea and vomiting when they take it on an empty stomach. You are getting too much zinc if you develop an upset stomach, diarrhea, cramps, or a metallic taste in your mouth. Taking excessive amounts of zinc will cause a tilt in your delicate mineral balance and may lead to a relative copper deficiency, as zinc and copper have to stay in balance with one another.

Silica

When talking about the skin, it's impossible not to bring up silica, which is found in every skin cell of your body. And remember, the skin is the largest organ of the body (no matter what the guys say). Silica is different from silicone, which is used in breast implants. Silica is natural, and remarkably, the human body contains about 7 grams of silica, which is quite a bit.

Silica is essential to your body's daily chemical actions and reactions. Silica maintains the strength of your pipeline (your blood vessels), so it's a great con-

MOTHER NATURE'S FIRST-AID KIT

If you have diabetes, you will benefit from having a few items in your first-aid kit. I've made a list of natural and conventional treatments in case you have a cut and want to treat it before it becomes a complication. Here's what you need to have:

CONVENTIONAL	NATURAL ALTERNATIVE
Hydrogen peroxide	Normal saline
Antifungal cream (Lotrisone, Tinactin, Micatin)	Grapefruit seed oil
Antimicrobial ointment (Neosporin, bacitracin)	Tea tree or tamanu oil
Hydrocortisone steroid cream (for itching/redness)	Florasone (natural nonsteroid)
Eucerin, Aquaphor	Aloe vera or shea butter
Anti-itch creams	Lavender essential oil
Mederma (prevent scarring)	Fresh *Aloe vera* (from the plant)
Metal foot scraper	Pumice stone
Antibacterial soap	Geranium soap

sideration for people with heart disease. Plus, silica keeps your skin and hair looking more youthful. If you have very dry hair, you could be deficient in this mineral. Silica helps maintain the integrity of the skin, so I believe it could speed wound healing. If you have hemorrhoids, it could help you too.

Food sources rich in silica include beets, leafy vegetables, and brown rice, but these are not going to be enough to replenish a deficiency of silica.

HOW TO SUPPLEMENT WITH SILICA. If you buy Cellfood's liquid silica you can supplement with it orally, and also squirt some on a cotton pad to apply to any areas that are painful (like hemorrhoids). Follow label directions. Supplements that contain horsetail (*Equisetum arvense*) are also a rich source of silica. Dosage is about 1,000 milligrams up to three times daily.

DRUG MUGGERS OF SILICA. This is not established.

CAUTION. Silica acts a bit like a diuretic, so ask your doctor if silica is right for you and whether you need any special monitoring of your electrolytes, especially potassium. Silica supplements are not recommended for people who take lithium or other drugs that are affected by diuretics. Also, if you happen to buy horsetail extract, make sure it says *Equisetum arvense* on the label, not its highly toxic relative, the marsh horsetail called *Equisetum palustre*.

OVER-THE-COUNTER AIDS TO RELIEVE MINOR SKIN IRRITATIONS

Sometimes we get into things we shouldn't, such as poison ivy or thorns. We can also develop allergic reactions to medications, food, or bites and stings of insects, such as mosquitoes, bees, wasps, and other flying creatures that carry nasty stuff to inject into us. It's inevitable that you will touch something, eat something, or get into something that causes your skin to become irritated. When that happens, it may help you to have the following list so that you will know your options. These products do not require a prescription. They are easily found at your local pharmacy or supermarket. You can count on these to short-circuit some of the misery caused by minor skin irritations, cuts, scrapes, and bites.

AVEENO BATH. Imagine soaking in oatmeal (but don't add blueberries and cream). The packets of natural colloidal oatmeal are intended to be sprinkled into your bath water so you can soak your irritations away. This soak helps itchy skin, rashes, eczema, insect bites, and poison ivy/oak or sumac.

CALAMINE. This is the pink lotion traditionally used for chicken pox and poison ivy lesions. It's a skin protectant that dries oozing and weeping sores, while relieving minor pain and itching. The Calamine Plus version is stronger because it contains pramoxine, a substance that numbs irritations, along with the calamine. Remember, though, if you have a skin irritation that becomes infected, see your doctor.

HYDROCORTISONE. There are dozens of creams, ointments, sprays, and roll-on products containing this steroid, which helps control itching, redness, and inflammation associated with skin rashes, eczema, psoriasis, bug bites, poison ivy, and seborrheic dermatitis.

DOMEBORO. This is powdered aluminum that you mix with water to make a compress, dressing, or soak. It acts as an astringent on the skin and can soothe skin rashes, bug bites, athlete's foot, or irritation from poison ivy, poison oak, or poison sumac.

SARNA SENSITIVE. This lotion contains pramoxine, a substance that basically numbs irritations and relieves itching for minor skin irritations. Sarna's original version is very cooling because it contains menthol and camphor.

BEDSORES ARE BAD

Bedsores, also known as pressure sores, pressure ulcers, or decubitus ulcers, develop when the weight of your body or bone squeezes your skin against the surface of the bed. This is what happened with poor Dottie, the woman I mentioned at the beginning of this chapter who lost both her arms and legs because of complications from diabetes.

Bedsores usually happen to people who are bedridden or wheelchair bound, and they occur on the tailbone, hips, shoulder blades, heels, elbows, and other weight-bearing parts of the body where there are bones and very little skin. Sometimes a sore forms within hours, sometimes days.

I've seen my share of bedsores because I worked in nursing homes for many years, and sadly about 15 to 20 percent of people in long-term care facilities develop these during their stay. This statistic makes me so angry! If this happens to you or to someone you love in a nursing home, speak up immediately, as by law, the staff is supposed to be trained to prevent these.

Some doctors near Lake Como in Italy looked at whether it was helpful to give older people with pressure sores some extra nutrition consisting of a formula enriched with protein, arginine, zinc, and vitamin C. I'm not surprised to hear that they saw their patients heal more quickly than did the patients on a nonenriched nutrition formula. Their work was published in the June 2009 issue of the *Journal of the American Geriatrics Society.*

Having poor circulation—and people with diabetes have poor circulation—increases your risk for these awful skin ulcers. So do numbness, neuropathy, and excessive moisture or perspiration.

Bedsores are dangerous and involve your whole body. The sore may begin as a reddened, sensitive patch of skin and then eventually forms an open sore or ulcer that digs its way deeper into your muscle or bone. If left untreated, a bedsore may lead to cellulitis or a chronic infection. They are dangerous because the wound may lead to death of your tissue—gangrene.

The best way to avoid them is to move around as much as you can, and to keep your blood flowing. If you are bedridden, an egg crate mattress may help take the pressure off. Also, splints or special cushions help redistribute your weight more evenly. This will help prevent the pressure from causing your skin to break in one isolated spot. Medical supply stores and some compound pharmacies may carry specially designed pads or anatomically shaped cushions. It's best to prevent pressure ulcers, of course, so frequently inspect the skin of anyone you love who is bedridden.

PART 5

MOVING BEYOND DIABETES: YOUR PATH TO FULL RECOVERY

12 Diabetes without Drugs: Steps 1, 2, and 3

I put my heart and soul into this book, and I believe that you will make the necessary changes in your life to finish strong. If you are like most people diagnosed with diabetes or prediabetes, you have probably already jumped on the bandwagon of prescription medications in an effort to reduce your blood sugar. People with diabetes are usually made aware of (and prescribed) countless medications that come with hefty price tags. And I don't just mean the out-of-pocket expense. I'm referring to the potential side effects and drug-mugging effects that can occur with pharmaceuticals.

It's true that medications can effectively bring down blood sugar, and I've written an entire chapter on that subject (see Chapter 5). But as effective as they are, they still have shortfalls. For instance, medications do not repair your beta cells, the cells in your pancreas that make insulin, nor do they help you regenerate healthy new beta cells.

Diabetic medications are like a missile aimed at one thing—bringing blood sugar down. Fine, but Mother Nature's medicine cabinet actually gives us plants that repair and regenerate beta cells. If that's a surprise, hold on, because many of the healthy options I will share with you in this chapter have received serious scientific study and have proven themselves with good results. There's a good chance you've never heard about any of this from your physician.

Doctors mean well. After all, their training as medical doctors is designed to focus on disease, not on wellness. Western physicians are not taught in medical school about the many natural supplements, spices, foods, and superfoods that work remarkably well and are capable of doing amazing things prescription medicines are not capable of. Unfortunately, they also get tangled up in the perpetual media spin Big Pharma presents—meaning they have found the Midas touch and whatever they touch turns to gold.

Doctors are taught about drugs, drugs, drugs at seminars, lectures, medical journals, drug rep visits, and even on their TV at home. They get busy taking care of people, and they do what they were trained to do—treat the disease, rather than the person. It's a disease-care, not a healthcare, system. That's why you have sought out my book. Because you know I can help you. By incorporating natural supplements into a diabetes-friendly diet, you are increasing the likelihood for a longer, more physically comfortable life.

In this and the next two chapters, I will give you my 5-step plan for wellness.

STEP 1: DRINK GREEN DRINKS

Green drink is just another name for a super-cool superfood. And superfood is the term that some people use to describe a food that has a high content of phytonutrients (plant-based nutrients like beta-carotene, vitamin C, and so forth). As part of my natural plan for wellness, I've placed green drinks at the very top of my list. Why? *If you only do ONE thing, do this: Drink a green drink every day.*

Don't get excited; I'm not talking about margarita cocktails. I'm referring to the healthy sort of greens, the powdered supplements that you can buy at any health food store and online. Ideally, you could juice your own organic produce every morning. That would be my preference. However, I know real life sets in, and I know that most folks prefer a more convenient, quicker option. It's easier to mix some powder into a glass of water and instantly create a nutrition-packed drink.

These drinks are so nutrition packed that if you make this a daily habit and change nothing else, I still believe you will be able to enjoy better health in many ways. This is the number-one general health tonic that gives your body what it has been craving—essential vitamins, minerals, amino acids, enzymes, chlorophyll, micronutrients, and antioxidants.

Green drinks provide pretty much a one-two punch when it comes to cancer-proofing your pancreas (and all the rest of you, for that matter) and dousing all those rampant inflammatory chemicals that are sickening you. Ah, I've exhaled a sigh of satisfaction in telling you this because I honestly feel that high-quality green drinks offer you superb antioxidants, such as superoxide dismutase (SOD), one of the most powerful free-radical scavengers known to humankind.

If you honestly want to change your life and reverse the effects of diabetes, I think starting with greens is the best way to go. These types of drinks (assuming you have a high-quality brand) provide exponentially more nutrition than your Centrum and One-A-Day vitamins put together!

Drinking greens also provides an easy way to get your daily servings of fruits and vegetables. There's a good chance you are not getting your recommended

---

ARE YOU EATING ENOUGH VEGGIES?

Just because I'm advocating green drinks doesn't mean you're off the hook for fruits and veggies. You still need to make sure you're getting adequate amounts of whole, organic produce in your diet. A nifty new website from the Centers for Disease Control and Prevention and National Institutes of Health—www.fruitsandveggiesmatter.gov features a cool calculator that asks you your age, sex, and activity level and calculates your recommended daily requirements. On the basis of the information I put in, my recommended amounts are 2 cups of fruit and 2.5 cups of vegetables a day. They even tell you how to measure servings and cups of fruits and veggies.

---

amounts per day. Most people don't. So green drinks are a convenient way to deliver powerful antioxidants and phytochemicals that have been proven to support good health.

I believe these drinks are really the way to go. When your well-intended diabetes educator asks why, mention that I said that it douses inflammation and zaps free radicals. If they have a better natural idea, I'm all eyes and ears. Is this just me touting a supplement I sell? Absolutely not—I do *not* sell supplements. I just believe in their dense nutrition, and I've talked to enough people who have reversed deadly (even terminal) diseases using them.

I've also read enough scientific literature regarding the ingredients in these drinks to know that I will never let another day go by without drinking a high-quality brand of green drink. You can try it yourself for a month and see how you respond. When you go back for your routine lab work after a few months, everyone should be amazed at how you are recovering. I want you to take a look at what nutritional researchers have found inside some of the best green drinks on the market.

Spirulina

Spirulina is a single-celled blue-green algae that has been around for eons. If you viewed it with a microscope, you would see the beautiful bright blue-green spirals for which it is named. The green comes from chlorophyll, the blue color from an exotic pigment called phycocyanin, which is known to help stimulate the creation of more stem cells.

Spirulina is a rich source of protein—the highest concentration of protein found in any food, ranking in at 53 to 65 percent protein, and it's almost twice as easily absorbed as the protein found in beef. Spirulina is an incredible source of minerals, which are needed for pancreatic health and insulin sensitivity.

Spirulina is one supplement that gives you lots of potassium, calcium, chromium, iron, copper, zinc, magnesium, manganese, selenium, sodium, and phosphorus. It also has various powerful carotenoids, including beta-carotene, and lots of B vitamins, as well as vitamins E and K. The full spectrum of amino acids in spirulina also helps produce brain chemicals that ease depression.

Spirulina contains as much iron as red meat, and it also is loaded with eye-loving antioxidants, such as beta-carotene and zeaxanthin. It contains SOD, an important enzyme and strong antioxidant. After mother's milk, spirulina is the next-best source of gamma linolenic acid (GLA). GLA is an important essential fatty acid in your skin, and it helps reduce inflammation.

Spirulina also contains the mineral sulfur, which is important for your pancreas, liver, and immune system. Discerning taste buds easily detect the sulfur-like taste in the powdered supplements, but that just means your brand has sulfur-bearing amino acids, which help rid you of poisons in the body. It's okay.

Try Spirulina Pacifica supplements by Nutrex-Hawaii in 500 mg tablets; take 3 tablets twice daily to equal 3,000 mg (or 3 grams). Many vegetarians, athletes, or sufferers of various conditions take much more—up to 10 grams per day—but dosages like this should be approved by your healthcare provider. Spirulina is totally natural and normally does not cause any problem, even with higher dosages.

Spirulina has received a good deal of attention from research scientists. An article that appeared in the peer-reviewed journal *Current Pharmaceutical Biotechnology* in 2008 discussed the use of spirulina in managing people's health. In fact the summary (known as the abstract) was so off-the-charts positive about spirulina that I must quote most of it for you here.

Spirulina is a photosynthetic, filamentous, spiral-shaped, and multicellular edible microbe. It is nature's richest and most complete source of nutrition. Spirulina has a unique blend of nutrients that no single source can offer. The algae contains a wide spectrum of prophylactic and therapeutic nutrients that include B-complex vitamins, minerals, proteins, gamma-linolenic acid, and the super antioxidants, such as beta-carotene, vitamin E, trace elements, and a number of unexplored bioactive compounds. Because of its apparent ability to stimulate whole human physiology, spirulina exhibits therapeutic functions such as antioxidant, antibacterial, antiviral, anti-cancer, anti-inflammatory, antiallergic, and antidiabetic, plus a plethora of additional beneficial functions. Spirulina consumption appears to promote the growth of intestinal micro flora as well.

See? This is the real thing!

In an article published in the same journal in 2005, research scientists at Bundelkhand University in Jhansi, India, wrote: "Preparations (of spirulina) have been found to be active against several enveloped viruses including herpes virus, cytomegalovirus, influenza virus and HIV." Just so you know, an enveloped virus is one that has a tough, fatty outer covering so these type of virii are difficult to kill. These scientists wrote that spirulina could even stop cancer from spreading, protect tissues, and reduce toxins in the liver, kidneys, and testes because of it's antioxidant properties.

Chlorella Pyrenoidosa

Chlorella is another green superfood that supports your entire body and reduces blood sugar. Clorella is a single-celled algae that grows in the water just like spirulina. It gets its name from its high content of chlorophyll (a green plant pigment).

According to a study published in the *Journal of Medicinal Food*, the intake of chlorella was beneficial to study participants who were followed for a 16-week period. By affecting fat metabolism and insulin signaling pathways, chlorella caused a noticeable reduction in body fat percentage, serum total cholesterol, and fasting blood glucose levels. Amazing that this inexpensive green supplement (Chlorella) was able to lower blood sugar and positively affect major biochemical pathways in the body. Other research with chlorella has suggested antitumor effects and benefits for people with digestive disorders including ulcerative colitis. Not too shabby for being green. The brand used in this study was Sun Chlorella.

These drinks are the best way to cleanse the bowels and the entire digestive tract and to eliminate toxins from the liver and colon. What exactly are these supplements cleaning out? Lots of junk, such as pesticides, herbicides, alcohol from your liver, polychlorbiphenyls (PCBs), and heavy metals, such as cadmium, arsenic, lead, and mercury. Chlorophyll also can help eliminate digestive odors and improve immune function.

Barley Grass

Leaves of the barley plant have been used since the time of Ancient Egypt. They are bright green and look just like grass. The young shoots contain the highest amounts of nutrition and are high in vitamins C, E, and B_{12}, minerals, and healing phytochemicals.

Barley grass is known for is SOD, a powerful free-radical scavenger that may protect against cancer, inflammatory diseases, and even pancreatitis. I wouldn't make that kind of claim without seeing research that backs it up.

In 1998 scientists from Bucharest published an article in *Roumanian Archives of Microbiology & Immunology* detailing some important findings: By 1998, the researchers noted, other studies had already established that reactive oxygen species play an important role in reducing the presence of some of the chemicals that cause inflammation (cytokines such as tumor necrosis factor alpha). As you know, inflammation has been implicated in everything from arthritis to heart disease, as well as disease of the gastrointestinal tract. The scientists wrote that, on the basis of these findings and research showing that "many plant extracts contain substances with antioxidant properties," they examined the anti-inflammatory action of a green barley extract, commercially available as Natural SOD.

They concluded that Natural SOD works against inflammation. They also prepared and tested a purified green barley extract and concluded the extract's antioxidant and anti-inflammatory properties could qualify it as an efficient drug in the treatment of rheumatoid arthritis.

Other research on barley grass has uncovered some powerful chemicals that can help lower cholesterol, reduce inflammation, and protect against ulcers in the gut.

Researchers in Taiwan, for example, published a study that looked at 40 patients, both smokers and nonsmokers, with high LDL (low-density lipoprotein, the "bad" kind of cholesterol). All 40 people were given 15 grams of young barley leaf extract daily or a different herb (adlay) once a day for 4 weeks. The researchers found both the barley leaf extract and the other herb had positive action, but the barley leaf extract "had a stronger antioxidative effect on the prevention of LDL." They also found this antioxidant effect was even stronger for nonsmokers than for smokers. Their conclusion was supplementation with barley leaf could decrease blood fats and inhibit LDL oxidation in both smokers and nonsmokers. Pretty amazing stuff, and so sad it is not common knowledge in Western medicine.

In barley the gluten is in the stalk and head of the plant. In fact, I believe that's why the leaves are used—they are gluten-free. But if you are very sensitive to gluten, barley-containing green drinks may not be right for you. Read the label or track symptoms.

Taking Action

So how does all this translate into an action step you can take? It's easy. You can take spirulina on its own, chlorella on its own, or barley grass on its own. Often, green drink supplements contain a variety of these greens and combine them into one formula. That's fine, too. There are dozens of green supplement products available. Flavor differs greatly, and so does nutritional content.

What follows is an overview of just some of the other powerful healing ingredients included in commercial green drinks in addition to spirulina, chlorella, and barley grass. It will be helpful to review these before making your product selection.

PLANT EXTRACTS. These are from plants and fruits thought to contain powerful anticancer chemicals. Sometimes the label will show you exactly which extracts are included in the formula. For example, you might see the following on the label: Blueberry, pomegranate, broccoli, cherry, grape seed, green tea, cranberry, or tomato. The benefits of all these could fill a book. There are scads of research papers written about each of these substances.

In 2004, for example, scientists at Creighton University Medical Center in Omaha, Nebraska, published an article in *Biochemistry* about the benefits of six berry extracts: wild blueberry, bilberry, cranberry, elderberry, raspberry seeds, and strawberry. They looked at the extracts in terms of antioxidant efficacy and as compounds to prevent tumor growth. The scientists wrote: "Edible berry anthocyanins possess a broad spectrum of therapeutic and anticarcinogenic properties. Berries are rich in anthocyanins, compounds that provide pigmentation to fruits and serve as natural antioxidants." They also noted that many studies published earlier have shown "berry anthocyanins are beneficial in reducing age-associated oxidative stress, as well as in improving neuronal and cognitive brain function."

Other studies have found that green tea and broccoli extracts exhibit anticancer action, blueberry extract can protect the eyes, pomegranate protects the heart, and tomato protects the prostate.

This kind of information is all over the medical literature. It still escapes me why this information isn't more in the mainstream in America.

DIGESTIVE ENZYMES. These include amylase, lipase, and protease. They help you digest your meals and break them down into smaller particles, easing the burden on your pancreas, liver, and spleen. These enzymes as well as proteolytic enzymes, help your body in other ways by reducing allergies, inflammation, and pain-causing chemicals, such as bradykinins and prostaglandins.

Two plant-derived proteolytic enzymes in high-quality greens include bromelain (from pineapple) and papain (from papaya), both of which have been found to reduce pain and inflammation and aid digestion.

Scientists in Europe and Asia are far ahead of us here in the United States when it comes to studying and applying information on natural remedies. Scientists at University Hospital in Zürich, Switzerland, for example, published an article in 2001 in *BioDrugs* called "Therapy with Proteolytic Enzymes in Rheumatic Disorders." The enzymes they studied included bromelain and papain. They concluded, on the basis of both experiments and clinical data, that enzyme therapy can help individuals with rheumatic illness.

Earlier, in 1999, researchers in Germany published an article in German (in the journal *Wiener Medizinische Wochenschrift*), with a title that translates as "Reducing Pain by Oral Enzyme Therapy in Rheumatic Diseases." In the article, the researchers wrote (translated into English): "Proteolytic enzymes have analgesic effects, besides the well known anti-inflammatory and edema-reducing properties."

As you know, *edema* means swelling. These scientists concluded that patients with painful arthritis (including both osteoarthritis and rheumatoid arthritis) experienced the same amount of reduction in their pain when they were given enzymes (including bromelain and papain) as when they were given other pain relievers, such as nonsteroidal anti-inflammatory drugs (NSAIDS).

BIOFLAVONOIDS Rutin, quercetin, and hesperidin are remarkably strong antioxidants already used in many countries as medications to protect blood vessels, reduce varicose veins, and reduce allergies. These bioflavonoids may also lower bad LDL cholesterol, protect against cancer, and free radical damage to your pancreas.

Green Drinks, Superheroes

Whatever formula they come in, whether made from single green species or enhanced with other extracts or enzymes, green superfoods really are my superheroes, and I might be tempted to write pages and pages of love letters to them. But I'm already writing this whole book for you, so I am just going to share the essential basics about green drinks. Pay attention—this is the big finish on greens now.

Green superfoods are made up of nutrient-packed substances, straight from Mother Nature's kitchen on this green Earth. Sadly, they haven't made it into our Western culture because, for one thing, you won't find them packaged by McDonald's, and they don't taste like doughnuts. They taste like—drum roll please—greens! Well, greens with some added flavors depending on the brand, the product, and whether you mix them with juice or water.

But with their high content of vitamins and minerals, these superfoods can help correct imbalances in your diet. And as I said earlier, if you change only ONE behavior after reading my book, I hope it will be that you add green superfoods to your daily regimen, after you check with your doctor to make sure there are no possible bad interactions with any medications you're using now. And there shouldn't be, however, as your body functions more efficiently, you may notice more side effects from your medication (meaning you may need a dosage reduction or drug discontinuation). Anyone taking blood thinners (i.e., Coumadin, Plavix, or aspirin), should ask a physician about greens because of an interaction.

Below is a summary of what I have learned in my research on superfoods.

GREEN DRINKS. MAY PREVENT OR REVERSE TYPE 2 DIABETES BY PROTECTING THE PANCREAS AND INSULIN-PRODUCING CELLS. How phenomenal is that?! And good, solid scientific research supports this statement.

One major study, published in the *Journal of Medicinal Food* in 2001 was aptly called "Role of Spirulina in the Control of Glycemia and Lipidemia in Type 2 Diabetes Mellitus." The summary of the study by scientists in India began with this sentence: "Spirulina, with its high concentration of functional nutrients, is emerging as an important therapeutic food." Interesting. These scientists set out to evaluate the role of spirulina in reducing both blood sugar and bad fats in people with type 2 diabetes. They looked at 25 people with type 2 diabetes and randomly assigned them to receive either 2 grams of spirulina per day or not to receive spirulina, and thus be the control group. The study lasted for 2 months.

After 2 months of receiving the spirulina supplements, the study participants had an "appreciable lowering of fasting blood glucose and postprandial blood glucose." (Postprandial means "after a meal.") In addition, the people who received the spirulina supplements showed "a significant reduction in (the) HbA(1c) [hemoglobin A1c] level," which means the spirulina also affected long-term glucose regulation. But wait, there's more!

The spirulina-supplemented group also had lowered levels of "bad" cholesterol (LDL) and a slight increase in the "good" cholesterol (HDL, high-density lipoprotein), as well as a reduction in total cholesterol. The researchers concluded: "These findings suggest the beneficial effect of spirulina supplementation in controlling blood glucose levels and in improving the lipid profile of subjects with type 2 diabetes mellitus."

I don't know about you, but I find that amazing! And I'm even more amazed that mainstream medicine in the United States still hasn't chosen to look more closely at such therapies.

MAY PROTECT EYESIGHT. Green drinks are chock-full of carotenoids, which support eye health. And lots of studies have found that carotenoids are good for the eyes. Good brands have dramatically higher amounts of beta-carotene compared with carrots, gram per gram.

SPARK ENERGY IN SOMEONE WHO HAS CHRONIC FATIGUE OR ANEMIA. These drinks contain B vitamins, which enable your powerhouses (mitochondria) to make ATP (adenosine triphosphate), an energy molecule.

IMPROVE THE GROWTH OF NAILS AND HAIR. These drinks are loaded with minerals that have been shown to beautify hair and nails. Minerals support glucose metabolism.

HELP BALANCE THYROID HORMONE LEVELS. These drinks could be useful for someone with hypothyroidism, Hashimoto's disease, or Graves' disease. Green drinks are packed with precious minerals such as natural iodine, selenium, and iron, along with an amino acid called tyrosine. Did you know that it takes tyrosine and iodine to form the active thyroid hormone T3?

MAY REDUCE INFECTIONS. Numerous well-designed clinical trials have concluded that blue-green algae has antiviral activity, possibly even against herpes and HIV.

MAY SERVE AS POWERFUL ANTICANCER COMPOUNDS. They contain vitamins, such as folic acid, as well as phytochemicals such as green tea extract and SOD, all of which have been shown to reduce risk for cancer.

MAY IMPROVE HAY FEVER AND ALLERGIES TO POLLEN AND MOLD. Spirulina and quercetin appear to block the production of interleukin-4, a chemical produced in our bodies that sparks some symptoms causeing us misery—including sneezing, runny nose, and itchy eyes, just to name a few.

MAY HELP IN THE FIGHT AGAINST CARDIOVASCULAR DISEASE. Spirulina, just one superfood in green drinks, is widely researched and has shown cardioprotective properties, so it is ideal for someone with heart disease or metabolic syndrome.

MAY REDUCE PAINFUL NEUROPATHY SYMPTOMS. Spirulina and chlorophyll are two chelators—meaning they help rid the body of heavy metal toxins, thereby reducing inflammation and pain.

MAY DISCOURAGE GROWTH OF PATHOGENIC BACTERIA IN THE GUT DUE TO THE HEALTH PROBIOTICS FOUND IN GREEN DRINKS. Not all green drinks contain probiotics, however, all green drinks will encourage your body to make it's own natural intestinal flora.

How to Supplement

I would like you to select one green drink supplement and use it daily for 1 month before you add any other supplement. Why the time lag? When you begin using one of these potent green drinks, there's every reason to expect that your body will start to run much more efficiently. When this happens, you may notice changes in your metabolism. The body needs time to heal, adjust, and rebirth new mitochondrial powerhouses and healthy cells. Just to give you a couple of examples, many people on greens may notice their blood pressure start to come down, or constipation clears up, or energy levels increase.

These kinds of changes are signs that you are getting healthier. As a result, the effect of medication may be stronger. A person taking antihypertensive medications, for example, may notice dizziness or lightheadedness. That's an indication perhaps that individual can reduce his or her dosage of medication. And that's good, right?

The problem comes if you don't wait out the 30 days and you start taking numerous supplements. You won't be able to easily tease out which supplement is causing what effect, and whether you need to reduce the medication dosage.

My comments are based on experience in watching hundreds of people take my advice for greens (I've written about it dozens of times) and gotten feedback. A good-quality brand can have a dramatic impact, and you need to allow it to begin normalizing your body before bringing in other supplements.

Follow label directions for the brand you choose. The dose is usually one scoop per day mixed in water. I really like the taste of the brands I use because they are almost minty. If yours tastes like freshly mowed grass, take it back and try a different brand (unless you happen to like the taste of freshly mowed grass).

Even with the best-tasting brands, you may have a little trouble adjusting to the flavor and texture at first. That's understandable. It takes time for your taste buds to adjust, but it is totally worth your commitment. Once you start seeing the results, you will start to crave your daily fix as I do (and as my husband does, who downs these daily, and only with water, not juice). Here are some hints to help you gently break in the green drinks if you just can't begin with a full serving as directed.

GO HALF WAY. Mix one-quarter or one-half of the recommended serving—rather than the full amount—into cold water.

ADD SOME FLAVOR. If you don't like the flavor and want it to taste sweeter, mix it with organic apple or grape juice for a few days. But then dilute the juice with more and more water each day until you get away from the juice altogether. The goal is to take these greens with filtered water if you can.

If not, juice is fine because the ultimate goal is to get the greens in, however you mix it. (Still, you really don't want to keep drinking sugary fruit drinks if you have diabetes.)

EASE INTO IT. Add just a little bit, say one or two teaspoonfuls into your water bottle. The fluid inside will turn greenish yellow, but it should still taste pretty much like water. Sip it all through the day. Build up your dosage after a few days.

REMEMBER, YOU ARE TO STAY ON THESE GREENS FOR 1 MONTH BEFORE BEGINNING ANOTHER NEW SUPPLEMENT.

TAKE CAPSULES. Some brands are available as capsule formulations.

Pick Your Greens Wisely

Be choosy when purchasing your formula. Read the label carefully. If you have trouble with your vision, ask someone to read it for you. The reason is you need to ensure your greens are free of artificial sweeteners. It's unfortunate, but many greens contain artificial sweeteners. Look for a product that is gluten and soy-free. These are not openly disclosed on the front label. You basically have to search it out on the ingredient list. Stevia is natural and okay to have. Also, try to find a product that is gluten-free and soy-free. Some of the best brands on the market include pure Hawaiian Spirulina by Nutrex-Hawaii, Boku Superfood, NanoGreens by Biopharmacy, and New Chapter's Berry Green. Marine Phytoplankton by Ocean's Alive is a different type of green that comes from the ocean. It's virtually tasteless and I notice a difference in energy within minutes.

STEP 2: TAKE A VITAMIN D SUPPLEMENT

After you've become comfortable with your greens and your new healthy diet of natural foods, I want you to add another supplement—vitamin D—specifically vitamin D_3, which is the best form of the nutrient.

According to one research study published in the *American Journal of Clinical Nutrition* in May 2004, this powerful antioxidant increases insulin sensitivity by up to 60 percent. That's better than the number-one diabetes drug used—metformin—which was able to get rid of blood sugar by a paltry 13 percent according to a *New England Journal of Medicine* study published in 1998.

In fact, vitamin D may be all some people with mild type 2 diabetes have to take. This vitamin is fatty, so it gets into certain parts of the body other antioxidants (such as vitamin C) cannot, namely the heart, brain, breasts, prostate, pancreas, and liver.

Vitamin D undergoes several conversions in the liver and the kidneys before it becomes an active hormone in your body called calcitriol. People with diabetes often have enzymatic changes that compromise their ability to activate the nutrient to its body-ready active form. This is why supplementation is even more important for the diabetic.

Because of all the research that's been done in recent years, I believe this is one of the most important nutrients you can take if you have diabetes. And most people who have diabetes are deficient in it. Did you realize using chemical sunscreens, especially those with SPF ratings greater than 8, basically prevent your body from creating healthy forms of vitamin D? I think this has contributed to the major epidemic of vitamin D deficiency in this country.

When most folks with diabetes—and probably most people in general—are tested with a simple blood test, they come up low on vitamin D. Just so you know, some of the symptoms of vitamin D deficiency include muscle aches, muscle weakness, fatigue, and bone pain.

Michael Holick, MD, PhD, who is a recipient of the National Institutes of Health's General Clinical Research Center Excellence in Clinical Research Award, as well as the Pauling Award (among many others), is an expert on and leading advocate for the importance of vitamin D. His groundbreaking review article published in the *New England Journal of Medicine* in July 2007 turned national attention to Dr. Holick's work and to the tremendous implications of vitamin D deficiency.

Vitamin D deficiency leaves millions of children and adults at risk for numerous diseases and disorders, according to Dr. Holick. His article concluded that despite all our modern technology, vitamin D deficiency is one of the most "commonly unrecognized medical conditions, a condition that leaves millions at risk of developing not only osteoporosis and fractures but also numerous serious and often fatal diseases, including several common cancers, autoimmune diseases, infectious diseases, and heart disease."

Of particular interest to those reading this book: Dr. Holick found 74 studies suggesting vitamin D supplementation in children reduces the risk of type 1 diabetes! Don't say I didn't tell you so.

In fact, while I was reading Dr. Holick's article in the *New England Journal of Medicine*, out of curiosity I did an online search for research articles published *just* in this one journal on the relationship between vitamin D and diabetes. The result? Some 203 articles in that journal alone made the connection between vitamin D and diabetes.

When I searched the entire database (www.pubmed.gov) of medical literature for the same connection, take a guess at how many articles came up . . . 1,225.

An article published in the June 2009 issue of *Nutrition Research Review* said that several clinical studies show vitamin D improves insulin sensitivity, even in people with normal blood sugar ranges. While researchers don't yet know exactly why this is the case, researchers say there is "substantial evidence" pointing to vitamin D and insulin sensitivity.

I agree with Dr. Holick's assessment—and that of other clinicians who say we are suffering from an epidemic of low vitamin D. True, the sun can help your body activate vitamin D, but as we age, our skin loses its natural ability to turn sunlight into enough of the active forms of vitamin D our bodies need.

Many people in America have been brainwashed that sunlight is awful and they are sun-phobic and slather on chemical sunscreens that block the ability to create active vitamin D. Other people have genetic problems that prevent them from getting enough natural vitamin D. Vitamin D is one of my favorite nutrients because it has even shown potential for helping people fighting various forms of cancer.

In short, I just want you to follow my advice by adding vitamin D to your supplement regimen. It makes excellent health sense. Vitamin D is on my list because it obviously helps people who have pancreas disorders, prediabetes, diabetes, or metabolic syndrome. People with a high risk for pancreatitis or pancreatic cancer can also benefit. The American Cancer Society estimated 32,000 new cases of pancreatic cancer would be diagnosed in 2007, with about the same number of people dying from it that year as well.

In a groundbreaking study led by Halcyon Skinner, PhD, of the Northwestern University School of Medicine, in collaboration with colleagues from the Harvard School of Public Health, Brigham and Women's Hospital, Harvard Medical School, and Dana-Farber Cancer Institute, researchers found for one group of study participants, vitamin D consumption cut the risk of pancreatic cancer in half. This is important because unlike many other cancers, pancreatic cancer does not really have a good screening test, so early detection is hard to come by. People who are diagnosed with pancreatic cancer are, sadly, often diagnosed at a terminal stage.

As outlined in Chapter 6, I suggest your doctor ascertain your blood levels of vitamin D to make sure you are in the healthy range. The optimal range in the body today is 60 to 90 ng/mL (nanograms per milliliter)—also expressed as

25 to 200 nmol/L (nanomoles per liter) by some labs. If I could have my way, I'd ask you to make sure you keep your blood levels above 60 ng/mL year-round, not just in the summer, especially if you are female, because doing so protects you to some extent from breast cancer.

You can even measure vitamin D levels yourself with a home test kit that runs about $65, which can be purchased from various outlets. (See "Vitamin D" in my Resources section on page 378.) You can also ask your doctor to order a blood test that measures the circulating form of vitamin D called 25-hydroxyvitamin D_3.

If your doctor finds you are vitamin D deficient, he or she will probably recommend a drug version of vitamin D. But I'd prefer you take an over-the-counter supplement. The drugs are the wrong form (they are D_2) and the OTC versions are better because they're the D_3. D_3 is natural. D_2 is not. Take about 5,000 IU per day or even more until levels are optimal. You'll have to work with your physician to determine what your maintenance level should be after that. Again, take D_3, not D_2 (drugs).

Vitamin D Overview

So let's review. Here are some benefits to using vitamin D that you don't get from the typical prescription medication. In addition to helping with blood sugar control, vitamin D helps you:

- Absorb calcium, which staves off osteoporosis and maintains blood pressure).
- Possibly reduce the effects of seasonal affective disorder, also known as winter blues because it results from reduced daylight hours and reduced sun exposure.
- Improve rheumatic pain and muscle weakness.
- Potentially lower your overall risk for certain cancers, such as colon, prostate, and breast cancers.
- Potentially protect against hearing loss. (Many scientific articles have been published on the connection between low levels of vitamin D and the ravages of aging, including hearing loss.)

How to Supplement

The best form of vitamin D to take is vitamin D_3, also known as cholecalciferol. If your supplement says anything else (including D_2), you probably have an inferior form. Cod liver oil (liquid or softgel) is your best source for vitamin D, or you can just buy plain capsules of cholecalciferol.

Take approximately 4,000 to 5,000 IU per day for 2 weeks, and then reduce the dosage to 2,000 IU every day for another month or indefinitely if your doctor approves.

If you have reduced liver or kidney function, please ask your doctor whether these dosages are right for you, because people with impaired liver or kidney function make less biologically active vitamin D than those with normal function. They also have difficulty clearing supplements from the body, although supplements are easier on their system compared to drug versions of vitamin D, which tax the liver and kidneys.

Stay on the vitamin D for 1 month (along with the green drinks) to give your body time to adjust before adding any other supplements.

Vitamin D_3 is sold nationwide at health food stores. There are dozens of excellent brands, among them Pure Encapsulations, GNC, Source Naturals, and Doctor's Best. There are physician-formulas, too, like D_3 which can be obtained through Xymogen, Thorne Research or Metagenics.

Allergy Research Group produces a natural source of vitamin D_3 derived from the lanolin of sheep's wool. If you have trouble swallowing pills and want a liquid, or if you want to start them young take Carlson Baby D Drops. Read the label carefully, this is very concentrated so you only need a few drops.

Concerned about Overdose?

Some experts warn that vitamin D can build up in the bloodstream and become toxic, but it honestly takes an awful lot for this to happen. The dosages I suggest may be higher than the United States recommended daily intake; however, for most people they are not enough to create an overdose situation, so don't stress. Follow your doctor's advice and supervision. With so many researchers now calling for higher amounts of vitamin D, your doctor will undoubtedly agree you should be taking these higher amounts.

Please know that many medications actually deplete your body of cholecalciferol (vitamin D_3). The drug-nutrient depletion effect is something I've termed the drug-mugger effect. It happens when you take a medication that robs your body of a needed nutrient. It's especially important to take a supplement to replace that lost nutrient.

In the meantime, here's a list of drug muggers—both prescription and over-the-counter medications—that are capable over time of wiping out your body's stash of vitamin D:

Acid blockers

    Ranitidine (Zantac)

    Cimetidine (Tagamet)

    Nizatidine (Axid)

    Famotidine (Pepcid and
        Pepcid Complete)

    Omeprazole (Prilosec OTC)

    Esomeprazole (Nexium)

    Pantoprazole (Protonix)

    Rabeprazole (Aciphex)

Antacids (Maalox, Amphogel,
    Gaviscon)

Anticonvulsants (phenytoin,
    phenobarbital, primidone,
    ethosuximide, carbamaze-
    pine, gabapentin, valproic
    acid and possibly pregabalin
    [Lyrica])

Budesonide (Rhinocort)

Butalbital-containing drugs
    (Fiorinal, Fioricet)

Calcium-channel blockers
    (verapamil [Calan, Isoptin],
    amlodipine [Norvasc], nife-
    dipine [Procardia, Adalat],
    diltiazem [Cardizem], felo-
    dipine [Plendil])

Cholestyramine (Questran)

Colestipol (Colestid)

Flunisolide (Nasarel,
    Nasalide)

Fluticasone (Flonase)

Ketoconazole

Isoniazid

Laxatives that contain magne-
    sium, such as magnesium
    citrate or milk of magnesia

Mineral oil

Olestra (fat substitute often
    used in "light" potato chips)

Orlistat (Alli, Xenical)

Over-the-counter diet aids and
    fat blockers (e.g., kidney
    bean extract or starch neu-
    tralizer)

Raloxifene (Evista)

Rifampin (Rifadin)

Steroids (dexamethasone,
    hydrocortisone, fluticasone,
    methylprednisolone, pred-
    nisone)

Stimulant laxatives

Valproic acid (Depakote,
    Depakene)

Statin cholesterol drugs

STEP 3: GET MORE FIBER

Fiber won't raise blood glucose, but it will help control blood glucose spikes. Fiber is fantastic, especially for seniors. The most important part about fiber is taking it slow. If you increase your fiber intake too quickly, it will cause stomach upset. There's good research to support the importance of including fiber in your diet.

Researchers in Naples, Italy, published an important article in the December 1991 issue of *Diabetes Care*. They mentioned that prior studies had repeatedly shown a high-carbohydrate diet increases insulin and triglyceride levels in the blood and can also wreak havoc with blood sugar control after eating. They then noted, "much of the controversy between advocates and detractors of dietary carbohydrate can be settled by taking into account dietary fiber." Several studies have shown, wrote the Italian researchers, that the unhealthful effects of a high-carbohydrate diet (in terms of metabolism) disappear for diabetic patients when they increase fiber along with those carbohydrates.

The researchers noted studies have shown, in particular, a high-carbohydrate/high-fiber diet "significantly improves" blood sugar control and reduces cholesterol levels in people with diabetes. In addition, they found a high-carbohydrate/high-fiber diet does not increase plasma insulin or triglycerides, despite the increase in carbs. The key element making the difference here is obviously the fiber. Very cool.

The Italian researchers concluded while recommendations to people with diabetes should include a diet low in cholesterol and saturated fat (to prevent cardiovascular disease), diabetics should *also* add in fiber-rich foods and foods rich in unsaturated fat in their place.

Fiber naturally occurs in fruits, vegetables, grains, and beans. There is no fiber in meat, seafood, dairy products, eggs, or fats. Americans get about 15 grams of fiber in a typical day's diet. However, experts say we all need is about 25 to 40 grams daily. They suggest women need about 25 grams of daily fiber, while men need about 30 grams per day. And it's a good idea to make sure about 20 to 30 percent of your daily intake comes from soluble fiber.

Dietary fiber is usually classified as insoluble or soluble. It has to do with whether the fiber dissolves in water. Many foods contain a little bit of both types of fiber. We need both of these kinds, and they both fill us up without adding calories. Here are examples of the two types, although the foods in each list may have both types of fiber.

Insoluble fiber enables you to have regular bowel movements, prevents constipation, removes toxic waste that might otherwise linger in the colon, and helps balance pH in the intestines, which neutralizes cancer-causing substances released by microbes.

Insoluble fiber is typically found in whole wheat products (okay as long as you are not gluten intolerant), corn bran, skins on fruits (like grapes, apples, and pears), and in vegetables, especially dark, green leafy ones, brussels sprouts, green beans, carrots, celery, green beans, and flaxseed. Beets are another source of soluble fiber and the pectin they contain is great at binding toxins and heavy metals.

Soluble fiber helps prevent blood sugar spikes after you eat and delays gastric emptying time. It may also help you feel full, so you won't overeat. In addition, soluble fiber can help you maintain healthy ratios of cholesterol (lower the bad LDLs). As a result, it may reduce the risk of heart disease, a frequent complication of diabetes.

Good food sources of soluble fiber include rice and rice cereals, pasta, oatmeal, cornmeal, barley, papaya, quinoa, and soy. Vegetables are also good sources of soluble fiber. Some examples are carrots, yams, sweet potatoes, turnips, pumpkins, and mushrooms.

It's important to get your fiber from different sources, such as vegetables, fruit, nuts, seeds, beans, and grains, such as oatmeal. That's more important than dosage. More specifically, I'm happier to hear you are getting more fiber in your diet by eating a variety of those foods I just mentioned, than if you tell me you are supplementing with Metamucil. You might be wondering why.

When you eat fiber from vegetables, it can help you reduce blood pressure and homocysteine (an amino acid in the blood linked with an increased risk of cardiovascular disease). When you eat fiber from grains, you may enjoy a lower body mass index overall, and when you get fiber from fruit, it may help decrease your blood pressure.

With fiber from nuts, seeds, and some dried fruits, people with diabetes may enjoy lower blood sugar levels and lower levels of "bad" LDL cholesterol. Another obvious reason to eat your fiber, rather than supplement with it, is the other health benefits from these types of foods, including vitamins, enzymes, minerals, and many healing phytochemicals (plant substances) and antioxidants. You don't get all those benefits from a pill or powder supplement, I assure you. Also, fiber supplements tend to bind up your medications and supplements, preventing you from getting the effect of the medications you're taking. So please get your fiber from foods, and vary the source of it. In any event, get some fiber into your diet every day.

If you insist on a fiber supplement, I want you to take one called guggul, which is helpful to diabetics. Guggul is an herbal extract from resin of the *Commiphora mukul* tree. On the basis of the principles of Indian ayurvedic medicine, people all over Asia have been using it for centuries for all sorts of conditions affecting the heart and circulation. There is also an association with relieving pain of arthritis.

Guggul is also associated with lowering blood sugar, so holistic doctors sometimes consider using it in the treatment of their patients with diabetes. Guggul is at the top of my list for fiber supplements, if you *must* supplement. The reason is twofold. For one, it could replace that statin cholesterol drug. Second, it reduces an inflammatory chemical called C-reactive protein. Inflammatory chemicals hurt the body, and this particular one targets the heart.

Guggul is sold at health food stores. A typical dosage range is 75 to 250 milligrams one to three times daily. Look for a product standardized to about 2.5 percent guggulsterones. (Seriously, that's what the active substance is called.)

Always take fiber supplements 2 to 4 hours away from all your other medications and supplements, or they will cause your medications to rush through your intestinal tract too quickly to be properly absorbed. If you follow this nutritional plan for a couple of months, then you are ready to proceed to the next chapter, where I tell you exactly what nutritional supplements work to repair your pancreas, mop up dangerous free radicals, and support your health in many ways beyond diabetes.

Be kind to yourself—what you are doing takes courage. It's much easier to eat garbage and take a few pills every day than it is to clean up your kitchen cabinet, eat better, and learn to incorporate healthy supplements. Kudos to you for wanting to!

13 Natural Ways to Reduce Blood Sugar: Step 4

The best way to reverse diabetes is by coming at it from all angles. By that I mean lowering blood sugar as well as lowering inflammatory chemicals, reducing free-radical damage, and losing weight.

You are already well on your way to possibly reversing diabetes if you read the previous chapter and began implementing steps 1, 2, and 3. So, in order, you began by taking a green superfood supplement, then taking a vitamin D_3 supplement, and are now paying attention to getting more healthy fiber in your diet.

You are now ready for step number 4. If you're reading ahead that's fine, too. It's good to be prepared for what's coming up. If you're not quite ready for step 4, but looking for more that you can do, start paying attention now to constructing a healthier kitchen. Read how to do that in Chapter 16. (Some of the first things to do include avoiding white flour, white sugar, and white table salt.)

Treating—and, in my opinion, reversing the causes of and damage from—diabetes is not just a numbers game to see how fast you can reduce fasting blood sugars and A1c levels. As you've learned throughout my book, I have secret weapons, namely natural vitamins, antioxidants, herbs, and other dietary supplements, that can add comfort to your life, reduce neuropathy, improve eyesight, boost your energy reserves, and protect your heart, kidneys, and precious legs. In this chapter, I've outlined the very best supplements that not only reduce blood sugar but also protect all of these precious aspects of your health.

Step 4 consists of selecting, with your doctor's help, a natural supplement or supplements that can help you reduce your blood sugar. To keep things simple and clear, I am sharing only the supplements that have been well studied (not necessarily well advertised), so you will have many to choose from. If one doesn't fit well in your current regimen, try another. You should ask your doctor whether a particular supplement is right for you, and be mindful that natural medicines carry risks, such as side effects and allergies, just as conventional medicines do.

What's right for you may not be right for your friend. I want you to pay special attention to this:

Herbal remedies should be treated with respect because they have phar-macologic effects.

I know herbal remedies are attractive because their side effects are usually less daunting than those of medications, but depending on your own body chemistry and the particular supplements and prescription medications you are taking, they still can affect your body in a detrimental way, especially if you choose poor-quality supplements or you integrate too many supplements all at once.

SENSIBLE SUPPLEMENTING: START LOW AND GO SLOW

I am not a doctor. I am only trying to help guide you to natural approaches. One more thing: Many of the nutrients in this chapter have powerful and broad effects on the body, so while controlling your blood sugar may be the focus of the supplement, depending on the supplement, you may also notice improved hair and nail growth, more energy, less joint pain, some weight loss, more refreshing sleep, no more constipation, and so on.

I've done the best I can to research the best (and safest) supplements I would take myself. Should you take them all? Ye gads, no! You would be swallowing pills all day long, and you would become toxic and hypoglycemic.

A sensible approach to integrating supplements is to try one new supplement every few weeks or once a month. That way, you can see what kind of effect it has on your blood sugar and your general health. If you do well with it, kick it up a notch and bring in one more new supplement at that point. Look, it took you years to develop diabetes. It's okay if it takes a few months to find a good supplement regimen, so pace yourself.

Another reason not to hurry is that if you add two or three supplements at once and begin to experience a side effect, such as stomach upset, you won't know which supplement to blame. Then you'll have to stop them all, slowing the process of your improvement. Bringing in two or three supplements at once could cause a dangerous hypoglycemic reaction. I really don't like those pesky disclaimers, but now is a good time to give you one, because I want to keep you safe and also make sure you understand where I am coming from.

RULES OF SAFE SUPPLEMENTING

When taking supplements, it's best to have some general guidelines. It's possible you will be taking nutriceuticals for the first time as you read my book, so I need to give you the best advice about taking them. Generally speaking you should follow these tips.

TAKE SUPPLEMENTS WITH FOOD OR A SNACK. There are exceptions, and those will be noted on your product label or in this book.

INTRODUCE ONE SUPPLEMENT AT A TIME. See whether you develop side effects, such as dizziness, easy bruising, headache, diarrhea, gastrointestinal upset, or any other reaction. Wait several weeks before beginning another supplement. Take note if that new one causes any side effects. If you are supersensitive, you may want to keep a log and note the time you took your supplement and what happened within a few hours that evening or the next day.

TAKE THE LOWEST EFFECTIVE DOSAGE. For example, some product labels will advise, "Take one or two capsules twice daily." I suggest you start with one capsule once daily and then increase that to twice daily after a week or two, whenever you feel you have adjusted well enough to proceed. Then, keep going up the staircase with your dosage if you are tolerating it well and noticing beneficial effects. Remember, start low and go slow. And ask your doctor's advice if you think anything about the supplement or dosage doesn't feel quite right.

CHECK THE EXPIRATION DATE. Health food store workers have a lot of responsibilities, and sometimes they don't pull expired supplements off the shelf in a timely manner. Before purchasing, make sure your product is well within the expiration date.

LOOK FOR LOT NUMBERS. It's a sign of quality and purity. A lot number refers to the batch that was produced. This is more or less a sign that your product is tested for quality assurance. If there is ever a recall for contamination, the lot number of your product serves as identification so that you will know to stop taking it. (If you don't know what a lot number looks like, ask your pharmacist to show you.)

TAKE THE ACTIVE VERSIONS OF VITAMINS. For example, buy active, usable forms of vitamins that your body can readily incorporate into the cells. How will you know which forms are best? You'll have to educate yourself, and I'm going to help you do that. For example, vitamin B_{12} as cyanocobalamin is okay to take, and millions of people take this B vitamin; however, the body-ready active form is significantly better. It's called methyl B_{12} or methylcobalamin.

Another example of this is with coenzyme Q10, which is good, but the active, body-ready form called ubiquinol is better for some people, especially those older than 50, because it is more readily absorbed. If you can't find active vitamins, it's not a deal breaker, but if you can find them, they're better for you in the long run.

PAY ATTENTION TO QUALITY. Do what you can to make sure your supplement contains the ingredients it should. Think of herbs, for example, as plant-derived medications. They have widespread effects in the body, and they have side effects too. So whenever you take an herbal supplement, treat it as you would a prescription drug and note whether you develop side effects or odd symptoms. Also, be aware some proprietary blends are pulling the wool over your eyes and the tablets within the bottle don't contain what the label says.

The best way to ensure quality is to always stick with reputable brands that are widely available, not obscure formulas that are sold only on someone's Web site.

GOOD THINGS WILL HAPPEN TO YOU

The supplements I am about to share with you actually work for most people, and they work very well. So I want to caution you right now if you try some of my suggestions, you should do so with blessings and supervision from your doctor. That's because the supplements might reduce your blood sugar level too quickly. Although reducing your blood sugar levels is exactly what you want to do if you have diabetes, reducing it *too quickly* or by *too much* will cause dangerous blood sugar swings or hypoglycemia. And we don't want that.

Work closely with your doctor and keep track of your blood glucose levels. As they improve, work with your doctor to reduce medication dosage. The goal is to one day get off your medications completely and just rely on healthy nutrition and exercise (and supplements if they are appropriate for you).

It's all about balance, which is why I believe in natural supplements. Life itself is all about balance—night and day, hot and cold, and yes, life and death. So let's focus on the life part and living fully. That's what Mother Nature is all about. Just look around you. Even yeast has a strong life force. So do you!

I wrote this book to help you consider natural approaches as options for taking care of yourself, and getting healthier. I should remind you again as you eat better, take healthy supplements, and exercise, your blood sugar will come down naturally, whether or not you take medications. Yay! But this also means it could come down even further if you take medication, including insulin. That makes sense, right? I'm talking about a possible drug and supplement reaction, because drugs and supplements *both* lower blood sugar.

THE INCREASING SPOTLIGHT ON CINNAMON

There's new evidence that cinnamon can be helpful in regulating blood sugar. Cinnamon stimulates the production of glucose-burning enzymes and increases the effectiveness of insulin, according to the USDA Beltsville Human Nutrition Research Center in Maryland. The center found that taking between ¼ and 1 teaspoon of cinnamon—the same kind you buy at the supermarket—every day helps control blood sugar levels.

Another research study published in the *Journal of the American Board of Family Medicine* followed two groups who received usual care for their diabetes, with one group also taking 1-gram capsules of cinnamon for 90 days. The study found that the group that supplemented with cinnamon reduced their levels of A1c twice as much as the group that did not take the caps.

People who use insulin and also take natural supplements that reduce blood sugar (chromium or resveratrol, for example) *must* remain under close medical supervision since their insulin dosage will need to be reduced as blood sugar drops.

FIND THE NATURAL SUPPLEMENTS RIGHT FOR YOU

Step 4 gives you lots of choices. You will have to pick from the following pages which supplements are right for you. There should be a discussion between you and your physician to make these decisions. I've taken great care to ensure every compound I recommend has been scientifically studied and tested in humans, so you can feel confident taking them.

In this book I have outlined the very best supplements that can help lower blood sugar and improve general health. They come straight from Mother Nature's medicine cabinet. That said, remember I always want you to discuss any changes to what you take—be it over-the-counter, or herbal—with your personal physician. I want you to go very slowly, pick only *one* of the dietary supplements listed in this section, and begin it only after your body (and blood glucose levels) have adjusted to the powerful greens and the vitamin D you began taking in earlier steps.

If you are stabilized on insulin or you have blood sugar levels that tend to seesaw, then please be sure to take extra cautionary measures while implementing new supplements. For example, make sure to monitor your blood glucose daily (or more often) if necessary; carry tubes of cake frosting in your pocket or purse in case you feel your blood sugar starting to drop quickly. I'm not trying to scare you. I'm trying to keep you safe because I feel confident the supplements I recommend to you really work.

So if you've been using a calendar, you should be on month 3 by the time you choose your first supplement from the pages that follow. I've sorted them alphabetically, so read through *all* of them before deciding (with your doctor) which supplement is the right one for you to start with.

I'm going to say all this one more time; it's that important. Once you begin a supplement in this section, stay on it for at least a month. Remember, these really do work for some people. You need to move forward very slowly to avoid dangerous hypoglycemic swings. You should also be mindful as your body gets healthier, it starts to work more efficiently, so you may need reductions in your medication dosages. Again, you know what I'm going to say, but I will say it anyway you should not discontinue your prescription medication without getting your doctor's blessing. After a month on one of these, you can add another one if you need more help.

Here are the best choices to reverse diabetes without drugs.

Aloe Vera

You've probably used the gel from the spiky green *Aloe vera* plant as a remedy for minor burns or itchy skin. But *Aloe vera* has a wonderful effect on your general health and may be the very best colon cleanser known to humankind, other than strong coffee. Drinking *Aloe vera* juice—sold at health food stores nationwide— can help relieve indigestion, constipation, bladder infections, and stomach ulcers.

Aloe vera contains a sugar called D-mannose. Don't worry, this kind of sugar doesn't negatively impact diabetes. D-mannose could help you overcome cystitis and chronic urinary tract infections, which are common in people with diabetes. It works by unsticking the infectious germ *Escherichia coli* from your bladder. You can buy supplements of pure D-mannose, by the way, or just enjoy its naturally occurring form in *Aloe vera*. Glucomannan, another ingredient in aloe, is a fiber thought to help reduce triglycerides and promote weight loss.

Aloe is a rich source of protein, enzymes, calcium, selenium, magnesium, zinc, and vitamins A and E. *Aloe vera* contains amino acids (protein's building blocks), which are essential for muscle and skin health. (Remember your skin is the largest organ in your body.) *Aloe vera* helps your liver spark production of glutathione, which is a strong antioxidant. The combination of mannose, gluco-mannan, and all these nutrients helps to deliver life-sustaining nutrients and oxygen to your cells and revitalize your heart, brain, legs, eyes, pancreas, and kidneys.

WHAT THIS HERB DOES. According to some Japanese studies published in the *Journal of Ethnopharmacology*, *Aloe vera* appears to reduce blood sugar and triglycerides in some people. Diabetics who drank *Aloe vera* juice for about 42 days experienced a 40 percent reduction in blood sugar and in triglycerides. *Aloe vera* juice is tasteless, so you will see it added into some of my recipes in Chapter 17. It adds tons of nutrition without affecting taste.

Here are some other actions that have been documented scientifically. *Aloe vera* extract:

- Helps reduce neuropathic pain, as it contains a lot of vitamin B_{12}. *Aloe vera* is one of the only vegetarian sources of vitamin B_{12}, which protects the coating around nerves (myelin sheath).
- Increases circulation because it contains a boatload of vitamin C, which promotes healthy arteries. When your blood vessels are strong and elastic, you have better bloodflow.
- Improves wound healing. This effect is from the vitamin C, zinc, and selenium, is a perk that may help prevent dangerous foot infections and bedsores.
- Regulates cholesterol ratios because it contains natural phytosterols (plant sterols). These can help reduce cholesterol and triglyceride absorption in the gut.
- Reduces the need for kidney dialysis. To get this effect, you need to take *Aloe vera* extract (about 500 milligrams daily) along with an immune-boosting fiber called arabinogalactan (500 milligrams daily).

HOW TO SUPPLEMENT. Fresh *Aloe vera* is best but you need to make sure you have the correct, edible variety. Sometimes, you can buy the leaves at grocery stores. If your plant is large, you can fillet it and eat fresh *Aloe vera* gel from the inside of the leaves. I used to do this and put it in my smoothies every morning. The most convenient way is to buy bottled *Aloe vera* gel or dried oral supplements. Look for organic brands that are enzymatically stabilized but avoid those that contain thickeners like carageenan, guar gum, or xanthan gum. If aloe has a thickener in it, it's possibly 99% water, 1% aloe, hence the need for a thickener. Shockingly, the label may still say 100% Aloe Vera. Follow label directions. One brand that you can take as a capsule instead of a liquid is New Chapter's Aloe

Vera Force. I trust their quality. Also Aloe Vera 100 by www.Goodcausewell ness.com is fantastic.

You can also integrate the gel into smoothies and other recipes. (See Chapter 17.) Another way to supplement is to buy dried *Aloe vera* powder. Take about 700 to 1,500 milligrams per day (or follow directions on the label). Supplements labeled "mannose extract" also contain acemannan, one of the primary carbo-hydrates extracted from the *Aloe vera* plant. This is fine to take as well, though I prefer whole aloe leaf supplements because you get more of the active ingredi-ents from the plant.

SIDE EFFECTS AND CAUTIONS. Allergies to *Aloe vera* are rare but can occur. One easy way to help identify whether you are allergic to *Aloe vera* juice is to simply smear some of the liquid on your inner arm or chest. Note whether you develop a rash or redness from it. Check every few hours. If you do not have any problems, chances are pretty good you can safely take it. It is generally well toler-ated. If you notice diarrhea, stomach cramps, or nausea, cut down on the dosage until you are tolerating it better.

Curcumin (Extract of *Curcuma longa*)

The bright yellow color of turmeric spice, found in many Indian dishes, comes from the compound curcumin. Curcumin is related to ginger and has been used as medicine for centuries. Hundreds of scientific papers testify to curcumin's potential benefits, including its ability to improve insulin sensitivity and reduce inflammatory chemicals that target the pancreas, heart, and kidneys.

Curcumin is also sold commercially in the United States without a prescrip-tion in supplemental form, and I have recommended this botanical for many years because it is a strong anti-inflammatory.

I was delighted to read a thrilling new study the other day, published by sci-entists at the MD Anderson Cancer Center in Houston in the January 2009 issue of *International Journal of Biochemistry and Cell Biology.* The title of the article shows what the scientists have found: "Potential Therapeutic Effects of Cur-cumin, the Anti-Inflammatory Agent, against Neurodegenerative, Cardiovascu-lar, Pulmonary, Metabolic, Autoimmune and Neoplastic Diseases."

What they're saying in that title is in the medical literature, curcumin is an accepted anti-inflammatory compound. Their study looked into whether cur-cumin could offer healing effects in the other diseases they cite. (Neoplastic means diseases of abnormal growth of cells, including cancer.) I love this article and would love to talk with these researchers, because they are saying in a peer-reviewed journal what I have been saying for a long time: Time-honored natural treatments are ignored by practitioners of Western medicine. In the article the researchers go on to say:

> *This is not the case, however, with curcumin, a yellow-pigment substance and component of turmeric (Curcuma longa), which was identified more than a century ago. For centuries it has been known that turmeric exhibits anti-inflammatory activity . . . The process of inflammation has been shown to play a major role in most chronic illnesses, including neurodegenerative, cardiovascular, pulmonary, metabolic, autoimmune and neoplastic diseases. In the current review, we provide evidence for the potential role of curcumin in the prevention and treatment of various proinflammatory chronic diseases. These features, combined with the pharmacological safety and negligible cost, render curcumin an attractive agent to explore further.*

I'm quoting extensively from summary (abstract) here, because I wanted you to read what the researchers themselves wrote.

In one study, lab animals showed improved insulin sensitivity and better glucose tolerance. Curcumin is also known to reduce pain and inflammation in people who have pancreatitis. And because it has anticancer properties, it makes sense that this herb might help reduce your risk for pancreatic cancer.

WHAT THIS HERB DOES. Curcumin has an amazing number of beneficial actions:

- It helps relieve painful neuropathies. One study found curcumin could reduce pain from neuropathy by causing the release of disease-associated proteins produced by a mutated gene. Curcumin has also shown promise in animal studies as a neuroprotective agent in diabetic neuropathy and central nervous system diseases.
- It may protect memory. Researchers are examining curcumin's effect on people with Alzheimer's disease, which if you recall from Chapter 2, is sometimes called Type 3 Diabetes.
- Studies suggest curcumin might increase levels of glutathione, a powerful free-radical scavenger that helps relieve neuropathy, helps eliminate toxins in the body, and helps protect the pancreas.
- It may reduce inflammation and pain, particularly postsurgical pain.

HOW TO SUPPLEMENT. You should be cooking with turmeric spice, which provides many active ingredients (including curcumin), and also you can take curcumin as an extract by itself, where it will be labeled as "standardized extract of *Curcuma longa*" or turmeric extract. Take 500 to 1,000 milligrams once or twice daily to lower blood sugar or improve insulin sensitivity. Higher dosages are often used for pancreatitis.

Curcumin is poorly absorbed by the body, which means supplements may not have strong activity. For this reason, some supplements are bound to black pepper extract (bioperine), and this is designed to help the curcumin get into the cells better. I like this combination, even though some experts feel it is more irritating to the gastrointestinal lining. If you are confident with the brand you are taking, stick with it. If you want to try a new brand, here are a few I recommend.

Super Curcumin with BioPerine by Life Extension. This has 800 milligrams pure curcumin in each capsule, along with piperine to help you with absorption. It is free of common allergens and is standardized to 95 percent pure curcuminoids.

Meriva by Thorne Research. This high-quality brand uses phosphatidylcholine (PC) to carry the curcumin deep into your cell. PC not only serves to carry curcumin in but has beneficial effects on your brain, liver, and pancreas. Meriva contains other plant-based herbs, so this multitasking formula may offer you powerful pain-relieving strength without fear of gastrointestinal bleeding or addiction (common with prescribed pain relievers).

Turmeric Force by New Chapter. This product is standardized for high purity and concentration, providing the world's first and only full-spectrum turmeric extract. It is suspended in pure olive oil.

SIDE EFFECTS AND CAUTIONS. This supplement is generally well tolerated. Sometimes curcumin, especially if it contains black pepper extract, may cause a harmless bitter taste in the mouth. It should not be used by people who have any kind of stomach ulcers or obstructions, such as gallstones or bile duct blockages. Long-term use may contribute to ulcer formation in the stomach. Hypoglycemia is a theoretical possibility when curcumin is used along with diabetic drugs.

Fenugreek (*Trigonella foenum-graecum*)

The herb fenugreek is one of the most impressive natural substances helpful for people with diabetes. Native to southeastern Asia, India, and the Mediterranean, fenugreek is a spice often used in curry. Also called Greek hay, the herb has been prized for centuries for its flavor, as well as its medicinal properties.

Women from India seem to have the most beautiful hair. During my research, I learned that fenugreek seeds are sometimes mixed with yogurt and used as a conditioner for their hair. I've put that on my to-try list, but what's most important about fenugreek is it contains powerful healing substances, including apigenin, genistein, quercetin, rutin, selenium, and kaempferol. Fenugreek also increases levels of superoxide dismutase (SOD), which squashes toxic free radicals in the body.

Today, you can buy fenugreek seed as a spice and cook with it, or you can buy fenugreek supplements that are thought to promote healthy blood sugar and cholesterol levels. Fenugreek is a strong antioxidant, so it's good at guarding your healthy cells from free-radical assault. It lowers blood sugar much the same way that drugs in the class of sulfonylureas (such as glyburide) do.

A study on teaching mothers to include micronutrient-rich and energy-dense complementary foods when preparing meals for their children was published in the *Indian Journal of Pediatrics* in January 2009. The only leafy green vegetable included in the study? Yep, fenugreek. Pretty impressive.

WHAT THIS HERB DOES. Here's what fenugreek delivers:

- It's a powerful antioxidant, thanks to it's ability to raise SOD levels. SOD is an enzyme that appears to have remarkable abilities to neutralize free radicals, so it could very well be protective against cancer and tumor formation.
- Containing quercetin and kaempferol compounds, fenugreek may be protective against cancers, such as pancreatic cancer. One 8-year study found three flavonols (kaempferol, quercetin, and myricetin) reduced the risk of pancreatic cancer by 23 percent, especially in current smokers.
- Researchers are now examining the potential of fenugreek seeds to protect against breast and prostate cancers, because preliminary research done in petri dishes (not with lab animals) suggests a positive effect.
- It may prevent varicose veins because it contains the bioflavonoid rutin, an antioxidant that improves the strength of capillaries and veins. Rutin is taken by people who tend to bleed or bruise easily, who want to increase circulation and strengthen blood vessels.
- It may protect against metabolic syndrome by regulating blood pressure, blood sugar, and cholesterol.
- Because it contains trigonelline (which, by the way, gives coffee that delicious

aroma and familiar, slightly bitter taste), fenugreek may protect against neuropathy. Trigonelline protects the nerves because it is an antioxidant, and according to one study, it may also prevent nasty bacteria from sticking to your teeth. (So it just might reduce dental cavities as well.)

- It may help lactating mothers secrete milk, which is very helpful if you've just had a baby and the creek is dry.
- One study showed an association between taking fenugreek seeds regularly and improved cholesterol ratios, as well as a reduced risk of heart attack.
- It helps you lose weight because fenugreek seeds are rich in dietary fiber, so it delays gastric emptying and after-eating sugar spikes.

HOW TO SUPPLEMENT. Fenugreek is a commonly eaten food. Seeds, however, are bitter. Taking supplements is best. If you opt for capsules, take about 1,220 milligrams two or three times daily. If you have cardiovascular issues and take heart medications, ask your doctor whether this supplement is right for you. If so, stick to very low dosages—about 600 milligrams once or twice daily. Over time, and with your physician's approval and supervision, you can always increase the dose, but as we always say in the pharmacy world, "start low and go slow." Nature's Way makes one good brand, sold widely at most health food stores and select pharmacies. GNC health food stores also sell a good-quality version that is an oral capsule called Nature's Fingerprint Fenugreek.

You can also grow fenugreek at home. It's easy. The seeds are planted in late spring and are ready to use in 2 or 3 months. You can also sprout the seeds to put into salads for a spicy taste. Another way to use the seeds is to soak a few of them (about ¼ of a teaspoonful) in water overnight. In the morning, drink just the water (not the seeds). The seeds are bitter.

SIDE EFFECTS AND CAUTIONS. Lowered blood sugar is an expected effect of using fenugreek, but this can be troublesome if you combine it with medications and do not monitor yourself properly. Make sure you see your doctor regularly to supervise your regimen. In rodents, fenugreek stimulates uterine contractions.

Fenugreek is a dietary fiber, and as with all fiber (including oatmeal), you have to space this supplement away from your other medications by a few hours. Finally, fenugreek may reduce the level of potassium in your body, which could affect your heart rhythm. This effect is far more pronounced if you also take diuretics, certain steroids, heart medications, and other potassium-lowering drugs. Finally, fenugreek is a bit of a natural blood thinner so if you take anticoagulant meds (Heparin, Coumadin, Plavix, etc.) check with your doctor.

Gymnema Sylvestre

Gymnema sylvestre is a woody climbing plant that grows throughout India and has been used by holistic physicians there for treating diabetes for nearly 2 millennia (as in 2,000 years and counting). I bet you haven't heard of it from your doctor, though. It's also called gurmarbooti, or gurmar, which means "sugar destroyer."

They've known about this herb for years overseas, where it's serious diabetic medication. Here in the United States, it's just a dietary supplement, no prescription required. Gymnema is a powerful herb for lowering blood sugar, and it seems to offer some support for the health of your pancreas as well. Gymnema also neutralizes the taste of sugar in your mouth, so it can help with that insatiable sweet tooth and carb cravings.

The first hint for Western science that extracts from the *Gymnema sylvestre* plant could help diabetics came more than 80 years ago when the leaves proved to reduce glucose in the urine of people with the disease. (Numerous well-designed clinical trials have shown that GS can reduce fasting blood sugar, postprandial [after-eating] blood sugar, and hemoglobin A1c, a measure of blood sugar levels.)

I'm excited to share the next study with people who have type 1 diabetes, because the results were equally impressive. In this study researchers looked at 27 people with type 1 diabetes, for time periods ranging from 2 months to 30 months, to see whether giving them 400 milligrams daily of GS4, a water-soluble extract of the leaves of *Gymnema sylvestre*, would help their condition. What they found is amazing. They found insulin requirements, blood glucose, A1c counts, glycosylated plasma protein (a protein with a sugar molecule attached to it that serves as way to measure glucose control), and serum lipids all came down to almost normal levels with the *Gymnema* and stayed there, when they checked 10 to 12 months later.

The coolest part is that there was an increase in C-peptide levels in the study participants. C-peptide is a peptide test often used with diabetics to indicate whether a person is producing insulin, and if so, roughly how much they're producing. So the findings basically mean insulin production was being restored, probably because of the regeneration and repair of beta cells. How amazing is that!

The control group—a similar group that took a dummy pill—did not show any of these types of improvements and worsened over the study period. No major adverse effects were reported either. So if you think you need insulin forever and ever, think again. It is possible that even if you require injections now, you may get to do away with those needles once and for all.

WHAT THIS HERB DOES. Gymnema is a pretty amazing all-around performer:

- It regenerates beta cells so your pancreas can make insulin. This could lead to your body increasing insulin levels on its own.
- It has been shown to lower serum cholesterol and triglycerides.
- It may be able to suppress your craving for sweets.
- By regenerating beta cells, it may be able to slightly offset damage done by the foods you used to eat. More specifically, it may be able to reverse damage done by alloxan, the contaminant used in bleaching agents that make white flour, and all those white-flour goodies that people eat (of course, not you). Information on alloxan is on page 3.
- It has antibacterial effects against some nasty critters like *Pseudomonas aeruginosa* and *Staphylococcus aureus*. It kills other germs as well. Why is this so important? Think of dangerous diseases such as pneumonia, endocarditis, meningitis, foodborne diseases, methicillin-resistant *Staphylococcus aureus* (MRSA), and sepsis.
- It helps enzymes in your body that cause your cells to actually take up the insulin and use it; this means your adrenal glands don't have to work so hard and neither does your liver.

HOW TO SUPPLEMENT. Take 250 to 1,000 milligrams total daily—in divided doses. So you could be taking 500 milligrams twice daily or 260 milligrams three times daily. You want your product to say it contains about 75 percent gymnemic acids or it is standardized to 25 percent gymnemic acid. There are quality brands at many health food stores, including WholeFoods, GNC, and Vitamin Shoppe.

SIDE EFFECTS AND CAUTIONS. Lowered blood sugar is an expected effect, but this can be troublesome if you combine it with medications that do the same and fail to monitor yourself properly. So make sure you confer with your doctor and show your doctor your results. This herb is remarkably well tolerated in normal dosages. Stick to the lowest effective dose for you, however.

Holy Basil (*Ocimum sanctum*)

In traditional Indian ayurvedic medicine, holy basil (*Ocimum sanctum*) is known as tulsi. Tulsi means "the incomparable one." The herb is native to India but grows all around the world.

Holy basil is one of the most incredible herbs to use if your goal is to take back control of your body from the ravages of diabetes. Holy basil can improve the functioning of beta cells in your pancreas, and that helps you produce more insulin. Some of the healing essential oils, such as eugenol, caryophyllene, and oleanoic acid, come from the leaves of the holy basil. It also contains ursolic acid and apigenin, two other chemicals that are thought to have antioxidant, anticancer, and anti-inflammatory properties. Eugenol eases neuropathic pain.

In one small clinical trial done in India and published in the *International Journal of Clinical Pharmacology*, about 40 patients with type 2 diabetes stopped their medication 7 days before beginning treatment with holy basil. Then they were given holy basil leaves for another 5 days before the main part of the study began. At this point, half were randomly given 2.5 grams of powdered holy basil leaf daily. The other half (20 people) got a placebo for 4 weeks, and then were "crossed over" into receiving the same amount of holy basil as the other 20 participants for an additional 4 weeks.

The results? Stellar! For the first group, after the first 4 weeks, their average fasting sugar levels *decreased* from just over 134 to about 100. Then, when that first group was put on a placebo for 4 weeks, their fasting sugar levels went back up to a bit over 115.

The researchers concluded: "Overall, mean fasting blood glucose was 21 mg/dl lower in the holy basil group. There were no adverse effects reported by those taking the holy basil or the placebo." Wow, medicines from my pharmacy don't have that good a track record and safety profile.

WHAT THIS HERB DOES. Holy basil just keeps on giving:

- It may have an antidepressant effect on the brain.
- It has strong anti-inflammatory activities and works by suppressing pain chemicals called prostaglandins. Similar to COX-2 inhibitor drugs (Celebrex). It could help with arthritis. One small animal study suggests holy basil has about the same pain-relieving quality as one aspirin.
- It's a powerful antioxidant, so it can help prevent the damage to your cells and organs caused by free radicals.
- It may protect the heart against damage from chemotherapy drugs, such as adriamycin. (If you're undergoing treatment for cancer, ask your oncologist about this.)
- It helps with metabolic syndrome because it has been proven to decrease blood pressure, cholesterol, and triglycerides in some people, and it lowers blood sugar.
- It has antimicrobial effects.
- It is well known for helping people cope with heartburn and bloating. Holy basil may have significant antiulcer activity by reducing the effect of peptic

acid on the delicate stomach lining. (If you have ulcers, talk to your gastro-enterologist about using this herb.)

- It may help people with chronic, inflammation-based respiratory conditions such as asthma.

HOW TO SUPPLEMENT. There is no typical dose for holy basil, but in the one human study, 2.5 grams of a dried leaf powder was used once per day on an empty stomach. One good brand that I've tried is New Chapter's Supercritical Holy Basil, sold at most health food stores. This high-quality brand contains 2 percent ursolic acid, an extract of holy basil, and provides 400 milligrams per capsule. The dosage for Supercritical Holy Basil is two capsules daily, which can be taken with or without meals. If it were me, I'd take one in the morning and one in the evening to enjoy continuous effects throughout the day. There are other brands that may be effective, but I really like this one, so try to hunt it down.

You can also get a milder effect by drinking tulsi tea and I recommend 1 cup daily.

SIDE EFFECTS AND CAUTIONS. Holy basil may theoretically interact with dia-betic medication and enhance the blood sugar–lowering effect. Monitor blood sugar closely and make sure your physician knows of any unusual changes and can advise you about adjusting your medications accordingly. Holy basil is different than Sweet Basil, the herb you find in the produce section at your supermarket. It's fine (and advised) to eat fresh basil as well as supplement with holy basil herb.

Lipoic Acid

Lipoic acid naturally occurs in the body. It's a fatty acid that works both in and around every cell in the human body. Your body uses it to produce energy, and in fact, lipoic acid is capable of converting glucose (blood sugar) into energy molecules.

Supplements that contain lipoic acid are known to reduce blood sugar. The good studies have been done using intravenous forms of lipoic acid, so it's hard to say whether an oral supplement will give you the same excellent effect. A 2006 study, however, concluded oral administration of alpha lipoic acid, at least in the short term (in the case of the study, twice daily over 4 weeks) increased insulin sensitivity in people with type 2 diabetes.

Lipoic acid has also been associated with relief from painful neuropathy complications of diabetes. One study of 328 people, published in the journal *Diabetes* in 1997, concluded that 600 milligrams of alpha lipoic acid given daily intravenously for 3 weeks was safe and effective at reducing symptoms of diabetic peripheral neuropathy.

In another study, published in the journal *Hormones* in 2006, oral treatment with 800 milligrams per day for 4 months seemed to improve cardiac autonomic dysfunction in patients who had non–insulin-dependent diabetes, a form of type 2 diabetes.

Lipoic acid happens to also be a powerful substance that activates antioxidant pathways in the body. Antioxidants squash dangerous free-radical compounds. Lipoic acid works at a molecular level by rejuvenating your mitochondrial powerhouses via the PGC-1 chemical that I discussed in chapter 3. It can penetrate both water and fat-loving cells, so it goes everywhere, like your brain, heart, and pancreas.

Another interesting tidbit about lipoic acid is that it can recycle other important antioxidant substances, such as vitamins C and E and glutathione, so they can go around your body and keep cleaning up. Even though tiny amounts of lipoic acid are found in many foods, there are higher amounts in kidney, heart, liver, spinach, broccoli, and yeast extract. Unfortunately, the lipoic acid molecule is bonded so tightly that it's difficult for your body to absorb it, which is why I recommend supplementation for people, especially diabetics.

The best part about lipoic acid is that it spurs your mitochondria (your cellular powerhouses) to work for you, so you can dump out fat and sugar from your cells. This may be an overlooked way of reversing insulin resistance, and you can say you read it here first.

WHAT THIS NUTRIENT DOES. When lipoic acid goes to work for you, it accomplishes a lot:

- It's brilliant at reducing nerve pain so it can help people with painful neuropathies. In mild cases, it may be all you need to stop the pain.
- It contains two substances (thiol groups) that latch on to dangerous metals in the body and brain, so it acts a bit like a chelating agent. This is good, as it may be able to clear your body of mercury and other harmful metals. This could mean reduced risk of Alzheimer's disease and Parkinson's.
- It penetrates the brain and protects brain cells from free-radical damage. This may help you preserve memory and function, possibly even after a stroke.
- It boosts thyroid hormone, so it can give you energy and help you lose weight.
- It seems to nourish nerves that supply the heart and may improve certain types of heart palpitations.
- It eases fine lines and wrinkles and is found in many creams.

HOW TO SUPPLEMENT. Supplements of lipoic acid vary greatly. The R form is the biologically active component (natural to our body) that imparts lipoic acid's phenomenal effects and its ability to drive up glutathione levels, which help your liver detoxify.

The S form is synthetically produced in a lab and is not as biologically active. Typical alpha lipoic acid supplements consist of both versions, meaning the R and S forms, in a 50/50 ratio. So if you buy a 50-milligram alpha lipoic acid supplement, then you are getting only 25 milligrams of the biologically active R form. That is why I recommend that you take R-lipoic acid over alpha lipoic acid. It may be a bit of a hunt to find it, but worth the effort.

Your body is better able to utilize the R form. Some companies, such as Xymogen (a physician-exclusive manufacturer), offer sustained-release formulas of alpha lipoic acid that continue to work for hours after you've swallowed the tablet. This is certainly an option if your doctor recommends it. I've used the brand ALAMax CR, and it worked well. But be warned, it makes your urine smell like asparagus! That's quite harmless, but possibly embarrassing.

If you opt for R-lipoic acid, take 100 milligrams two to four times daily. If you select alpha lipoic acid, take twice what you would take for the R version. (So if you were taking 100 milligrams of R-lipoic acid, and you switched to alpha lipoic acid, then you'd need to take 200 milligrams to get the same effect.) Take these supplement two or three times daily. These supplements are best taken on an empty stomach, 1 hour before meals or 2 hours after. Here are the brands that I have taken and can safely recommend for you.

Super R Lipoic Acid by Life Extension. I like this brand because it is extremely usable in the body and very pure. It goes to work much faster than other brands because it has a special delivery system. It is also the R form of lipoic acid, so it's quite potent, and it comes as 300-milligram capsules. This is a good dose, so I recommend it often for people with diabetes, especially those with painful neuropathies. You could take this once or twice daily with a meal. And it's a vegetarian formula.

R Lipoic Acid by Source Naturals. This is another strong version providing R-lipoic acid. This is a 50-milligram dose, and you can take it several times a day to maintain beneficial effects. It's inexpensive and easy to find—sold widely at most health food stores.

R Lipoic Acid by Country Life. This one provides 100 milligrams of R-lipoic acid per capsule.

Thiocid by Thorne Research. This provides 300 milligrams of R-lipoic acid. I took this brand on and off for many years. It's very pure.

ALAMax CR by Xymogen. The controlled-release version of alpha lipoic acid keeps the supplement around longer in your bloodstream. It is alpha, though, not R, but very high quality. It provides 300 milligrams per tablet.

SIDE EFFECTS AND CAUTIONS. Because lipoic acid reduces blood sugar, you may need to reduce the dosage of your insulin, metformin, glyburide, or other diabetic medication. Also, alpha lipoic acid and R-lipoic acid may boost thyroid levels, and this could mean that you need a lower dose of Armour Thyroid, Synthroid (levothyroxine), or other thyroid medication. Lipoic acid's effect on a person's thyroid is very individual. It may not be wise to use in someone with Grave's Disease (overactive thyroid) or someone taking the drug methimazole. Because lipoic acid seems to slightly boost thryoid function, I think it can be helpful for those with Hasimoto's and hypothyroidism.

Also, when shopping for supplements, read labels closely. I am talking here about alpha *lipoic* acid, not alpha *linoleic* acid. These are two entirely different supplements.

Resveratrol

Resveratrol is a powerful antioxidant found in cacao, red grapes, berries, and red wine. It is one amazing extract that has been the subject of hundreds of scientific papers. This chemical is released naturally by plants. Resveratrol supplements, sometimes known as the wine pill, ironically come not from wine but from the Japanese knotweed plant.

Initial studies of resveratrol were done on animals, but resveratrol and newly derived compounds made from it are now being tested in ongoing human clinical trials. This could take some time.

It's being tested in humans now because of the remarkable findings from the studies on animals (mice and rats). One study even showed that mice fed a high-fat diet and also given resveratrol were able to live out a normal lifespan, avoiding both heart disease and diabetes. Their bodies were more sensitive to insulin, and they were more mobile.

The medical literature is now beginning to reflect the remarkable potential of resveratrol. An article published in the August-September journal of *The International Journal of Biochemistry and Cell Biology* noted the "anticancer effects" of resveratrol, observing that these come from suppressing the growth of cancer cells. The article even mentions cancers of the colon, breast, liver, pancreas, stomach, intestines, rectum, and prostate, as well as lymphoma, myeloma, and neuroblastoma, "have been improved by the use of resveratrol."

(In this case researchers were studying cells from these cancers in petri dishes.)

I feel there is enough substantial evidence to suggest resveratrol supplements to help you reduce risk for cancer, inflammatory disorders, heart attack, and diabetic complications. The reason I've included it here is that resveratrol uniquely targets a molecule in the body mentioned earlier on in the book, called PGC-1 alpha. You can learn all about PGC-1 alpha in Chapter 3 if you'd like more science behind my recommendations.

The point here is that resveratrol promotes a better work ethic in your mitochondria, the cellular powerhouses that help you detoxify. You might say that resveratrol does good housekeeping on your cells, just like curcumin and lipoic acid. The better your powerhouses work, the healthier you are and the less likely to come down with a dreadful metabolic disorder. Lazy, old mitochondria emit more free radicals, which damage your cells. So resveratrol is one of the most important supplements a diabetic should consider.

Resveratrol is a strong antioxidant, and it's true that it's found in red wine because grape skins are a source of resveratrol. But here's the part that some consumers don't know. The content of resveratrol varies widely from grape to grape, and it depends on growing conditions of the grapes and how the wine is stored, processed, and packaged. *If the wine isn't made with organic grapes, it may contain no resveratrol at all.*

You'd also have to drink about 100 bottles of wine per day to get the same amount of resveratrol used in those animal studies mentioned earlier. That's why you can't rationalize drinking red wine as a "supplement." In fact, if you overdo it, it's downright dangerous, because alcohol is a primary cause for pancreatitis and pancreatic or liver cancer. Please see my rant about alcohol in Chapter 4. And sorry if I just smashed your excuse for a nightcap. It's because I really care.

WHAT THIS PLANT EXTRACT DOES. Resveratrol promotes many healthy actions in the body.

- It may improve thyroid function and protect against thyroid cancer.
- It may be able to help you attain the right cholesterol ratio—the relationship between "good" (HDL, high-density lipoprotein) and "bad" (LDL, low-density lipoprotein) cholesterol.
- It may reduce your risk for heart attack and stroke.
- It may protect your eyes from glaucoma and other diseases that lead to blindness.
- It may improve insulin sensitivity.

- It may help reduce arthritic pain.
- It may relieve symptoms, such as pain and fatigue, of certain autoimmune disorders, such as rheumatoid arthritis and multiple sclerosis.
- It thins the blood, so it improves bloodflow and circulation to the hands and feet.
- Animal studies seem to indicate it prevents neuronal cell death, so it even has potential to prevent or slow the progression of Alzheimer's disease and other neurologically based diseases.
- It's a powerful free-radical scavenger, so it may have potential for the prevention or treatment of cancer.

HOW TO SUPPLEMENT. Choosing high-quality supplements is extremely important. After all, resveratrol is one of the most important nutrients you can take if you have type 2 diabetes. So I am a bit fussy about what you consume.

Please know that regular resveratrol has a very low rate of absorption in the body. Most of it, about 75 percent of it, leaves your body through the urine and feces. Whatever does get absorbed hangs around for only a few minutes. Keep this in mind when you are choosing brands, and don't be afraid to ask your doctor to order special brands for you. Some of the best brands are sold only through doctors' offices.

Take about 100 milligrams of resveratrol once or twice daily. You want a product made from a standardized root extract of *Polygonum cuspidatum*. This is the Latin term for the Chinese herb hu zhang, commonly known as Japanese knotweed, so you will frequently see this on the label.

Here are some of the better brands I've come across:

Xymogen's Resveratin has a unique long-acting form. Their formula uses a more stable and active form of resveratrol, which your body readily takes up and puts to action. This company uses a methylated form of resveratrol. For the consumer, this translates to higher activity. Because this product is sold only through practitioners, please see my Resources on page 378 for information on how to buy it.

Resveratrol 100 by Jarrow is 100 percent trans resveratrol. This potent product is body-ready and easy to incorporate. It is pretty easy to find at health food stores and online.

Transmax Trans-Resveratrol by Biotivia, a very pure product often used in clinical trials, contains pure trans resveratrol. It is not genetically modified, nor does it contain any fillers. I appreciate that this company posts its certificate of purity on its Web site.

Polyresveratrol by Thorne Research contains pure resveratrol, along with other active ingredients that sweep away free radicals. These include green tea, grape seed, and pterostilbene (one of the active components in resveratrol). This is another physician favorite. You can buy it online or through Thorne Research. See my Resources on page 378 for purchasing information.

Longevinex 100 mg containing 100 milligrams of trans resveratrol.

SIDE EFFECTS AND CAUTIONS. Resveratrol is usually well tolerated in low dosages. Some people have reported the following side effects: stomach cramps, nausea, diarrhea, insomnia, joint pain, numbness/tingling in the hands or feet, heart palpitations, and a buzz like a caffeine rush. These side effects most often occur when the dosage is high or the quality of the product is poor.

I need to make you aware that choosing good-quality resveratrol supplements is important. The job of picking out a supplement gets confusing because companies don't always disclose the amount of active resveratrol—a substance called trans resveratrol or trans-R—in their product in relation to the total weight of the product. So when you shop for this supplement, you'll see notations such as the number 50, or a percentage such as 50 percent or 70 percent and so on. This refers to the amount of resveratrol in the product compared to the total weight of the product. The higher the number, the more potent the product.

Some products use fillers, such as emodin, to take up space. It can spark diarrhea in most people, unless of course you have a cast-iron stomach. To ensure you get a pure, authentic brand of resveratrol, stick to those I've mentioned above, or ask the manufacturer of a company whose other products you have used to good effect to provide you with a certificate of authorization. Make sure the product is fresh (always check the expiration date), and the test confirming purity was done at an independent lab.

Reputable companies will not mind at all faxing or mailing their certificates of purity if you call and ask. There is more information at the Web site www.resveratrol.info.

Stevia (Honorable Mention)

Stevia is actually a naturally occurring sweetener derived from the plant *Stevia rebaudiana*. I am giving it an honorable mention here because this chapter is devoted to products that can help you reduce blood sugar. Stevia is just amazing because it can sweeten up your food and beverages, and it actually has the ability to lower blood sugar by acting directly on the beta cells of your pancreas to help you release insulin.

You can find stevia at any health food store. It is sold as a sweetener in liquid extracts, as well as in pretty little packets under various brand names. Stevia is one of my all-time favorite ways to help you sweeten up your foods and not upset your blood sugar. If anything, it may help to reduce it. To read more about stevia, turn to page 298.

METABOLIC GLUCOSE FORMULA

This one-of-a-kind formula combines some of the natural herbal extracts that I have been talking about in this chapter, such as resveratrol, curcumin, *gymnema sylvestre*, vitamin D_3, R-lipoic acid, and chromium.

These ingredients, as you have seen, have been clinically proven to help maintain healthy blood glucose levels, and make it easier for your body to beat free-radical damage and burn fat. You can try one nutrient at a time, or you can try this combination supplement, which can multitask for you.

With continued use, it's fair to say that you might experience the following benefits from Metabolic Glucose Formula:

- Reduced blood glucose
- Fewer cravings for sweets
- More energy
- Faster fat-burning potential
- Easier ability to lose weight
- Improved wound healing time
- Fewer nerve pain sensations
- Improved insulin sensitivity
- Reduced cholesterol and blood pressure

Metabolic Glucose Formula is sold nationwide at a popular weight loss clinic called Metabolic Research Center. Their program seeks to help you lose weight by balancing important hormones in the body such as estrogen, progesterone, insulin, DHEA, thyroid, and so on. This product is also sold online at www.emetabolic.com.

The Magic of Minerals: Step 5

You may not think you are stressed, but in this crazy world of ours, you probably are. Certainly, if you have prediabetes or diabetes, your body is under constant stress. Stress can lead to mineral deficiencies, and when this happens, maintaining blood sugar at reasonable levels becomes more difficult.

Minerals are an inexpensive and easy way to support your natural metabolism and improve your blood sugar levels. In fact, without healthy minerals, your immune system takes a hit, and you are more likely to catch a cold or flu; you can't produce enough thyroid hormone, which contributes to insulin resistance; your heart may not beat in proper rhythm; and you feel weak and tired. Minerals are essential to good health, and to life itself.

There are two basic types of minerals, macrominerals and trace minerals. The macrominerals, as their name implies, means we need a lot of—sodium, calcium, magnesium, phosphorus, and strontium.

Microminerals, also called trace minerals, account for only a few grams of body weight. We need microscopic amounts, hence the name. In the body, trace minerals serve as helpers. And for the diabetic they are very helpful indeed. Trace minerals include iron, zinc, vanadium, chromium, manganese, copper, and iodine.

Significant amounts of minerals are lost during food processing. To see just how much is lost, check out "Potential Mineral Loss in Food Processing" on page 282. This comes from the book *Staying Healthy with Nutrition: The Complete Guide to Diet and Nutritional Medicine* by Elson M. Haas. I think this chart says it all. The authors and publisher have been kind enough to let me share it with you in my book.

If I had to put money on it, I'd bet you don't ingest sufficient amounts of healthy minerals on a daily basis. I'm also guessing that you probably get excess amounts of one particular mineral, namely sodium. You get this by shaking regular white table salt (sodium chloride) onto your foods and in just about every processed food that passes your lips. White table salt is virtually deficient in almost all the minerals your pancreas craves. You can read my full exposé on salt in Chapter 9.

POTENTIAL MINERAL LOSS IN FOOD PROCESSING

WHEAT MILLING		REFINING SUGAR CANE	
MINERAL	LOSS	MINERAL	LOSS
Manganese	88%	Magnesium	99%
Chromium	87%	Zinc	98%
Magnesium	80%	Chromium	93%
Sodium	78%	Manganese	93%
Potassium	77%	Cobalt	88%
Iron	76%	Copper	83%
Zinc	72%		
Phosphorus	71%		
Copper	63%		
Calcium	60%		
Molybdenum	60%		
Cobalt	50%		

Data in this table has been compiled from information found in Henry Schroeder, MD, *The Trace Elements and Man.*

The best way for you to get important minerals is by eating a healthy diet that is rich in dark green, leafy vegetables. Another easy and simple way is to drink a green supplement, as I've asked you to do in Chapter 12. Green drink supplements are made from superfoods, such as chlorella and spirulina. These provide exponentially more minerals than any other supplement you could take, plus they come in a natural form that your cells readily absorb.

Minerals improve insulin sensitivity so they help your body incorporate all the sugar into the cells that would otherwise slosh around and damage your kidneys, eyes, and brain.

I realize many people sell oral supplements that contain minerals. There is nothing necessarily bad about taking multimineral supplements. It's just that many of them come in forms difficult for your body to absorb, so they can cause a lot of side effects. Also, sometimes the ratio of minerals in a particular formula pushes your personal mineral balance out of kilter; so again, I am happier if you eat foods rich in minerals, or you supplement with greens that come from Mother Nature and get powdered up for you into a dietary supplement.

MINERALS TO NORMALIZE BLOOD SUGAR

Let's talk about the most important minerals you need to keep your blood sugar normal.

Chromium

Chromium is one of the most useful trace minerals for diabetes because it helps turn carbs into energy. It may also stabilize blood sugar and reduce carb cravings.

In people with type 2 diabetes who are deficient in chromium, supplementation works by increasing insulin (which ultimately contributes to weight loss) and by helping to steady spikes in blood sugar that occur after mealtimes. And this little fact about chromium is key for people with diabetes: The mineral could influence thyroid function because it helps you convert inactive thyroid hormone to active hormone (T3), and that helps determine your fat-burning capabilities. As you know, low thyroid hormone could contribute to weight gain and type 2 diabetes. People with hypoglycemia may also use chromium for this stabilizing effect on blood sugars.

Studies have shown a deficiency of chromium can contribute to your cholesterol being too high. One study showed that when participants were given chromium, they experienced a reduction in harmful lipoproteins and an increase in HDLs (high-density lipoprotein). So even though chromium is best known for its ability to help shut down sweet-tooth cravings and to stabilize blood sugar, it can also improve cholesterol ratios.

Studies conducted by major hospitals and universities show chromium supplementation can help people reduce body fat, stabilize blood sugar, increase muscle growth, and decrease elevated cholesterol levels. Researchers saw these effects especially in people who were deficient in chromium to begin with. They didn't see these effects when giving more chromium in supplement form to people who already had sufficient levels.

HOW TO SUPPLEMENT. Most supplements are made of chromium picolinate. Chromium polynicotinate, however, has been recommended by the U.S. National Research Council as the preferred form of chromium supplement because of its easy absorption and superior activity in the body. The polynicotinate form of chromium is more effective than other types of chromium supplements sold in health food stores because it binds the elemental chromium to niacin (vitamin B_3). This provides a biologically active form of chromium, which is easily used by the body.

You will often see labels on chromium supplements as Chromium GTF. The GTF stands for glucose tolerance factor. A few reputable supplements include Natural Factors, Chromium GTF Chelate 500mcg tabs; Jarrow Formulas, Chromium GTF 200mcg caps; and Bluebonnet Nutrition, GTF Chromium 200mg V caps.

The recommended dosage is 100 to 200 micrograms one to three times daily. Never exceed 1,000 micrograms per day, because doing so could damage your kidneys over time, and it could cause a relative deficiency of other minerals. Taking ibuprofen, aspirin, or naproxen may increase the absorption of chromium in the body.

CAUTION. Taking a chromium supplement could decrease your blood sugar, which is a good thing. But if you also take blood sugar–lowering medications or other supplements for that purpose, you could experience dangerous hypoglycemia, which could cause a diabetic coma. Chromium is generally well tolerated, but check with your doctor about whether it is right for you, as some people have experienced side effects such as dizziness, faintness, fatigue, appetite loss, or unexplained bruising.

Magnesium

The essential mineral magnesium helps stabilize heart rhythm, helps reduce depression and pain, and helps form thyroid hormone. It is an incredible mineral needed for good health across the board. A deficiency in magnesium can contribute to type 2 diabetes and create complications for your very hardworking and loyal heart.

Americans may be low in magnesium for several reasons. For one, processing foods causes the mineral to be stripped away. Also, the soils in which our food is grown, on the whole, are often deficient in magnesium. Foods rich in magnesium include unrefined grains, nuts, and green vegetables. Green, leafy vegetables are particularly good sources of magnesium because they contain high levels of chlorophyll (as does the green superfood I want you to drink daily).

Many medications are drug muggers for magnesium, so when you take certain diuretics, blood pressure pills, steroids, estrogens, or diabetic medications (sulfonamides, which are sulfa based), you may end up with a magnesium deficiency from the drug-mugging effect.

Finally, people try to bone up with calcium and prevent osteoporosis, but some experts feel supplementing with calcium drives magnesium out of the body more easily. The two minerals sort of compete. The take-home point is magnesium can do wonders for a person with diabetes. (If you take a calcium supplement, it's a good idea to also take a magnesium supplement.)

In fact, a study published in 2009 concluded for people with type 2 diabetes, magnesium deficiency can be extremely harmful to kidney function. Supplementing with this mineral may improve the activity of insulin in the body. Another important benefit to people with diabetes or metabolic syndrome is magnesium's effect on the heart. It can help strengthen arteries, improve heart contractility, and promote healthier cholesterol ratios. It may also relieve leg cramps and muscle spasms, and of course increase bone strength. One more impressive benefit is magnesium's ability to help a person "chill out." It has a calming effect on people with anxiety.

Some symptoms of magnesium deficiency include, not surprisingly, agitation and anxiety, restless legs syndrome, sleep disorders, low blood pressure, abnormal heart rhythms, muscle spasm and weakness, difficulty falling or staying asleep, and poor nail growth. Some scientists even believe magnesium deficiency may contribute to seizures.

HOW TO SUPPLEMENT. Adults should take approximately 100 to 200 milligrams once or twice daily. Some people find that they can tolerate a bit more. However, take more only with your physician's approval, because people with liver or kidney problems (which include many people with diabetes) may end up with magnesium toxicity.

The best forms of magnesium are the chelate or glycinate forms, which are sold at health food stores. You want your magnesium to be bound to an amino acid such as aspartate, malate, or glycinate, because these forms are less likely—if at all—to cause diarrhea, one traditional side effect of magnesium.

Be careful at the pharmacy, and don't get those green bottles of magnesium citrate, because those will make you go in a hurry. They are laxatives. Also be aware that too much magnesium can cause nausea, appetite loss, diarrhea, drowsiness, weakness, low blood pressure, or abnormal heart rhythm.

I believe in mineral supplementation because the human body requires minerals, and, as I mentioned earlier, the soil may be depleted of minerals. Superfoods come from the ocean rather than land where the soils are depleted. Ocean plants absorb minerals of the ocean and turn them into a form of minerals that your body readily takes up. It's an efficient way of getting minerals into your body quickly. That's why I mentioned a marine-derived green in Chapter 000 called Ocean's Alive Marine Phytoplankton. Two other reputable brands of magnesium are Dr. Stephen Sinatra's Advanced BioSolutions Broad Spectrum Magnesium or Doctor's Best High Absorption Magnesium.

Iron

Iron is a metal that is essential to most life forms, including human. It is one of the most abundant metals on the planet. In our body, iron gets involved in many enzyme reactions, and it helps deliver oxygen to each and every cell. Without enough iron, your body starves for oxygen.

About two-thirds of the iron in the human body is found in hemoglobin, the protein in red blood cells that carries oxygen to our tissues. So as you can see, iron is integral to your good health.

Your ability to store iron is controlled, in part, by the health of your intestinal system. This is one more reason to eat healthy, nutritious foods. If you become deficient in iron, your cells will starve for oxygen and suffocate until they start to die off. Eventually, cell death results in lowered immunity, weakness, and fatigue.

Iron deficiency can also lower levels of active thyroid hormone (T3) because you need iron to convert inactive thyroid hormone (T4) to its active, useful form (T3). Iron deficiency is particularly bad for people with diabetes because it contributes to hypothyroidism. Recall from Chapter 6 that people with hypothyroidism are more likely to experience diabetes because they can't dump out all the fat and sugar in their cells; their metabolism is sluggish. Just for the record, iron is not the only mineral that affects the thyroid. So do zinc and selenium.

Other symptoms that might alert you to an iron deficiency include feeling cranky and depressed or having trouble concentrating. Your nails may break easily, and your heart may beat like crazy after hardly any exertion at all. Many

WHAT THE NUMBERS MEAN

When doctors measure your iron using the serum ferritin blood test, the full range differs for men and women.

Male: 12 to 300 ng/mL
Female: 12 to 150 ng/mL

The lower you are within the normal range, the more likely you are to experience symptoms of iron deficiency. The general goal to shoot for is somewhere between 70 and 90. When ferritin is low, you will become hypothyroid at the cellular level, which in turn exacerbates diabetes. This is fully explained in Chapter 6.

other disorders and mineral deficiencies can cause similar symptoms, so teasing out a true iron deficiency is not always easy. Doctors in the know order a blood test called serum ferritin, which gives them an idea of whether your stash of iron is healthy. If found to be low, supplements (along with green drinks containing spirulina) may very well be in order for you.

It takes only a few months of iron supplementation to breathe life back into an individual who is deficient, and in people with diabetes, a little iron can make a big difference to their health.

And one more very important consideration: Drug muggers that rob your body of valuable iron include acid-blocking drugs (used for reflux and heartburn) as well as aspirin, many antibiotics, some diuretics, and popular anti-inflammatories, such as ibuprofen and naproxen. A shocker is that some diabetic medications (particularly the sulfonylureas) are also drug muggers of this important mineral.

HOW TO SUPPLEMENT. Unless a blood test shows you are deficient in iron, I prefer that you get your iron from green drinks or black strap molasses. Some of the ingredients in greens include spirulina, which contains 2,000 times the amount of iron as compared to spinach. Don't worry, that's still safe and actually considered healthy.

Getting iron from food is much easier on the stomach. Some foods with rich sources of iron include lean meats (preferably free range), liver, eggs, green leafy vegetables (kale, spinach, turnip greens), whole grain breads, raisins, and molasses.

Iron exists in two forms: heme and nonheme. Heme iron is found in animal foods, such as beef, chicken, turkey, pork, and seafood. The body can get the nonheme form of iron from nuts, beans, fruits, vegetables, and grains. Foods that contain vitamin C (like citrus fruits) lend a helping hand by boosting your ability to take up iron from your foods.

If you do require an iron dietary supplement, then stick to those brands that are easily digested, or you could wind up with constipation and stomach cramping. The better brands of iron, which are less likely to cause gastrointestinal side effects, include Iron Glycinate, and Nu-Iron (Nifere)x (iron polysaccharide complex), and they are sold at most pharmacies and some health food stores.

Dosage is about 150 milligrams daily, taken with food, for 2 or 3 months or as your physician suggests. It may take that long for you to notice improvement in your symptoms and an increase in your blood's iron levels. I don't recommend taking ferrous-sulfate brands of iron, but these are still sometimes recommended

---

SALT SECRET

Healthy salts support thyroid function and improve blood sugar numbers. I carry my own saltshaker so I can put healthy, unadulterated sea salt on my food, instead of cheap table salt, which is void of healthy minerals.

Buy yourself a little cylinder-shaped plastic or metal pill container at any pharmacy or camping store. Make sure it is airtight. The one I have is metal, and it fits right on my key ring so I can take it everywhere I go. Read page 333 to learn about the healthiest salts on Earth that not only make your food taste better but also have the ability to improve your health.

---

by physicians, perhaps because they are so easy to find, and they are inexpensive. If you take this form, I suggest that you take a little bit of vitamin E with it, because some research suggests that this vitamin is depleted by ferrous sulfate.

Harmless green discoloration of the stool often occurs with iron supplementation. (Tell your friends you're doing your part and "going green.")

Iron accumulation can be dangerous for tots, so be sure to lock up your medicine cabinet when young children are present. One more note of caution: Some types of liquid iron can stain or blacken teeth in adults and children, specifically animal-based (heme) forms. The *vegetable-based* (nonheme) forms of liquid iron should not do this. Just to be on the safe side, it's best to brush your teeth immediately afterward if you take liquid iron supplements.

Vanadium

The body needs only tiny amounts of the trace mineral vanadium. There's no doubt in my mind a deficiency of vanadium can contribute to diabetes and affect insulin sensitivity; however, I'm not convinced people with diabetes are actually deficient. It's easy to maintain your warehouse of vanadium in the body through diet.

It is true that low levels of this mineral have been associated with high cholesterol and high blood glucose, at least in animal studies. Vanadium supplementation may make your body more sensitive to the insulin in your blood, so it can help reduce blood sugar and send glucose to your muscles, where it's needed.

Some people have rushed to embrace vanadium as a supplement for everyone with diabetes, but this is based only on animal studies (on rats, to be specific). Supplements may be able to reduce bad LDL (low-density lipoprotein) cholesterol, which is associated with hardening of the arteries, and also appear to reduce the need for insulin in both type 1 and type 2 diabetes.

I think this supplement is good for you, if you are shown to be deficient in vanadium. Supplements probably won't help that much if you are not deficient, and could contribute to kidney problems. Foods that contain vanadium include whole grains, seafood, seeds, mushrooms, dill, olive oil, beans, carrots, greens, garlic, lettuce, and pepper.

HOW TO SUPPLEMENT. I prefer that individuals take vanadium as part of a trace mineral supplement rather than an isolated supplement all by itself. Trace minerals contain other minerals that help vanadium, such as chromium, zinc, manganese, and magnesium. Another reason is that your diet might provide you with 20 to 60 micrograms per day, where a supplement may be as high as 100 milligrams. That's quite a bit, and may shock your system. So I usually don't suggest that you take that much unless your doctor wants you to, and you are monitored by blood tests for any red-flag changes.

In summary, minerals are absolutely essential to pancreatic health and insulin sensitivity. Rather than taking single minerals, it is fine with me if you take a single supplement with various minerals in it. I'm thinking of an all-in-one formula. I've found several high quality formulas that offer you minerals in the best form. They are Dr. Dave's Magic Minerals available online at www. stages-of-life.com; Jarrow Formula's Mineral Balance at most health food stores; and Biomins by Thorne Research, which is magnesium stearate-free, at www.thorne.com.

PART 6

RECIPES AND KITCHEN TIPS

15 Eat Sweets without Suffering

Americans have an insatiable sweet tooth, downing about 90 to 180 pounds of the sweet stuff every year per person! Worldwide, the mass consumption of refined sugar and dangerous additives like high-fructose corn syrup (HFCS) is creating an epidemic of obesity, autoimmune disorders, digestive disorders, thyroid problems, diabetes, and the triple threat called metabolic syndrome—dangerously high cholesterol, high blood sugar, and high blood pressure, often in conjunction with excess pounds.

With this epidemic of malnourished and oversugared citizens, I think it's high time we reevaluate our belief system about food and the addiction we all have to gooey desserts and processed foods in general. If we don't make changes in the kitchen and use safer ways to sweeten our foods, we will continue to lose our quality of life and die younger. Fortunately, the changes that I'm recommending here are good for you, and they taste great. You will eventually stop craving so much sweet stuff once you get used to eating better sugars. It may take a few weeks, so be patient.

Later on in this chapter, I promise to classify the most popular sugars available as either "good," "better," or "best" so you'll have delicious, healthy alternatives that add sweetness to your life without causing you to suffer. This chapter also includes information about the popular glycemic index diet, which many diabetics follow. I don't agree with this diet, and I'll tell you why. For now, let's take a closer look at the sweetest poisons.

HOW DOES SUGAR BEHAVE IN THE BODY?

Let's get something straight right now. Sugar is not the bad guy in diabetes that everyone makes it out to be. We need some sugar to help us think, and I don't want a bunch of people reading this book and becoming sugar-phobic. Diabetes and other related problems, such as metabolic syndrome, hyperglycemia, and insulin resistance, are really about your body's *response* to sugar and its inability to process sugar correctly.

With all of that understood, I want to move on now to white, refined sugar, which is different from the kind of sugar that occurs naturally in nature. White, refined sugar is heavily processed, and it's a lot sweeter than Mother Nature's sugars. This type of crystal is sold everywhere in large bags in supermarkets.

White, refined sugar is the kind of chemical that actually promotes diabetes. It suppresses the immune system by causing the pancreas to secrete abnormally large quantities of insulin to break down the sugar. Insulin stays in the bloodstream long after it is needed and proceeds to suppress an important immune-boosting hormone called growth hormone. Don't worry; this suppression doesn't mean you will shrink, but you might get repeated infections.

Excess sugar is stored in the liver in the form of glycogen. But your liver can only store so much. It will balloon until its capacity is overwhelmed. Then sugar floods your bloodstream in the form of fatty acids, which are then stored in the "inactive" areas of your body—in other words, stored fat. This leads to thicker thighs, a bigger bottom, and that spare tire that some people confuse with love handles.

Fat is literally the excess energy (or calories, which are a measure of energy) you have taken in, energy that your body doesn't need, so it stores it in case of famine. This is another example of how miraculous our bodies are, and how in modern times, with all our conveniences, we are upsetting our bodies' survival-oriented mechanisms.

Anyway, back to our story of fatty acids. After the fatty acids are stored in the "inactive" (ahem) areas, these dangerous substances are distributed to more active organs, such as your heart and kidneys, which eventually start to fall apart on you because you're asking them to work beyond what they can do.

Think of an exhausted factory worker being pushed and pushed to work until she drops. Or a marathoner who is asked to run another marathon without rest. That's what happens to your heart and kidneys when you work them too hard by eating more than your body needs. Your brain gets in the picture as well. Memory starts to slip, simple arithmetic problems become difficult, and you can't recall what you ate for dinner last night, or the name of whomever or whatchamacallit. Sugar makes you dumb.

Sugar also destroys the natural healthy bacteria that normally reside in your gut. Without a healthy camp of beneficial bacteria, your body is unable to make B vitamins and worse, you become infected with the fungus *Candida albicans*. This whole cascade leads to fatigue, depression, nerve damage, confusion, and dozens of other symptoms that each commands its own prescription drug to fix. Eat too

SUGAR BY ANY OTHER NAME

If you're doing your best to limit your sugar intake, you'll want to read all product labels carefully. What are you looking for? Alas, it's not enough to simply look for sugar. You need to keep an eye out for these items as well:

Sucrose—another name for sugar, the refined, crystallized white stuff in your sugar bowl. (Chemically, sugar is a combination of glucose and fructose.)

Dextrose—actually pure glucose, a simple sugar made of only one molecule

Lactose—a simple sugar from milk

Maltose—a simple sugar from starch, usually grains

Maltodextrin—a manufactured sugar from maltose and dextrose

Brown sugar—the refined sugar coated with molasses or colored with caramel

Raw sugar—a less-refined white sugar with a small amount of molasses remaining

Fructose—a simple sugar from fruit

Corn syrup—a manufactured syrup made from corn, containing varying proportions of glucose, maltose, and dextrose

High-fructose corn syrup—a highly concentrated corn syrup of predominantly fructose

White grape juice—a highly purified fructose solution (Virtually no other nutrients are present.)

many gooey cinnamon buns, and ultimately you become a walking pharmacy.

Just when you thought it couldn't get any worse, it does. That's because sugar is a drug mugger of minerals in your body. Seriously.

Drug muggers are drugs (or any substance) that rob your body of essential nutrients you need to survive and to enjoy good health. For example, statin cholesterol drugs mug coenzyme Q10 from the body, causing fatigue and muscle cramps; birth control pills mug magnesium, zinc, and B vitamins, leading to depression and hypothyroidism; and so on. Your diabetic medicine could be a strong drug mugger of several nutrients, including vitamin B_{12}.

I think it's important for you to know that sugar is a drug mugger of many minerals essential in protecting you from diabetes. White refined sugar appears to be a strong drug mugger of:

- Chromium, which helps you maintain proper blood sugar levels
- Zinc, which plays a role in the synthesis, secretion, and storage of insulin
- Magnesium, which improves insulin sensitivity and maintains blood pressure

- B vitamins, which guard you against nerve damage and painful neuropathies
- Potassium, which helps regulate blood pressure and heartbeat
- Calcium, which works in tandem with vitamin D to prevent diabetes

We also need these minerals that we have been mugged of to maintain healthy bones and teeth.

Sugar also changes the acid-to-alkaline ratio in your bloodstream, making it more acidic. With all the acid that sugar creates, your acid-to-alkaline ratio is thrown out of kilter. Your body will do what it can to bring harmony back and raise the pH to a higher level of alkalinity. It robs minerals from your bones and teeth to bring back the acid-to-alkaline ratio in the blood. This is why some experts believe eating sugar every day contributes to brittle bones and tooth decay.

But even with all of these problems associated with white refined sugar, I'd choose it over those artificial sweeteners, which tend to poke holes in your brain. (I'll go into details about that later in the chapter.)

NOT ALL SUGARS ARE CREATED EQUAL

Your body can't avoid consuming some sugars. In fact, you need carbohydrates and certain sugars for your very survival because your cells break these down and turn the glucose into energy for you. Sugars are a natural part of many of the foods you eat, including fruits and vegetables. Sugars found in processed foods or that you add to your foods are another matter, however. Some are relatively healthy, and others are not so good for you. What follows is an overview of different kinds of sugar—the good, the better, the best . . . and the not-so-good.

GOOD SWEETENERS

TURBINADO SUGAR is also called raw sugar. In the United Kingdom and overseas it's sometimes known as demarara. Turbinado sugar is created when sugar cane is slowly boiled down, leaving a beautiful golden crystal that still contains molasses.

FRUIT JUICE CONCENTRATE is made from fruit juice that has its water content reduced. When water is added back to it, the taste is not exactly the same.

EVAPORATED CANE JUICE is the sweet liquid that comes from the sugar cane before all the refining and bleaching takes place to turn it into white sugar crystals. This sweetener retains some of the natural nutrients found in sugar cane.

AGAVE SYRUP is a sweetener that resembles honey, but there are no animals or insects involved. It is extracted from a spiky plant that looks similar to *Aloe* *vera*. The sweet extract is purified and can be used in cold beverages or in cooking because it dissolves easily.

Unfortunately, there are now reports that many brands of agave syrup are heated and refined. Manufacturers are not designating this on the label, so you think it's pure and unprocessed, but your product may be heated to high temperatures for long periods of time. Even more disturbing, ingredient data show that it contains a lot of fructose, about 90 percent fructose and 10 percent glucose.

Some nutritional experts now feel that agave syrup is just as bad as high-fructose corn syrup, but I do not feel quite this strongly. Agave syrup does not normally spike your blood sugar (it's fairly low on the glycemic index), plus it's less processed than white, refined sugar. And in my book, a lot better than HFCS.

I do feel, however, that because of its high fructose content, agave may tax your liver and deplete you of minerals, as do other refined sugars. High fructose has also been associated with insulin resistance, so if these reports prove to be true, I will have to take agave syrup off this list completely. For now, I use it in my own home on occasion, and I have listed it in several recipes. Use it sparingly and for the most part, stick to better sugars or natural ones like maple syrup, honey, or black strap molasses.

BETTER SWEETENERS

MAPLE SYRUP comes from the sap of maple trees. It takes about 10 gallons of sap to make 1 quart of maple syrup. Be careful when purchasing, as there are many artificial, look-alike products. You want 100 percent pure maple syrup. It will say that on the label, and it's not inexpensive. Available at supermarkets.

BROWN RICE SYRUP is a grain-based sweetener, but it comes from rice, not corn. Rice syrup is produced by cooking together brown rice flour (or starch) along with some enzymes, which might at times be genetically modified. The result is a syrup that gets filtered and evaporated and is often used in energy bars and health food products. This grain-derived sweetener is fine to use if you are gluten-free. Available at most health food stores.

HONEY is the sweet nectar that bees make. It's really bee regurgitation, if you want the freaky truth. I like honey. Its primary constituents are fructose and glucose, and the ratio is similar to the type of HFCS used in soda (about 55 percent and 45 percent, respectively).

One tablespoon of honey ranks at 55 out of 100 on the glycemic index. (I discuss the glycemic index later in this chapter.) Even though this is relatively high on the glycemic index scale, I've classified honey as one of the better sweeteners because it comes from nature and many pure, unadulterated raw versions of honey contain healthful enzymes and minerals that support immune function and fight cancer. For example, Manuka honey from New Zealand tastes great, and when applied externally to wounds, it appears to speed healing and prevent dangerous staph infections because it has antibacterial properties.

A 2006 Israeli study that was published in the journal *Medical Oncology* showed LifeMel honey could reduce anemia in 64 percent of individuals undergoing chemotherapy. It also decreased the incidence of severe, life-threatening neutropenia (a disorder of the blood that causes abnormally low white counts), which often occurs with chemotherapy. So, no doubt honey has health benefits as compared to refined white sugar.

The honey story gets a little sticky, however, because commercial farmers often heat and process honey. When that's done, you lose all these beneficial compounds. Processed honey is what's most commonly sold in grocery stores, so it's worth going to the farmer's market or to health food stores (or online) to purchase your honey. Because the two honey products mentioned above have been scientifically validated, I've included them in my resource section so you can find them easily.

BEST SWEETENERS

COCONUT SUGAR is just evaporated coconut sap. I use this sugar in my home. It has the texture of brown sugar, but it is truly one of the best choices for a health-conscious person because it is rich in phosphorus, potassium, and other minerals. I don't really advocate the glycemic index measuring system, but if you want to know, coconut sugar ranks in at 35, compared to cane sugar, which is 68. I found an organic brand online. It's called Coconut Palm Sugar and is available at www.livesuperfoods.com.

MUSCOVADO SUGAR is unrefined sugar straight from the sugar cane that looks like rich brown crystals, thanks to all the nutritional molasses. The texture is similar to that of brown sugar, but it's more nutritious and less refined. Around the world, it may be called moist sugar or Barbados sugar. Unlike white sugar, this type retains many minerals, including magnesium, potassium, calcium, and iron. Be careful cooking with it—its moistness may make your recipes too wet.

STEVIA. Stevia is harvested from the plant *Stevia rebaudiana*, which is native to South America. It belongs to the genus *Chrysanthemum*, which is part of the daisy family. The leaves of *Stevia rebaudiana* have been used for centuries as sweeteners for bitter medicines and teas. You can use fresh Stevia, in fact, is such an incredible sweetener and has so much going for it in terms of health benefits that I'm going to go into a great more detail below. For now, I want to continue this overview of sugars.

SUGARS YOU SHOULDN'T USE

Now that you know which sugars you can safely use (sparingly please), let's focus on the ones you should do your best to avoid.

XYLITOL is a synthetic sugar-alcohol that is heavily processed and promoted to prevent tooth decay. It is not the same thing as naturally occurring xylan, which is found in corn, as well as many fruits and vegetables in tiny amounts.

Xylitol is known to cause diarrhea fairly quickly in individuals who are sensitive to it. So is a similar sugar alcohol called sorbitol. You'll find these wanna-be sugars in candy and gum, so kids take in a lot of it. Xylitol is pitched as a healthy sugar substitute, but in my book, it's far from healthy, because it is hydrogenated and processed; I think you should avoid it.

HIGH-FRUCTOSE CORN SYRUP is a man-made form of sugar that is heavily refined.

BROWN SUGAR is sugar made from sugar cane, but not as far along in the refining process. The real thing still contains some healthy, mineral-laden molasses. Be aware, however, that many brands are just white, refined sugar with dark molasses added back in. Coconut sugar or muscovado sugar could easily be substituted for brown sugar, and you would get far more health benefits.

ARTIFICIAL SWEETENERS are, well, artificial, and your body has trouble breaking them down. I will go into a great deal of detail about a couple of artificial sweeteners—aspartame and sucralose—later in this chapter.

SUGAR'S MORE SINFUL SISTER— HIGH-FRUCTOSE CORN SYRUP

High-fructose corn syrup (HFCS) is really the marriage of fructose (a simple plant sugar) and glucose (another simple sugar). Either way, both are "simple" sugars, and as you have heard me say many times, all the food you eat should be complex versus simple. This doesn't mean I'm asking you to solve a jigsaw puzzle to make breakfast; it's a matter of chemistry. The more complex the sugar or carbohydrate, the more nutritious it is—it's as simple as that.

The ratio of fructose to glucose differs, depending on the type of food it is being used to sweeten. Some forms of HFCS are 90 percent fructose, 10 percent glucose. The type of HFCS used in soda pop is usually 55 percent fructose, 45 percent glucose.

HFCS is found in candy bars, soda pop, baked goods, spaghetti sauce, salad dressings, ketchup, and thousands of other foods at your supermarket. Yes, thousands. The average American consumes about 12 teaspoons of HFCS every day. *I absolutely believe this additive is a major cause for the growing number of diabetics in our country.* And that's the simple and sad truth.

HFCS is such a cheap sweetener to produce, food manufacturers justify its use in virtually everything. HFCS is disgustingly sweet, and it blends easier into beverages than table sugar. In January 2009, the FDA came out and said that HFCS used in soda pop is natural and safe. That floored me, because the research I have read suggests just the opposite.

Since it took brain-dead health officials about 20 years to decide that trans fats can kill you, do you believe what they say about HFCS now? *HFCS is a highly reactive substance that can spur the production of free radicals in your body.*

Free radicals act like loose cannons inside of you. They seek out and destroy healthy cells and take out as many as they can. Free radicals attack the pancreas, and studies prove it is exactly this type of free-radical oxidative damage that leads to diabetes and pancreatitis, and to many other disorders, too!

In 2009, the peer-reviewed journal *Obesity* published a study that made my dreams come true. Several research scientists in Saudi Arabia wrote an article titled "Diabetes of the Liver: The Link between Nonalcoholic Fatty Liver Disease and HFCS-55." The title says it all. It makes the link between a specific type of liver disease, which is not caused by drinking alcohol (nonalcoholic fatty liver disease or NAFLD), and high-fructose corn syrup. The 55 just designates one type of HFCS.

There is tremendous information in this one study, but I'll spare you the cellular and bioscientific complexities and just cut to the chase. These scientists concluded from their studies examining both *in vitro* (or test tube) and *in vivo* (or live human) individuals whose diet included 20 percent of calories from HFCS showed signs of fatty liver disease and even disruption on a cellular level (mitochondrial disruption). These scientists concluded that this version of HFCS may well contribute to the disease process of nonalcoholic fatty liver disease.

If that Saudi Arabian study on one form of HFCS doesn't do it for you, how about this one? Scientists at the University of Pennsylvania in Philadelphia have been looking closely at the effects of fructose and glucose on human metabolism. In a 2004 study published in the peer-reviewed *Journal of Clinical Endocrinology and Metabolism*, researchers concluded: "Because insulin and leptin, and possibly ghrelin, function as key signals to the central nervous system in the long-term regulation of energy balance, decreases of circulating insulin and leptin and increased ghrelin concentrations, as demonstrated in this study, could lead to increased caloric intake and ultimately contribute to weight gain and obesity during chronic consumption of diets high in fructose."

Translation: Eat fructose in any form (including and especially in HFCS), and your body makes less leptin (the "feel-full" hormone) and less insulin, making it impossible for you to know when you feel full, and leading you to overeat ("increased caloric intake") and gain weight. Essentially, the hormone leptin is suppressed, and the cycle of misery, weight gain, and diabetes is set in motion. Please see discussion on leptin in Chapter 3.

On August 23, 2007, yet another study was reported on at the 234th national meeting of the American Chemical Society. During the symposium "Food Bioactives and Nutraceuticals: Production, Chemistry, Analysis, and Health Effects," Chi-Tang Ho, PhD, professor of food science at Rutgers University in New Brunswick, New Jersey, spoke on his chemical tests of 11 different carbonated drinks containing HFCS.

Dr. Ho found "astonishingly high" levels of reactive carbonyls in those beverages. These are compounds associated with fructose and glucose that are essentially loose cannons in the bloodstream, substances that cause tissue damage! Interestingly, Dr. Ho found that these same compounds (reactive carbonyls) that appear to set off the chain of tissue damage in the body are not present in table sugar. In table sugar, fructose and glucose molecules are "bound" and thus more chemically stable than the HFCS molecules, which are "unbound."

Here's the fascinating part: Dr. Ho and other researchers have found that reactive carbonyls are also elevated in the blood of people with diabetes, and are linked to complications of diabetes. *Hello!* Dr. Ho estimated that a single can of soda contains about five times the concentration of reactive carbonyls than the concentration found in the blood of an adult person with diabetes.

Interestingly, Dr. Ho and his associates also found that adding epigallocatechin gallate, a compound found in tea, to drinks containing HFCS may help lower the levels of reactive carbonyls, in some cases by half. I have a better idea: Drink tea and forget about the sugary carbonated beverages!

Do you see now why consuming soda is not a good idea?

The bad news about HFCS doesn't stop there, however. Emerging research conducted at the Institute for Agriculture and Trade Policy found traces of mercury (a manufacturing contaminant) in HFCS. So some types of HFCS could be tainted with heavy metal poison that attacks the brain and kidneys. And this is deemed safe by the FDA? Hmmm, I wasn't born yesterday. One study I read revealed about 30 percent of foods in the supermarket contain HFCS that is contaminated with mercury. So it's very difficult to avoid this poison if you continue to eat boxed or processed foods and drinks.

This conversation prompts the question, "Is plain fructose any better?" Yes, I think that fructose is somewhat cleaner than HFCS, technically speaking. But fructose is still a "simple" sugar. It's a plant sugar, also made from corn. Crystalline fructose is a different story, though. I don't recommend that one because, according to the site www.Sugar.org, crystalline fructose is "produced by allowing the fructose to crystallize from a fructose-enriched corn syrup." In addition, this substance—which sounds like it comes from Superman's planet—also contains arsenic, albeit 1 mg/kg (milligram per kilogram) maximum. Still, it's arsenic, so it's verifiably poison!

WHAT ABOUT FRUIT JUICE?

I'd prefer that you eat your fruit rather than drink it. Some juices contain HFCS, some don't. You'll have to become a label sleuth and read the ingredients list to know which are clean. Mothers have problems with their kids when it comes to juice because the kids want all the sweet stuff that is only 10 percent juice, while the rest of the mixture is laden with HFCS, preservatives, and artificial colorants. Some of the red juices contain bug juice too, in the form of carmine, a natural colorant that comes from crushed-up beetle bugs. It is considered a natural colorant—aren't bugs natural? Most red-colored yogurt, candy, and beverages are dyed with boiled-up bug colorants.

With all the sugar and HFCS that some of these juices contain, is it any wonder that your kids are running around in circles all over the house, unable to concentrate? No worries, your doctor can give you another chemical (Ritalin) to negate the effects of high-octane sweeteners and other food additives. Am I saying juice boxes and HFCS-containing foods can contribute to attention deficit disorder or childhood obesity? Yes, I am, but there are certainly other factors involved, too.

Mothers, let me ask you this: Would you ever let your child sit down and eat 8 apples or 2 pounds of grapes at one sitting? I didn't think so. I didn't let my kids do that, either, but that's the approximate equivalent of one juice box (6.8 ounces, give or take). It's a heck of a lot of sugar, and it can increase the risk for diabetes.

According to a study published in the journal *Diabetes Care* in 2008, just one serving of fruit juice per day increased the risk for developing type 2 diabetes in women. There's an easy way to break your child of sugary juices and sodas. Water them down. It's easy. Just keep adding water over the course of 10 days until they don't like it anymore. They'll never even know why, and what they don't know won't hurt them.

Obviously, selecting 100 percent juice drinks for your family is better than the garbage juices that only contain small amounts of juice and a lot of other additives. But as I suggested earlier, it's better to eat the apple rather than drinking apple juice because then you get all the good fiber, which aids digestion. Juice boxes don't give you any fiber.

As the age old saying goes, "An apple a day keeps the doctor away." It doesn't say, "An apple juice box a day keeps the doctor away." Further, a real, organic, fresh apple also happens to contain a healthy substance called malic acid, which can relax muscles. In fact, malic acid is so fantastic at relieving muscle pain that people with fibromyalgia take supplements of malic acid.

PUT STEVIA AT THE TOP OF THE LIST

Now let's go back and take a look at the one sweetener you need to pay special attention to if you have any form of diabetes or any issues with blood sugar control—stevia.

The leaves of the stevia plant contain glycosides, a group of organic plant compounds that taste sweet but have zero calories. The leaf extract that is commercially marketed is actually one of the active steviosides in this plant, and it's about 200 to 300 times sweeter than sugar. When buying products, you'll find that the label will just say "stevia," or it will go by brand names such as Sweet Leaf and Only Sweet.

The stevia plant's leaves, the aqueous extract of the leaves, and purified steviosides are all used as sweeteners. Once extracted, the stevia herb is converted to a sweet white powder. Stevia may be a new word to you, but people overseas have used it for centuries. It can sweeten anything you like, including coffee and tea, and you can also bake with it; however, when converting the recipe you need to be aware that the conversion to sugar is *not* the same. One Web site offers a conversion chart. (See www.steviainfo.com/?page=equivalency_chart.)

Stevia is completely free of calories and carbohydrates, plus it's zero on the glycemic index, which means that it will not spike your blood sugar the way white, refined sugar does. It also means that it's safe for people who have diabetes as well as those concerned about *Candida*. I think it's your healthiest alternative to both sugar and artificial sweeteners because besides being sweet, it can help you balance blood sugar and lose weight.

As of today in the United States, stevia is not allowed to be sold as a food additive, though it is considered safe as a dietary supplement. But the Japanese have been using stevia in foods and soft drinks for many years. It's even in their Coca-Cola.

Stevia is the perfect sweetener for people with diabetes or hypoglycemia because it does not cause blood glucose levels to spike or fluctuate. It is considered safe, too, and has been well documented in scientific studies. Not only is it safe, but it's nutritious. The herb has been found to have a stabilizing effect on blood glucose, but ironically it is not allowed to be promoted for that purpose, whereas a patented, chemically altered version called Truvia is! (The United States just recently approved Truvia for use in foods as a sweetener in December 2008.) Some things just make you go *hmmm*.

Not only does stevia help control blood sugar, but it has other scientifically documented health benefits as well:

- It may be able to alleviate heartburn.
- It may be able to lower blood pressure.
- It seems to improve glucose tolerance in people with high blood sugar.

You can buy stevia plants anywhere you find other edible herbs (like grocery stores or nurseries). It's sometimes called Sweet Herb. Pull a few leaves off and steep with tea or chop into a salad or some rice.

How to Supplement

Buy liquid stevia extracts that are standardized to contain the active steviosides, which are one of the compounds in stevia known to promote health benefits. I would like your product to be alcohol-free, since alcohol can damage the pancreas.

If taken as a dietary supplement, follow directions on the label for your liquid extract. It's usually about five to 15 drops taken once or twice daily in water.

Some brands offer flavored stevia (like cherry, root beer, or vanilla), and that's just fine to use as a sweetener in your coffee, tea, or dessert.

You can also buy stevia in powdered form to use as a sweetener in your foods and beverages daily. You'll find the sweeteners at health food stores and even some supermarkets.

Pure and naturally occurring stevia as described in this section is *not* the same as Coca-Cola's Truvia, or Pepsi's PureVia. Both are proprietary sweeteners based on an extract of stevia. Stevia comes from nature; Truvia only begins with nature.

ARTIFICIAL SWEETENERS: NOTHING SWEET ABOUT THEM

I think artificial sweeteners are like nonprescription drugs because they produce effects in your body and also have undesirable side effects. They are human-made chemicals, and they have to get FDA approval to be sold, just like prescription drugs.

It shocks me that these chemicals—which have been conspicuously tied to cancer and serious neurological disorders—are approved by the FDA, our supposed health watchdog, and sold to the masses as if they were a healthy substitute for sugar. These are dangerous chemicals, and they should never be ingested as far as I'm concerned, especially if you're diabetic.

If you truly understand that diabetes is not a disease of high blood sugar, but rather one of free-radical damage, you will see that these chemicals only add to the amount of free-radical damage you have. Although your blood sugar numbers may appear to be good, these chemicals actually worsen your condition over the long haul. As a class, they are known collectively as excitotoxins.

Simply put, these chemicals stimulate a cell so much that they basically excite it to death. Sometimes the cause is related to how the excitotoxin changes the fluid balance in the body, causing brain cells to swell up with fluid and die. You don't know this is happening at first because millions of healthy cells have to die before the target organ malfunctions, finally alerting you to damage in your body. Excitotoxins are also implicated in migraines in susceptible people.

Let's meet the sweeteners that come in those pretty packets, and then I'll tell you why you should avoid them.

ACESULFAME-K, marketed as Sunette and Sweet One, was one of the first FDA-approved artificial sweeteners, and was hardly even tested.

SACCHARIN is actually benzoic sulfinide. It comes in the pink packet sold by the brand name Sweet'N Low.

ASPARTAME is the substance in the blue packet sold by several brand names such as NutraSweet and Equal. It is known overseas in other countries as Canderel. Approximately 40 percent of aspartame is broken down into the amino acid aspartic acid (also known as aspartate), an excitotoxin.

SUCRALOSE comes in yellow packets and is sold under the brand name Splenda.

TAGATOSE, better known by its brand name Naturlose, is a low-calorie sweetener that comes from a sugar that naturally occurs in dairy and whey. You especially want to avoid this one if you have allergies to casein (milk). The makers claim preliminary studies prove that it's helpful for type 2 diabetics because it prevents blood sugar spikes, but the data is very preliminary.

TRUVIA has everyone raving because they think that it is stevia. It irritates me that natural stevia was banned years ago, but now that a company has found a way to slightly modify it, make it taste less bitter by altering it, and patent it (and therefore profit from it), suddenly everyone is trying to sell it to you.

Truvia, PureVia, or some form of this sweetener will soon be found in thousands of foods and beverages across America.

Truvia is not stevia; don't say I didn't warn you. Truvia is the brand name given to a patented synthetic chemical that came from rebiana. Rebiana is one of many naturally occurring sweet chemicals that come from the stevia leaf. To make Truvia, scientists combined rebiana with another chemical called erythritol, which is a sugar alcohol. The sweetener is FDA approved because the manufacturer was able to create a unique molecule that is patentable according to laws set forth by the U.S. Patent and Trademark Office.

Regardless, I think you should just buy stevia, the natural sweetener that comes from a plant, not its lab-created (dysfunctional) cousin. I am frustrated because the FDA is unwilling to approve the use of natural stevia in our foods, yet they're quick to approve this modified version as a food additive and paint it as completely natural to millions of naïve consumers. Is it safe? Probably but it's too soon to give you 100% assurance. Ask me again in 5 years. And just FYI, we are the guinea pigs.

Generally speaking, I think Truvia is better than the other artificial sweeteners on this list, but I'd prefer you just use stevia until we know more about Truvia.

What about sugar alcohols, such as sorbitol, erythritol, and xylitol? I don't like these either because they are processed, unnatural sweeteners and in some cases (like sorbitol) have been linked to diarrhea, stomach cramps, and severe weight loss. It annoys me that these are found in sugar-free products aimed at people with diabetes and also at kids. These sugars are not natural or healthy in my book.

So to summarize the story of sugars and sweeteners, our love for sugar started out with plain sugar cane, and then a few natural derivatives like molasses and turbinado sugar came into the marketplace. Then someone came along and screwed with healthy, plain sugar from the Earth and turned it into nutritionally naked white, refined sugar. Enter high-fructose corn syrup, to launch a more vicious assault to the pancreas.

Now we have artificial sweeteners, supposedly better than HFCS and white, refined sugar. But what was wrong with nature's sugar cane? It's enough to flummox anyone. Even the most intelligent of people don't know which packet to use, or which sugar to buy. Hopefully, I've given you enough information to know that the closer it is to nature—*and the further it is from a laboratory*—the better it is for your body.

It's a Bucket of Bad News for Artificial Sweeteners

Let me simplify it by grouping all the artificial sweeteners listed above into one giant bucket. What do all of them have in common? They are either partially (in the cases of Truvia, PureVia, and Naturlose) or completely (for all the rest) foreign to nature and not easily processed by the human body. Artificial—that's the key word here. The human body does not know how to unstick artificial sweeteners from cells where they lodge and cause a vibration of sorts; that's why they are classified as excitotoxins by scientists. They "excite" the cell to death.

I believe—and there is a lot of documentation—that there are real dangers associated with some of these synthetic chemicals, especially the ones that have been out for years. The newer ones don't have long-term studies on them and appear to be less modified. The dangers range from behavioral disorders in children to epilepsy and cancer. I want to give you as much information here as possible, because I realize that you may take some flack from your diabetes educator when you return to a meeting and state that you have made a decision to stop consuming artificial sweeteners (against their advice). You need to be armed with knowledge, and you need to feel at peace with your decision.

Let's talk about aspartame for a moment, because that one is incredibly popular. This ingredient is FDA approved, but it took many years for that to happen. Here is the story.

Aspartame was discovered in 1965 by James M. Schlatter, PhD, a chemist working for G.D. Searle & Company. While working on an antiulcer drug, he licked his finger, which had the compound aspartame on it, and realized it had an extremely sweet taste.

Aspartame was tested for safety in human consumption, but during these tests, scientists discovered that aspartame might cause brain tumors in rats, which are also mammals (as we are). Because of these findings, the FDA would not approve its use as a food additive.

Fifteen years after Dr. Schlatter discovered aspartame's sweetness—in 1980—the FDA held a Public Board of Inquiry, asking independent advisors to look into the link between aspartame and cancer of the brain. While the board found no direct link, the members still advised against approving aspartame for use as a food additive because of some still-fishy cases of cancer in laboratory rats.

In 1981, President Ronald Reagan appointed Arthur Hayes as the FDA commissioner, and Hayes approved aspartame for use as an additive in dry foods. This was 16 years after it was discovered. In 1983 (18 years after it was discovered), the FDA approved the use of aspartame in carbonated drinks and desserts, including ice cream, frozen yogurt, and baked goods. According to Hayes, a study had been done in Japan that pointed to aspartame's safety.

Still, think about it. The FDA refused to approve aspartame for many years because they found it to be dangerous. At high enough temperatures aspartame releases a chemical (methanol) that ultimately breaks down into formic acid and formaldehyde. Yes, formaldehyde! The same chemical used to preserve dead bodies. In the living, formaldehyde is a toxin that attacks the nervous system and may cause seizures.

While it is true that a combination of formaldehyde and methanol is a by-product of our body's metabolism, this is a naturally occurring process. By eating foods and drinks with aspartame in them, we risk being exposed to excessive levels of these otherwise naturally occurring by-products. Just as excess sugar overworks many of the body's organs, so do excess chemicals, such as aspartame, increasing levels of otherwise harmless by-products to a toxic level.

It's ironic to me that diabetic specialists advocate the use of aspartame when this ingredient has been linked to causing diabetes, which can also lead to diabetic retinopathy. Is it really worth the risk?

Aspartame could lower your body's store of a brain chemical called serotonin. Serotonin is one of your "happy" brain chemicals. When this natural, normal chemical becomes decreased, from long-term usage of aspartame, you may start to experience considerable mental and emotional changes including depression, panic attacks, agitation, anxiety, insomnia, hostility, and bipolar disorder. While the existing studies that link aspartame to these neurological problems have been done in animals only, I don't know about you, but I don't want to be the human subject that gives the evidence!

Sucralose (Splenda) is another incredibly popular sweetener. It is also an excitotoxin. This could shock you, but the blockbuster sweetener that is found in thousands of products is actually chemically related to the deadly pesticide known as DDT (dichlorodiphenyltrichloroethane).

True story: The compounds have similar chemical structures. (They share the same chlorinated base.) Splenda started out from sucrose, a natural sugar, only someone who wanted to patent a chemical and make millions of dollars took sucrose and messed with it. You don't really need to know details of the chemistry. But here's what they did: They made a patentable substance by replacing three natural hydroxyl groups with three chlorine atoms.

Marketers are brilliant because they know how to sell us stuff. Don't you enjoy the idea of eating something called Splenda, which conjures up yummy images and smiling faces? What if you asked for it by its real name? Watch your waitress's face when you say, "Could you get me some 1,6-Dichloro-1,6-dideoxy-beta-D-fructofuranosyl-4-chloro-4-deoxy-alpha-D-galactose for my coffee."

In animal studies, the sweetener was found to shrink the thymus gland, which you need to fight off infection. A number of scientific studies have also tied the sweetener to autoimmune diseases, migraines, and panic attacks. (Don't look now, but some forms of diabetes are autoimmune diseases.)

Clever marketing campaigns fooled people by leading them to believe that Splenda was naturally derived because it came from sucrose. Well, sure, they took a naturally occurring sugar and created a space-alien compound in the laboratory that they could patent. Sucrose is fine; its lab-created cousin sucralose is not, at least not in my book!

Additionally, sucralose is broken down in the body prior to elimination, and its metabolites are questionable in terms of their safety too. Because the makers rake in about $1.5 billion a year, do you think they want you to know this?

Finally—and I seriously do hate to burst your bubble—but artificial sweeteners fatten you up faster than natural sugars. According to a 2008 study in the journal *Obesity* researchers at the University of Texas Health Science Center in San Antonio looked at information from nearly 4,000 people who had participated in a 9-year study on obesity. The researchers followed this group of people for about 7 years and found something dramatic enough to write an article about for a scientific journal:

For people who were at a normal weight, the risk for becoming overweight or obese nearly doubled when they consumed more than 21 artificially sweetened beverages per week versus those who drank none. Almost DOUBLE! And overall, for those who drank the artificially sweetened beverages, their body mass index was almost 50 percent (47 percent) higher than those who didn't drink them! Need I say more?

THE GLYCEMIC INDEX DIET: IT'S A MIND GAME

One dietary strategy that many diabetics use is based on the glycemic index of food. The glycemic index (GI) is a way to ascertain how quickly foods raise your blood sugar. It was based on the initial findings and research of Phyllis A. Crapo, RD, from Stanford University, and then further developed by David A. Jenkins from the University of Toronto.

The theory is that certain foods, specifically complex carbohydrates that are digested more slowly in the body, do not spike blood sugar the way foods that are digested quickly tend to. Each food is assigned a number, based on how quickly it affects your blood sugar level. For example, long-grain white rice (like the Uncle Ben's kind), is ranked at 56 on the glycemic index, so the theory is that it is better to eat this than to eat wheat bread made with honey and salt (which ranks a 65 on the GI) because the rice turns into glucose more slowly. In this example, rice would have a lower GI than wheat bread.

The theory is that foods with a high GI drive blood glucose levels up fast, and should therefore be limited, or for some people avoided entirely. (To view the full glycemic index table and choose a comparative food, go to the Web site www. glycemicindex.com, developed and maintained by the Human Nutrition Unit, School of Molecular and Microbial Biosciences, University of Sydney, Australia.)

According to the GI method of dieting, choosing carbs that are low on the GI will cause only small fluctuations in your blood glucose and insulin levels. According to Dr. Crapo's research, eating this way will theoretically help you manage diabetes.

A lot of controversy is aimed at the GI diet and its overall effectiveness in the treatment of diabetes. The GI theory was pretty much obscure for decades until a marketing campaign resuscitated it among nutritionists and consumers. In 1999 the World Health Organization and the Food and Agriculture Organization subsequently recommended that people in industrialized countries base their diets on low-GI foods to stave off the most common diseases of affluence, such as coronary heart disease, diabetes, and obesity.

If the diet is intended to improve diabetic status or reduce cardiovascular insult (and it is), then I think it makes a good start for people who require insulin injections, but it is not a diet that I've ever recommended to anyone. Why? There are a number of reasons that following this diet is not ideal.

THE HASSLE OF LOOKING THINGS UP. You can drive yourself crazy tracking numbers and having to check charts to see if you can eat a food. This sort of stressing takes the joy out of eating, and it's virtually impossible to maintain.

REAL FOODS GET DISTORTED. The GI of a food is based on a single item, but we eat foods combined with others. The GI of white bread, for example, is 70, but the GI for pizza is 60 because the fat content of the cheese slows down the absorption of carbs. This in turn lowers the GI of pizza. So let's get this straight. According to the GI diet, pizza is better for you than white bread, and, for the record, it's also better for you than whole wheat bread. Oddly, the GI gives no ranking for cheese on its own.

No nutritionist in their right mind would agree with that kind of thinking, because eating lots of pizza increases your risk for obesity, heart attack, and other diabetic complications. Cheese also feeds *Candida albicans*, a yeast tied to diabetes. See how silly Dr. Crapo's theory can be when used this way?

FLAWED SCIENCE. I think the glycemic index is flawed from the get-go. The measurements cannot be easily replicated. In other words, if you test one group of people and measure their blood glucose after a particular meal, and then test another group of people with that same meal, you will never get the same results. Experts know that to be clinically valid, results should be reproducible.

PROVIDES LIMITED INFORMATION. The glycemic index theory does not tell you how much insulin your body needs to fully digest the meal. It tells you only how high your blood sugar may go after 2 hours. What about 1 hour later, or 4 hours?

BASED ON HEALTHY PEOPLE, NOT DIABETICS. The entire GI diet was based on what happened in the average *healthy* person, not a person with diabetes. People with diabetes often have high blood pressure, some degree of heart disease, some kidney function problems, and thicker, more sticky blood. They probably have high cholesterol as well.

The GI diet does not account for how food is metabolized in people with multiple—or comorbid, as they are called—conditions. A truly sensible diet would factor in these multiple conditions and advocate the use of foods with antioxidants and healing enzymes, vitamins, and minerals. These are foods that promote heart health and reduce inflammatory chemicals and free-radical damage.

COUNTERACT CARBS WITH VINEGAR

High-carb meals like white bread or rice can spike blood sugar. Vinegar can help blunt the spike in blood glucose that would normally occur with the ingestion of white rice or white bread. According to a 2004 article in *Diabetes Care*, just 2 tablespoons (30 mL) of vinegar taken before a starchy, high-carb meal can reduce the spike of blood glucose that normally occurs.

CAN BE MISLEADING. If you look at the list of foods that are good for you on the GI, you'll see many that actually contribute to obesity and disease. Many foods that are low on the GI are very high in carbohydrates, and all that extra starch will convert in your liver to cholesterol and get stored as body fat. Chocolate milk, for example, has a GI of 35, making it "better" for you than blueberries, which have a GI of 59. I'm not kidding. That's how it plays out in actual practice.

By glycemic index standards, some dairy-based foods, such as hard cheese, milk, and cream, are considered better than blueberries. Blueberries are, in fact, a superfood, and have been shown to help prevent life-threatening diabetic complications such as kidney failure and blindness. A 2009 study, for example, found that blueberries may improve metabolic syndrome (syndrome X) by burning off belly fat and helping improve fatty liver disease.

STUDIES DON'T SUPPORT THE DIET. Scientific studies, in fact, show that not everyone who strictly adheres to the GI diet fares well when it comes to lowering A1cs (glucose measurements). Researchers at Duke University in Durham, North Carolina, for example, published a study in 2008 that found a diet lower in carbs proved better in controlling glucose levels than did a diet based on the glycemic index.

I don't think the GI diet is the right choice for all people with diabetes. It may be a helpful guideline, but that's all it is—a guideline—not an actual diet. To be fair, according to a news release from the *Journal of the American Medical Association*, researchers evaluated the effects of a low-glycemic diet versus a high–cereal fiber diet on people who were taking diabetic medications. The low-glycemic index group were fed a diet that was rich in beans, peas, lentils, nuts, pasta, rice, pumpernickel bread, rye, quinoa, flaxseed, oatmeal, and oat bran. The high–cereal fiber diet group was given more brown foods, such as whole grain breads, breakfast cereals, brown rice, whole wheat bread, and crackers. In this case the low-glycemic index participants fared better and showed better reductions in A1c.

CHAPTER 16

Construct a Healthy Kitchen

The American Diabetes Association has said diabetes is a chronic disease that has no cure. I completely disagree with that statement as it relates to type 2 diabetes. I believe the cure is in your kitchen and on your plate.

Let me be perfectly clear up-front. When I talk about reversing diabetes, I'm talking about type 2 diabetes. Medical science does not yet have the answers for reversing type 1 diabetes, although research may change that picture in the not-too-distant future.

I believe that many metabolic disorders can be reversed, even cured in some cases, by making better food choices—eliminating gluten-containing grains and the casein in milk and dairy products, avoiding hormone-laden meats, dangerous oils, refined sugars, and processed foods. That pretty much limits what you can eat, right? Not necessarily. Healthy foods that have not been tampered with by industry can be even more delicious if you learn how to cook and season them properly.

Nevertheless, everything I say in this chapter will be of help to anyone with any kind of diabetes or other kind of blood sugar disorder. What you put in your mouth on a daily basis makes all the difference in the world in the progression of the disease.

People don't realize that food is a drug, and we are addicted to it. We are not what we eat, but we certainly will become what we eat. We need to think differently about food choices.

All of us—not just those faced with the challenge of diabetes—are fixated on what we should avoid eating, making those taboo foods even more desirable in an ironic way. Don't you want what you can't have?

Nevertheless, it *is* important to avoid eating certain foods, even if they are approved for you by your dietitian or sanctioned by the American Diabetes Association.

I know I seem to be taking on the American Diabetes Association a lot in this book. Actually, I admire their work and a great deal of what they do. I just take issue with some of their recommendations. I do give you the science—much of it new research—behind my disagreements with ADA recommendations throughout this book.

For now I'll tell you a true—and idiotic—story. It's about the Cosmo Club of Missouri, which held a fundraiser for diabetes research in January 2009. Their fundraiser attracted hundreds of people one morning for—are you sitting down?—"Pancakes and Sausage Saturday." This artery-clogging, home-cooked breakfast fundraiser was to raise money for research on diabetes. Is that hilarious or what? Two foods that contribute to diabetes and heart disease were served up to people in order to raise money for diabetic research! Hmm . . . maybe the research project should have begun right there.

The club supports many organizations and the funds raised from this event went to the Ronald McDonald House. Speaking of McDonald's, does it surprise you to know that children find food tastier when it's wrapped in McDonald's food paper? Yep, up to six times more appetizing according to a 2007 Stanford study published in the *Archives of Pediatrics and Adolescent Medicine*.

The kids participating in this study practically turned up their noses at the same exact foods when they were wrapped in plain paper. To give you an example of this "Happy Meal" mentality, 60 percent of the kids liked the McDonald's-branded french fries, whereas only 10 percent would touch them when served up in plain packaging.

Oh, the power of advertising and pretty paper. It works, or else the food and beverage industry wouldn't spend an estimated $10 billion a year to brainwash our kids. Why don't they spend that money to help parents learn how to feed kids healthy meals?

YOU HAVE THE POWER

People feel a lot of guilt about what they may have done to develop diabetes in the first place. But this kind of thinking is self-defeating. You *always* have a choice. Even after you develop diabetes, you still have choices.

You could choose today to start eating healthy foods and stop holding on to toxic myths that food advertisers would have you believe. I want you to feel encouraged and to stop blaming yourself for your condition. Enough is enough. You *can* change your belief systems about food and exercise. You have that kind of determination.

There is a lot of healing power in detoxification and good nutrition. Certainly weight is an important factor, but being heavy isn't the sole cause for diabetes.

Free-radical damage and inflammation also come into play. Skinny people also get diabetes because they are eating the same toxic foods as everyone else, just less of them. Is that a shocker?

Let's get back to the statement I made at the beginning of this chapter, that foods are drugs. I'm a pharmacist, and I know a drug when I see one. But don't take just my word for it. According to the World Health Organization, the word *drug* is broadly defined as any substance that, when absorbed into the body of a living organism, alters normal bodily function.

This means that food is a drug because it does, indeed, alter your bodily function. This also means that artificial sweeteners are too, and so are artificial colors, additives, and genetically modified products. Pretty much everything we put into our mouth could be considered a drug. So if food is a drug, that makes your kitchen a pharmacy. Let's construct a healthier kitchen that will help you deal with diabetes, shall we?

MAKE YOUR KITCHEN A FANTASTIC PHARMACY

The ancient Greek physician Hippocrates said *Let thy food be thy medicine, and let thy medicine be thy food*. Brilliant! So why has it all gone awry? As industry and technology has advanced, our foods have become toxic. Very toxic. The failure of modern medicine and the epidemic proportions of sick people give you an idea of just how toxic.

Some people just don't want to give up their greasy cheeseburgers, fries, and beer. Then they're shocked when the doctor wants to put them on three different medications, and they're angry about how much they have to spend at the pharmacy.

Tired of being a part of that grim picture? Then look at your plate. The problem is staring right back at you. You can construct a healthier body by paying attention to what goes on your plate and into your mouth. You can begin by constructing a healthier kitchen. The medical profession is quick to provide a pill for your ill rather than suggest a healthy diet filled with raw foods. It's up to you to eat wisely and become your own nutritionist and doctor.

Many diabetes educators and physicians promote the glycemic index diet or the diet promoted by the ADA. According to a study published in 2006 in the journal *Diabetes Care*, a low-fat vegan diet improved blood sugar control better than the ADA diet. All the research evidence tells me that a low-fat, vegan diet supports the body's own natural healing mechanisms and detoxification pathways.

Don't panic, however. If you're not ready to make a change that's that extreme, there are many positive changes you can make in your kitchen that will have a tremendous impact on how you feel and how your body manages blood sugar. And, I promise, you can make those changes without sacrificing taste. On the other hand, if you don't change your diet, your blood sugar rises, your weight climbs, and your doctor is unhappy. Enter the pills.

How can you fix chronic malnutrition with a pill? That is one of the underlying issues you are dealing with if you have chronic aches and pains, or metabolic disorders like diabetes. Tell me, how does medicine restore enzymes, vitamins, and minerals to your body and reverse diabetes? It doesn't, but raw natural foods and organic fruits and veggies can do just that.

I'm not saying you can't ever have a Pop-Tart again. I'm just advocating that you place limitations on these sorts of foods and tilt your diet in the healthier direction. Over the course of a few weeks—and that's really all it takes to experience some changes—you will break cravings for diabetes-promoting foods. I promise you. There'll come a point where you taste the Pop-Tart again, and you'll have to spit it out. It's because humans tend to follow their taste buds.

Industry keeps adding chemicals to our food so our brain registers it as tasty, but it's really not. It only seems that way because of all the additives, such as MSG. My goal is to allow you to tantalize your taste buds with good food that brings you joy and health, and doesn't compromise your health or fake you out with chemicals.

WHERE SHOULD YOU BEGIN?

I realize that a new lifestyle and adoption of drastically different eating habits sounds overwhelming. I've been there. I've done it myself. When I was a teenager, my parents owned ice-cream trucks, and they let me eat whatever I wanted. My idea of a good meal consisted of treasures that I could find in the trucks.

So I grew up eating a lot of ice cream, potato chips, beef jerky, pickles, soda pop, candy bars, Pixie sticks, and gum. I was athletic, so you could not tell my diet was terrible when you looked at me. But I'm sure the damage was taking place inside.

As a pharmacist, a parent, and a health-conscious adult, as well as your health coach right now, I truly understand all sides of this dietetic Rubik's Cube. I've had to raise my children and clean up my own body by eliminating processed food and toxic chemical additives. For the last 15 years or so, I've served fresh, whole organic foods that support, rather than suffocate, life.

So for some people, it may be easier *not* to dive into a healthy lifestyle right away because it may be too much at first. If you are hesitant, or concerned about staying committed to the program, just go slowly. Start by eliminating one or two dangerous food groups at a time. For example, make a plan to stop eating sugary breakfast cereal this week. Instead, have some herbal tea and a handful of almonds or walnuts, or fresh young coconut, blueberries, grapefruit, quinoa cereal, or a superfood shake (see my recipe for Almond-Papaya Smoothie on page 340).

At the same time, start steaming your vegetables, and when they are still crisp-tender (not fully cooked), drizzle them with healthy fats, such as grape seed oil instead of canola oil. After a week, you won't even miss your Frosted Flakes, and that oil switch you made will put you on the road to better health and will taste good too. I promise you.

Keep going. The following week, bring in a new vegetable like kale. Follow my recipe for Sun-Dried Tomato Kale on page 369. Every day, integrate a different green, leafy vegetable, and within a week or two, you will be positively craving the fresh ones. And those canned, processed vegetables will be history.

Who wants to eat asparagus that's been sitting in a can for a year anyway? Think about it. Fresh, organic food tastes better. Once you get started you will experience the new cues your body gives you to eat fresh, organic food.

We've all lost sight of what real food is. Today's generation of children think that food comes out of a box, a can, a microwave, or a drive-through.

If my dietary edits seem too difficult to implement, then try it this way. Go vegetarian (or vegan if you can) for just 24 hours. Once you've successfully done that, stretch the time frame. In a few days, try it again, and go for 48 hours.

I know many people crave meat, and that's okay with me. I don't think meat is necessarily bad, but it's not something I eat a lot of. I just ask you to be reasonable. Meat and fish are okay at times. Just buy the healthy types, like grass-fed, hormone-free beef, or wild-caught, cold-water seafood.

While preparing this section of my book, I spoke to chef Alan Roettinger, who knows all about healthy food. He's written a fantastic cookbook that teaches you how to use the *right* fats, not the bad fats. His book *Omega 3 Cuisine* contains healthy gourmet recipes that don't require you to diet and lose all the joy in your life.

He explained to me why so many people have problems when they try to change what they eat: "You know why diets don't work? Because they're no fun! The whole point of everything we do is to feel joy. Cooking and eating are prime examples of this—it's all about enjoyment. The challenge before each of us is to learn how to cook and eat so that we get maximum pleasure without sacrificing our health. (It's no fun if we start feeling bad). We can't outsource pleasure or health—it just doesn't work unless we're having it ourselves. So it's up to us to get it right. Fortunately, it's not that hard to figure out."

Chef Roettinger is 100 percent correct. One "challenge before all of us," he says, "is to learn how to cook and eat so that we get maximum pleasure." And having counseled thousands of patients over the years, I am aware of other challenges, too. Let's talk about how to overcome those now. I put them in the form of "edits" that you can make to your daily diet that should improve your general health status and help you keep your blood sugar under control.

E-D-I-T WHAT YOU EAT; DON'T D-I-E-T

It's not necessarily what you eat that causes diabetes, it's also what you *don't* eat. I don't believe in diets—they are destined to fail because they are usually restrictive. Don't diet; it's a waste of time. *Think about it: If you go "on" a diet, you have to come "off" a diet.*

You'll lose more weight if you EDIT what you eat, versus DIET. Look closely at those words; I only arranged the letters differently. D-I-E-T when rearranged spells E-D-I-T, see? Here's a closer look on how to edit food and create a healthier kitchen:

> **CHALLENGE.** *White refined sugar and artificial sweeteners, such as aspartame, saccharine, sucralose, tagatose, Truvia.*
> **THE EDIT.** Use natural sweeteners, such as dark agave, molasses, stevia, or unrefined coconut sugar.
>
> **CHALLENGE.** *White flour, all-purpose flour, self-rising flour, and dozens of other permutations of white flour.*
> **THE EDIT.** Rice, almond, walnut, coconut flour, or sorghum. If you want a transition flour before going to any of these, start with organic, unbleached 100 percent whole grain flour, then switch to rice flour, and then try the nut flours like almond flour.

CHALLENGE. *Iodized table salt (sodium chloride). This is more like an industrial chemical than a gourmet finishing salt.*

THE EDIT. Use unbleached Celtic sea salt or French grey sea salt. These types of sea salt have flavor and offer a rich source of minerals. Natural sea salts supply necessary minerals for your pancreas and your thyroid glands, such as chromium, iodine, magnesium, zinc, vanadium, iron, and so on.

CHALLENGE. *Snacks, usually potato chips, that contain fat substitutes like olestra. Many people advocate the use of this artificial ingredient as healthy, but research suggests this ingredient may— over time—contribute to heart disease, immune suppression, cancer, and diabetes. It may be associated with these problems through an indirect connection, the result of olestra depleting us of fat-soluble vitamins that protect us from these disorders.*

THE EDIT. Eat snacks, such as avocados or walnuts, that contain naturally occurring fats. If you are going to eat chips, go for those that are free of olestra, and preferably those that contain nothing but sea salt and healthy oils (sunflower, for example, not canola).

CHALLENGE. *Canned foods—sauces, vegetables, and fruits.*

THE EDIT. Replace with fresh or frozen foods, preferably organic, because canned foods have been processed and trucked in from far-away places. If you are in the habit of buying canned vegetables, switch to fresh ones. Beans are okay if canned because they save time and still give you some healthy nutrition. Just make sure that they are organic. Eden's brand is a good choice. Everything else you eat should be fresh or frozen.

CHALLENGE. *Prepared foods. If it comes in a prepackaged box, it needs to go. Read the labels, and on most processed foods you'll see an ingredients list that is extraordinarily long, with many unpronounceable words.*

THE EDIT. Get rid of them! All of them. Replace processed foods with fresh, organic foods, including almonds and walnuts, berries, and apples.

CHALLENGE. *Water containing chlorine and arsenic, which includes most tap water. Even low to moderate levels of arsenic in the water may be promoting diabetes. Consuming arsenic-tainted water can increase your risk for diabetes by fourfold, according to a study published in 2008 in the* Journal of the American Medical Association. *The researchers discovered that people with type 2 diabetes—the most prevalent form of the disease—had 26 percent higher levels of arsenic in their urine than people without type 2 diabetes.*

THE EDIT. Drink clean, filtered water. You can buy a variety of filters to attach to your sink or have one professionally installed. There are also companies that sell water alkalizers, which are beneficial.

CHALLENGE. *Soda pop—any commercial soda (other than plain seltzer or club soda)—because they contain large quantities of sugar and high-fructose corn syrup.*

THE EDIT. Drink my natural soda. You won't taste the difference, and it has two ingredients, not a dozen. You'll find the recipe on page 348.

CHALLENGE. *Potato chips—these often contain hydrogenated oils, which contain unhealthy trans fats.*

THE EDIT. Eat nuts—Brazil nuts, macadamia nuts, walnuts, almonds—and also seeds, such as hemp seeds, sunflower seeds, and pumpkin seeds. Raw or dry-roasted nuts are easy to find, and okay for some people, however if you soak your nuts in water, they will become much easier for you to digest. This is what I do at home: Cover the nuts with water and a pinch of salt, if you want. Leave them overnight, drain them, and then air dry. Refrigerate. They will keep a few days. Another way to get that salt fix is with dehydrated vegetable chips. Check labels carefully because even these sometimes contain unhealthy oils or sugar.

CHALLENGE. *Trans fat–laden oils, such as margarine, lard, shortening, bacon fat, and any product that contains hydrogenated or partially hydrogenated oil. These cause all sorts of metabolic problems and fuel the development of heart disease, obesity, and diabetes.*

THE EDIT. Grape seed oil; almond oil; extra-virgin, cold-pressed olive oil; or coconut oil.

CHALLENGE. *Candy bars, cookies, and Toaster Streudels. I know they're yummy, but they're not good for you.*
THE EDIT. Eat healthy energy bars, such as Boomi Bar, Larabar, or Mrs. Mays snacks.

CHALLENGE. *Pies and cakes. (Unless it's a birthday party. I'm not a complete party-pooper.)*
THE EDIT. Eat apples instead of apple pie, and colorful berries (raspberries, blueberries, cranberries), pineapple, pomegranate, oranges, kiwi, coconut, papaya, mango, and so on. I'd prefer that you eat your fruits withOUT extra sugar, in the raw-and-pure state.

CHALLENGE. *Factory-farmed commercial meat and poultry. These animals are usually riddled with parasites, bacteria, disease-causing hormones, and other chemicals. They are horribly mistreated and fed corn and soybeans, an unnatural diet. Many sick animals make it to your plate because they are prodded to do so, but that's another book. If you are interested in more reading about this important topic, consider reading* The Omnivore's Dilemma *by Michael Pollan.*
THE EDIT. Eat grass-fed, free-range, hormone-free meats from animals that have lived a more natural, happy life prior to slaughter. Limit consumption to no more than three servings per week. Call me neurotic if you want to, but if you are a red meat eater, I would advise that you eat steaks rather than hamburgers. A single hamburger may have up to 1,000 different cows ground up into it, while a steak comes from a single cow. The hamburger made from 1,000 animals greatly increases your risk of ingesting deadly microorganisms.

YOUR BODY NEEDS AN OIL CHANGE

You would never touch it again if you really knew what it was. I'm talking about trans fats, of course. You'll find trans fats aplenty in any processed food that contains hydrogenated fat or partially hydrogenated oil. These are refined, processed oils that are really just a greasy food additive.

This chemical has replaced pure butter and lard in baked goods and most deep-fried foods. (Think french fries.) Trans fats are made by taking a pure and natural liquid oil and treating (by cooking, or adding compounds) the chemicals in a lab to produce a thicker, fatty substance that remains solid at room temperature. Experts agree that trans fats raise our cholesterol and train our bodies to be fat.

Trans fats are lubricants; they're not food. The reason that trans fats are so popular in today's diet is because production of the substance is cheap, so it lowers food prices. Plus it extends the shelf life of foods, which saves a lot of money. Trans fats are not the same as essential fatty acids like the omega-3 fatty acids DHA and EPA. That's the understatement of the year. I'm all for those good fats because they are anti-inflammatory and helpful to people with diabetes or heart disease.

Other good fats include healthy oils, such as grape seed, hemp seed, olive oil, walnut oil, and almond oil. In fact, these types of healthy fats are crucial to good health. You need a certain amount of good fats in your diet to survive. But you need to pick healthy fats and oils. Even butter or ghee (clarified butter) is better than margarine, a trans fat cooked up in a lab.

It's actually best to avoid trans fats altogether because they raise levels of bad (LDL, low-density lipoprotein) cholesterol. I have read that eating just 5 grams of trans fat per day (the equivalent of just one doughnut) increases your risk for heart disease by 25 percent! Did you hear me? That's huge and likely accounts for the unprecedented rise in obesity and metabolic diseases.

Trans fats make you fat by leading to rapid weight gain and a spare tire around your middle. Trans fats have been linked to poor liver function, and guess what else? That's right—to diabetes as well. In Canada, producers are not legally allowed to dye trans fats to a yellow color as they do in America, and so Canadians who want to spread it on their toast use a white pastelike substance that Americans have named margarine. At least Canada is not deceptive about what they market. In Denmark, there have been laws in place against using trans fats in food since 2003.

In America, things have improved over the past few years, with the help of urging from the Harvard School of Public Health. According to the FDA, just changing the federal law so that manufacturers were required to list the amount of harmful trans fats in every packaged good, as of July 2006, helped Americans curb their risk of cardiovascular disease related to dietary trans fats, and conservatively saved an estimated $900 million to $1.8 billion a year in medical costs, lost productivity, and pain and suffering.

With statistics like that, does it shock you that health organizations allow for trans fats in your meal plan? I was recently reviewing the Exchange List for Meal Planning put out by the American Diabetes Association and the American Dietetic Association. Page 21 of this booklet lists protion sizes of certain foods, under the section called Saturated Fats List. Apparently, these organizations approve of bacon, bacon grease, chitlins (pig intestines), and lard for diabetics. Insane! These are exactly the types of foods that *cause* disease because they are loaded with bad fats, not to mention the fact that they also contain nitrates and other cancer-causing chemicals!

Eating these foods is the equivalent of bungee jumping without a rope. You just don't do it. Since fats are very different, I've decided to offer you an overview of oils classified as good, better, and best. Please adhere to these oils when cooking in the kitchen. They are all okay to use when following my recipes in Chapter 17. But first, a word about frying and bad oils.

Fried Food Fries Your Brain

One thing I've learned about cooking with oils is NOT TO! When you cook with an oil, you almost always ruin the innate health properties of the oil. Never fry your food either. One of the world's leading authorities on oil, Udo Erasmus, MD, author of *Fats That Heal and Fats That Kill*, took the time to teach me more about the good, the bad, and the ugly oils. He pioneered special methods for producing unrefined oils. These methods are still in use today by good-quality manufacturers of flax and other healthy, pure oils.

Dr. Erasmus says it best: "Frying your food fries your health. Tell your readers not to do it!" We discussed how many people refuse to make the necessary dietary and oil changes in their kitchen but rather want to rely on omega-3 fish oil supplements.

Dr. Erasmus goes on to explain that none of us can be healthy on supplements alone: "People make the mistake of thinking that a supplement will make up for eating the wrong fats, the kind found in processed and junk foods. People should avoid oils that are damaged by processing at the manufacturing level or by our own mistakes during food preparation, like heating them too much.

"Balance is extremely important. The ratio of omega-3 and omega-6 fatty acids should be about 2 to 1. This way, your dietary foundation of essential fatty acids is strong. Supplements may be used, but only if they are high quality, but they do not make up for a poor foundation.

THE SKINNY ON GOTHAM

New York City—also known as Gotham—took a bold step in December 2006 when its Board of Health voted to ban all trans fats from restaurant kitchens. They took this step after learning that there are at least 500 annual deaths in the city from cardiac arrest brought on by too many trans fats. What a wonderful Christmas present! Restaurants were given a deadline of July 2008 to comply, and New York City restaurants—including all the fast food restaurants—have been artificial trans fat–free since then! Gotham rules!

"Over the past 20-plus years we have worked with thousands of people and have seen powerful results on health, beauty, and performance, as well as weight management and a wide range of health parameters, including hormone function, bone strength, and inflammatory and autoimmune diseases."

While I was studying with Dr. Erasmus, it became clear we agree that people with diabetes are in desperate need of a "fuel shift." That is, they need to be burning their fuel (energy) from fats rather than all the carbs in the typical American diet. Those carbs lead to leptin resistance and insulin resistance. The body's resistance to these two hormones has an impact on the development of both diabetes and obesity. As you know by now, excess carbs in your diet are stored as fat in the body. So Dr. Erasmus is spot-on in my book.

The fewer nonnutritious carbohydrates that you consume, the more your body will burn up the fat it has stored in your liver and your waistline. Udo's Choice blend of pure omega oils can be found at virtually all health food stores nationwide.

I highly recommended Udo's Choice's blend of omega-3, -6, and -9 to promote cardiac health, but it's useful in the kitchen, too. Just mix it with a neutral-tasting oil (like grape seed or Bija's almond oil) and you suddenly have a clever way to promote good health while eating. Your kids won't even know the difference if you combine it well. And what they don't know won't hurt them.

Cheap Vegetable Oil—Just Say No!

It may take some getting used to, but you have to think of cooking oils as a health supplement. I'm not referring to those cheap plastic bottles of vegetable oil that you can buy at grocery stores. I'm referring to high-end, pure, unadulterated, unrefined nutritious oils. They are not that hard to find. In my local health food store, I buy Bija brand. Bija produces one of the most impressive (and organic) brands of healthy oils you will ever find. Their oils are pure, unfiltered, and unrefined, and some of them are quite exotic. I love healthy oils. This is one area of my kitchen that I do not compromise on. Bija oils are among the best in the world. They didn't pay me a dime to say that. It's just that I'm a bit of a connoisseur and I can *taste* the difference with their oils, which I recommend in many recipes in Chapter 17.

The point is, cheap vegetable oils are easy on the pocket, but they are dangerous to your health. From now on, I want you to use high-quality, unrefined oils that contain healthy nutrients, and that's the only kind of oil I want you to consume.

Please remember that when any oil is heated—even the good kind—and it begins to smoke, all of those precious nutrients are lost, and instead dangerous chemicals are released. Many of those chemicals have been tied to cancer. So no more frying. Take your frying pans out of your kitchen because you can't construct a healthier body if you insist on frying.

Sautéing is another practice that I think you should limit. In my home, I steam my veggies and greens in a stainless steel pan, or a steamer. I drain them (or dry them a bit in the case of spinach) and then I drizzle them with a pure and healthy oil. This is also the time to add your finishing salt or seasonings.

Sautéing in butter may taste good, but I'd prefer that you limit your intake of cow's milk products such as butter, cheese, and milk. If you must, use ghee, which is clarified butter. This one takes a higher temperature, and many people who are casein-sensitive seem to do okay with it. But it is dairy-derived so it's lower on my list of healthy oils. (I take a closer look at the problem with milk and dairy products in Chapter 4.)

Oils Are Not Created Equal

Not only are they *not* created equal, some of them are garbage with clever labels on them. It's just hard to tell what kind of oil you are getting based on a label. For example, take olive oil, since that is one of my healthy oil picks for you. Often, you see it with the words *cold-pressed* printed on the label. This is supposed to mean that the olives were squished without any heat, hence *cold* pressed. It's meant to make us think the oil is good for us, because heat destroys a lot of nutrition that is normally found in oil.

You don't want your oils to be heated during processing. But the cold-pressed term on the label means nothing to you as a consumer because currently, the use of the term is totally unregulated. Companies print that on the label to make us think the oil is good for us. Some of the companies actually do obtain their oil by using cold-pressed methods, but some don't. Unscrupulous companies advertise cold-pressed but still heat the oil to 450°F, and you wouldn't know it. There's just no guarantee.

The term *extra-virgin* is regulated, however. If a company prints extra-virgin on their label, it means that it's the first pressing of the oil. The oils are first squished into a paste, and then the oil is pressed from the paste. Again, it's the first pressing of the oil. If a manufacturer is inspected, and is found to not be doing that, there are penalties. But if it says *cold pressed* on the label, generally no one checks to see if they're actually doing it. It's a marketing ploy.

Expeller-pressed is another ploy. It's printed on the label to make you think it's something special, but it is meaningless. It's just referring to a type of extraction method.

When discussing healthy oils, I'd like to awaken you to a little-known fact. Oils change their chemical structure—and might become carcinogenic—as soon as they start to smoke. You never want to heat an oil to high temperatures, and I mean any kind of oil, with the exception of ghee, which can be heated to fairly high temperatures.

So think of oils as another health supplement and choose the sort of oil that offers you a lot of healthy essential fatty acids, such as omega-3, -6, and -9 fatty acids. Using something like Udo's Choice oil is so much healthier for you than using vegetable oils. So please, start integrating healthy oils in your kitchen today. Your body will thank you in remarkable ways.

OILS: THE GOOD, THE BETTER, AND THE BEST

The best way to use oils is to use different ones throughout the week. That way you will have a good balance of omega-3, omega-6, and omega-9 essential fatty acids.

You don't want to overdo one oil, for example flax oil, and use it exclusively, because that will cause you to run out of omega-6 in your body and spark symptoms. And likewise you don't want to exclusively use sunflower oil, because you will get too many omega-6s. The best way to enjoy healthy oils is simply to switch it up a little.

What follows are some of the best oils I think you should consume. In terms of brand names, it gets confusing. Here in American health food stores and grocery stores, I've decided that these are the better brands, based on the way they produce the oils: Bija's, Udo's Choice, Barleans, and Spectrum Naturals.

Good Oils

Here's the story on some good oils that you may enjoy.

SAFFLOWER. This oil comes from the safflower, a bright yellow, orange, or red flower that boasts long, spiny leaves. The extracted oil is rich in vitamin E and omega-6 fatty acids, which help you make prostaglandins. Don't heat this oil. Eat it cold, in salad dressing, for example, or you will lose the benefits.

SUNFLOWER. This oil comes from the beautiful sunflower, and the extracted oil happens to be high in vitamin E and low in bad saturated fats. Check for brands that contain both oleic acid and linoleic acid—two ingredients that appear to lower cholesterol and support heart health. As you read in Chapter 000, oleic acid affects your levels of GLP-1 in the very best way. You'll want to use this one cold as well. Don't heat it, because the polyunsaturated fats in it are damaged at high temperatures.

Better Oils

Two oils make the grade for everyday use.

COCONUT. This oil is a solid at room temperature, but don't worry. That doesn't make it a trans fat. It is virtually a superfood. It increases energy without spiking your blood sugar. You can cook with it, and it may even help you burn fat. One reason that I've placed coconut oil in the "better" category is because it is made up of smaller molecules of fatty acids (compared to those in olive and sunflower oil), which can be converted to energy quite quickly, rather than being stored for use later.

OLIVE. When choosing olive oil, go for the best. Get extra-virgin and cold-pressed, which means that the olives are tastier and they haven't been heated. Virgin olive oil is of lesser quality than extra virgin.

Before olive oil became such a big business, olives used to get squeezed into a paste, and then the oil was extracted. If you can find cold-pressed oils, there will be greater health benefits for you, because heating this oil destroys some of the nutrients.

Because of the higher demand for olive oil, there has been an influx of bogus oil. Some are cut with cheaper vegetable oils and mislabeled. The fraud is so bad with olive oil that some companies will sell you Italian lamp oil, called lampante. Because it's made in Italy, you may assume that it's good for you. This constitutes olive oil "trafficking," because it's so easy to doctor up cheap oil and filter it to clean it, then slap it with a pretty label.

Once you've tasted *real* olive oil, you won't touch the fakes. Better brands use olives that are hand-picked, as opposed to being mechanically harvested. The flavor will be better, and the content of healthy fatty acids, vitamin E, vitamin K, and cholesterol-busting phytosterols may be a little higher as well.

Best Oils

These oils are more expensive, but worth every penny.

GRAPE SEED. This oil is extracted from the seeds of grapes, and it is one of the most pleasant, light-tasting oils you'll ever find. I use this every day. High-quality brands have a light green tint to them. As you know, grapes give us many powerful antioxidants and heart-healthy compounds. This oil could actually raise your good HDL cholesterol too.

FLAXSEED. Bringing flaxseed oil into your diet could be the single most important health decision you make. The term *flax* usually refers to the plant, which grows annually and has beautiful little flowers on it.

Flax is cultivated for its fibers and its seeds. The seeds can be ground up or turned into flaxseed oil, also called linseed oil. It provides some essential fatty acids, which reduce inflammation, as well as vitamins, minerals, and the nutrient alpha linoleic acid.

Flaxseed oil has a light, nutty flavor, and I have it on the "best" list because it can help you reduce cholesterol, reduce inflammation and pain, raise energy, strengthen fingernails, and I believe it may even help improve vision.

This oil spoils quickly, so keep it in the fridge. You'll find it in the refrigerator section at your health food store for a reason. It's not meant to be heated. If you must warm it with your food, keep the temperature on low. Flax is a natural blood thinner, which is considered a good thing.

Using ground flaxseed in your diet and using flax oil are also great ways to reduce the body's burden of toxic types of estrogen, the kind that promote prostate and breast cancers.

AVOCADO. This oil comes from the fleshy green part of the avocado, not the seed. This fruit-based monounsaturated oil—yes, avocados are fruits, not vegetables—is a rich source of vitamins A, E, B_1, B_2, and D. Avocado oil is low in cholesterol and high in healthy essential fatty acids. Sometimes the oil is found in massage oil. It is wonderful for skin conditions such as psoriasis or eczema.

Avocado is a powerful liver and pancreatic cleanser because it contains one of the strongest antioxidants known to humankind—glutathione. Glutathione acts like an astringent because it helps your liver free your body of dangerous free radicals that crop up after digestion. Avocado oil can be used to sear, sauté, and deep fry. Higher temperatures don't affect its nutritional value, and it won't smoke. Just like grape seed oil, avocado oil may have beneficial effects on your cholesterol.

ALMOND. This oil comes from almond nuts, and it's an excellent substitute for butter. It has a nutty flavor. I like to use it because it's relatively neutral, so it's nice in salads, desserts, or sauces.

Almond extract is different from almond oil. The extract is concentrated and found in the flavoring section near the vanilla extract. The oil can be found online or at health food stores. It is incredibly rich in nutrients, just like the almond itself. It has a high smoke point, so of all the oils mentioned here, you can use almond oil (or grape seed oil) if you have to heat something to medium or medium high for a few minutes.

HEMP SEED. This oil provides good fats such as omega-3 fatty acids. It also contains linoleic acid and linolenic acid. Hemp has been around for eons and is nutritionally packed. I have included hemp seeds in many recipes, and the seeds are fairly easy to find. But most people don't realize there is an oil. It's fantastic for you because it a superfood. Hemp (and hemp seed oil) contain miraculous chlorophyll, which you read about in Chapter 12. It is a strong detoxifier. The color of this oil is a beautiful light green.

The essential fatty acids in hemp allow you to maintain a healthy body and mind. It is very low in saturated fats, only about 8 percent of total oil volume. I couldn't love hemp any more. I use it every day in my salads or as a finishing oil. It should not be heated to very high temperatures. I use a certified organic, cold-pressed brand by Nutiva found at most health food stores (not supermarkets). See www.nutiva.com.

Bad Oils: Do Not Use

While we're on the topic of fats and oils, there are several that you should put on your "never, ever" list.

MARGARINE AND FAKE BUTTER. Strictly avoid margarines and all products containing margarine, such as I Can't Believe It's Not Butter. Believe this: Margarine is nothing but thick white paste with some dye and chemicals added in.

Pretend butter spreads include products like Smart Balance. This last one claims to have zero trans fats, but on their Web site, it says that they have lowered the fat content "to limit trans fats to less than one-half gram per serving, thereby qualifying to claim zero trans fat content per serving." It's perfectly legal for them to claim zero, even though the product does have a small amount. In my opinion it's not a real food.

COTTONSEED OIL AND PROCESSED PALM OIL. Strictly avoid these two, but the extra-virgin red palm oil called dende is fine.

HYDROGENATED OR PARTIALLY HYDROGENATED FATS AND OILS. You'll have to read labels to find these in the ingredients list.

The take-home point is that the quality of your oils depends on how well a manufacturer has protected it from heat, light, and oxygen. You need to get picky with oils. The slippery stuff should be your best friend in the fight against diabetes. When used properly, oils provide your body with healthy essential fatty acids, which in turn squash the nasty fats and cholesterols that have invaded your cells. Think of them as supplements for your food.

HEALING FOODS Q AND A

You'll find much more about how to eat to keep your blood sugar under control throughout this book. And there are a number of great kitchen tips and tasty recipes in Chapter 17.

In the meantime, I think it might be helpful to answer some questions about healthy eating that you're likely to have right from the get-go.

Q: Should I buy "sugar-free" products?

A: No. They often contain unhealthy ingredients, such as artificial sweeteners like sucralose (Splenda) or aspartame (NutraSweet).

Q: What about products that say "no sugar added"? What does that really mean?

A: It means that the manufacturer has not actively placed sugar into the product; however, it may still be very high in other dangerous food additives, including artificial colors or high-fructose corn syrup, one of the all-time worst substances. Don't get me started on that one right now, but do check out Chapter 15 for my rant.

Q: Can sugar-free products help me lose weight?

A: No. They actually contribute to weight gain. Are you shocked? There is actually a lot of research on this. In 2008, for example, researchers at Purdue University demonstrated that artificial sweeteners not only fail to prevent weight gain, but they actually cause people to pack on the pounds. In another study, rats given yogurt sweetened with zero-calorie sugar substitutes ate more calories, gained more weight, and increased their body fat.

The thing is, real sugar—ideally raw cane sugar and unrefined nectars—raises your core body temperature as it provides calories and energy. Artificial sweeteners don't, leaving you as hungry as you were before you ate. I could go on and on about this one too, as the notion that sugar-free products can help you lose weight is one of my biggest pet peeves.

Q: Do portions matter?

A: Yes, big time. If you can learn to eat slower, your body will have adequate time to release leptin, one of your feel-full hormones, and this will help you control your portions and begin to lose weight. Always stop eating before you feel full. Wait 10 or 15 minutes, and you'll see that you are no longer hungry.

Q: Does the method of cooking really matter?

A: Yes. Grilling, baking, and steaming your foods is best. Also, sautéing your food (in healthy oils) is better than deep frying or smoking your food.

CONTROVERSIAL FOODS: CAN YOU EAT THESE GOODIES?

Now let's take a look at some specific foods that you may have some concerns about. Is it okay, for example, to drink coffee?

Yes, I think a cup or two of coffee is fine each day, but it depends what you put into it. Generally speaking, coffee beans, especially the green ones (versus roasted coffee beans), contain healthy antioxidants that may stave off heart disease, cancer, or other diseases driven by free-radical assault.

Please don't pour in white refined sugar, artificial sweeteners (like sucralose), or one of those liquid creamers that contain partially hydrogenated oils, emulsifiers, artificial flavors, and colors.

Companies that produce artificial creamers can be deceptive about how they present their products. I found that out last year after getting headaches shortly after consuming coffee sweetened with a liquid coffee creamer. I read the ingredient labels and saw sucralose was listed as an ingredient, but the product was not labeled as sugar-free. I avoid these fake sugars like the plague, so I was surprised to find it hidden in the small print. I called the makers and expressed my dismay, because I thought this was deceptive.

When products say "sugar-free" or "no sugar added," they usually contain these artificial sweeteners. Watch out for low-fat ice cream with a no-sugar-added label, for example.

When I asked people at the coffee creamer company why they did not disclose artificial sugar openly on their product, the representative said that they are within the laws set by the FDA and only have to label their product as sugar-free if it contains more than 0.5 grams of sugar per serving. Since this flavor combines sugar and sucralose, it did not exceed 0.5 grams of total sugar, so therefore it did not have to be labeled as sugar-free.

I am appalled that artificial sweeteners are used in hundreds of food products that are not labeled as sugar-free. It's shocking to me that a product I've been buying for years can suddenly change and begin including artificial sweeteners without openly saying so on the label.

So if you want to avoid sugar-free products, you may unknowingly still be consuming some sucralose because food manufacturers have laws to protect them, not you. And although you think you're only consuming the stuff in moderation, at the end of the day, you may have ingested quite a bit.

Here's the takeaway point here: Read labels if you want to find the hidden ingredient of sucralose or other artificial sweeteners. Don't trust food makers to disclose this information and alert you by telling you it's sugar-free. Remember, too, that many sugar-free foods are not healthy for people with diabetes.

Now let's get back to coffee for a minute. Scientific studies seem to show that coffee is fine. But it's probably best to limit your intake to a maximum of two cups of brewed coffee a day, assuming you don't suffer from anxiety, insomnia, a fast or irregular heartbeat, or any stomach problems, such as diarrhea or irritable bowel syndrome. So yes to coffee. Please buy organic and preferably fair trade.

Remember that too much caffeine will jolt the heart, cause insomnia, and raise blood pressure. (Actually, my preference is that you drink no more than one cup a day.) What about cream? Forget the artificial creamers. Use fresh almond, hemp, or goat milk instead.

What about Chocolate?

I'll make a deal with you. Eat only dark chocolate, not milk or white chocolate. If you consume brands that contain at least 60 percent cacao, then you are giving your body powerful heart-healthy antioxidants. White chocolate isn't even chocolate, it's just fat. I think people could easily justify one square of dark chocolate per day.

Besides being delicious, the melt-in-your-mouth luxury reduces your risk for heart attack and lowers blood sugar too. Chocolate contains proanthocyanidins, and scientists in Japan caused quite a stir when they came out with their findings on what happened when they fed chocolate to obese mice. Basically, the obese mice who ate the chocolate (cacao liquor proanthocyanidins) had lower blood sugar levels than the obese mice who weren't fed the proanthocyanidin-rich chocolate. The scientists concluded that foods or drinks made from cacao beans might be beneficial in preventing type 2 diabetes!

Is Wine a Thing of the Past?

Go ahead and enjoy a glass of wine, but only for special occasions. Limit this practice to once per month, please. Hey, I'm not an tyrant, I just let you have coffee and chocolate. Wine (and other alcoholic beverages) impairs your pancreas and liver function.

Alcohol is a powerful free-radical toxin and is a leading cause for pancreatitis and liver failure. If you are seeking the resveratrol that is found in some red wines, you're better off taking resveratrol supplements, because many red wines hardly even contain resveratrol. You'd have to drink hundreds of bottles of wine per day to get a meaningful dose of healthy resveratrol, so again, supplement, don't get sloshed.

This conversation about grapes reminds me of another point: You can also take grape seed extract or use grape seed oil for added health benefits. You won't be getting resveratrol, but you will be getting other antioxidants that have similar effects. And hooray, because these fruit-based options don't shut down your internal organs, nor will they make you slur your speech (or dance on tables).

RUN FROM FAST FOODS

Burger King, McDonald's, Taco Bell, KFC . . . forget about it. Aside from the fact that fast food is fattening and has bunches of additives in it, these foods often contain a boatload of MSG (monosodium glutamate).

Now, I'll understand if you succumb to one of their delcious sandwiches once or twice a year. Hey, it happens. (It even happened to me back in 2006.) But I don't want you to sustain yourself on this kind of grub. (Sorry, I can't bring myself to call it food.)

MSG is one of the worst and most pervasive food additives. It's an excitotoxin that overexcites your cells and causes excessive nerve firing. It's actually the free glutamate portion of MSG that causes the extra activity in glutamate-responsive tissues such as the brain, heart, nervous system, eyes, and pancreas.

A number of researchers and experts in the field maintain that MSG kills your body's cells, and damage occurs to an organ after millions of cells have died. You don't even know at first that this is happening. These same experts maintain that MSG also contributes to headaches, heart attacks, arrhythmias, nerve pain, memory loss, tremors, and conditions that include neurologic changes, which may be diagnosed as Alzheimer's, Parkinson's, or Lou Gehrig's diseases.

It's even possible that you've been given a terrible misdiagnosis, because your symptoms may just be related to the ingestion of processed foods and all of their dangerous additives, MSG being one of them. I'm not trying to go against what your doctor has told you now. I'm just saying this is something to consider.

The FDA insists that consuming MSG does not cause any problems, but they do state this on their Web site:

Abnormal function of glutamate receptors has been linked with certain neurological diseases, such as Alzheimer's disease and Huntington's chorea. Injections of glutamate in laboratory animals have resulted in damage to nerve cells in the brain.

It's almost impossible to avoid MSG if you eat any processed foods, because it's in almost all of them, and you are being deceived. Laws require that the ingredient monosodium glutamate be listed on the label, so food manufacturers have learned how to disguise MSG as something altogether different.

More specifically, food labels don't have to label ingredients that contain free glutamic acid, even though it's the main component of MSG. Some other aliases for MSG include hydrolyzed protein, yeast, gelatin, sodium caseinate, and auto-lyzed yeast. See, food manufacturers clean up their label and proudly display "no added MSG" to trick you, but the toxin may be in there in the form of free glutamic acid. They know it's in there, they just count on you to remain uneducated.

This is yet another reason I advocate consuming whole, fresh organic foods for most of your meals. I've prepared a longer list of the other names that MSG goes by. See "MSG Aliases" on page 336 so that you can avoid this silent killer additive.

YAY FOR YERBA MATÉ

If you are sensitive to the effects of coffee, or just want to avoid it, try a fabulous substitute called yerba maté. It's really an herb made from the leaves (and a few stems) of a rainforest tree native to South America. Yerba maté is revered as the "drink of the gods" and may increase your mental alertness, energy, immune function, and mental clarity.

Yerba mate has a trio of xanthene compounds—some caffeine, theobromine (a stimulant also found in chocolate), and small amounts of natural theophylline, which, believe it or not, is sold as a prescription drug for people with asthma. Yerba maté does not typically give people the jitters. People often find maté to offer a different "lift" than coffee. The different effect is probably due to the rich nutritional profile of yerba maté. It is much more than just a stimulant.

While visiting Sebastopol, California, I got to visit the first and only yerba maté café and enjoyed a fresh-made chai yerba maté latte. It was delicious, so much so that I bought some yerba maté to bring home. I enjoy it every day, instead of coffee. I've probably had a hundred cups of the stuff during the writing of this book. It's actually more of a tea than a coffee, and it contains 24 vitamins and minerals, 15 important amino acids, and a plethora of antioxidants to reduce free-radical damage to your pancreas.

If you visit Argentina or Paraguay, you will see people walking around sipping yerba maté out of hollow gourds, much the same way that Americans tote their cup of Starbucks. Yerba maté is sold in bags, just like coffee. To make it, use a French press, or a regular coffee maker. If it tastes bitter, it's because you've used boiling water—you only want to use hot water, not boiling.

Let it cool, okay? We don't want to heat up your mouth or esophagus too much. Be fancy like me, and make a yerba maté latte! Sweeten the brew with some honey or stevia and almond extract. Make a latte topping by frothing some almond milk or hemp milk. Information regarding yerba maté and where it is sold can be found at www.guayaki.com or by calling 888-482-9254.

WHY EAT RABBIT FOOD?

Fresh or frozen produce is good for you, no doubt. There have been several studies looking at the relationship between intake of fruits and vegetables and reduction in risk for heart disease. But in one study, published in the journal *Diabetes Care* (July 2008), researchers followed women who were part of the Nurses' Health Study. Begun in 1976 with 121,700 female registered nurses between the ages of 30 and 55 years from 11 different states, the Nurses' Health Study looked at their medical history and has followed their lifestyle, diet, and other health practices ever since. In the 2008 study, researchers found that the women who ate five or more servings of fruits and vegetables daily had a lower risk of developing type 2 diabetes than did their colleagues who did not eat the five or more servings of fruits and vegetables each day. That's good enough for me!

I would like you to eat organic vegetables, such as dark, leafy green lettuce, kale, and spinach. Eating more meals that contain natural, organic, raw plant foods will help increase the activity of enzymes in your gut, as well as antioxidants and other healing compounds in your body. I will share with you some of my favorite recipes in Chapter 17. For now, just know that veggies play a major role—along with exercise and supplements—in addressing, and potentially reversing, your condition.

NOT ALL SALTS ARE CREATED EQUAL

In Chapter 1, you learned why white refined flour is bad for you. Now let's talk about another white refined food—table salt. It is known chemically as sodium chloride. These are two minerals that we need for our very survival. Before you read on, I want to get something straight. I think a certain amount of sodium and chloride is important to you, but I don't think the best way to get it is through typical table salt, even though that is a good source.

What's the problem with typical table salt? This type of salt also happens to contain a mixture of potassium iodide, glucose, and synthetic anticaking compounds that keep the salt from sticking to itself so it will pour out easily. Table salt, as compared to healthy sea salt, is so refined that I view it as just another food additive. In fact, it's frequently used to deice highways.

Now there's someone with good business sense—take an industrial chemical and convince millions of Americans to eat it. Want to know just how clever this person was? According to the Environmental Literacy Council, sodium chloride (table salt) is so harmful to the environment that when it is dumped on the road to melt snow and ice, the melting water (with the sodium chloride in it) gets into vegetation and soil, and eventually even gets into some of our local waterways. Subsequently, anything growing in this salty soil can be harmed because the salt has the same effect on the plants as it does on us: High levels of sodium chloride in soil make it harder for the vegetation to absorb both water and nutrients. It's true. This, in turn, slows down plant growth, which affects the animals who depend on those plants, causing the animals to suffer from lack of food.

As if all this weren't shocking enough, when the soil gets so salty that it breaks down, other contaminants from the soil drain into the local rivers. Once the salt gets into lakes, rivers, and other bodies of fresh water, the salt builds up to such a high

MSG ALIASES

Trying your darnedest to avoid monosodium glutamate (MSG)? If you think that scrutinizing labels for monosodium glutamate or MSG is enough, you'd be mistaken. Manufacturers know that many people won't buy foods that contain MSG, so they've come up will all kinds of ways to disguise the presence of this chemical. Here's what to look for:

Autolyzed yeast

Calcium caseinate

Gelatin

Glutamate

Glutamic acid

Hydrolyzed protein

Monopotassium glutamate

Monosodium glutamate

Sodium caseinate

Textured protein

Yeast extract

Yeast food

Yeast nutrient

If you see any of these ingredients, be aware that they often contain some MSG or else create MSG as the food item is processed:

Flavors and flavorings

Seasonings

Natural flavors and flavorings

Natural pork flavoring

Natural beef flavoring

Natural chicken flavoring

Soy sauce

Soy protein

Bouillon

Stock

Broth

Malt extract or flavoring

Barley malt

Whey protein

Carrageenan

Maltodextrin

Cornstarch

Citric acid

Powdered milk

Anything ultrapasteurized

level of concentration that plants and other organisms that live in fresh water are harmed. All of this from the chemical in your saltshaker. Talk about "earth-shattering."

Heavily processed table salt is corrosive to everything it touches—your shoes, your dog's paws, your car, your organs . . . you get the picture. And yes, all of this from the same chemical as table salt! Who knew?

Now that you know all this, is there any wonder why your doctor tells you to cut down on salt intake? Too much regular table salt may cause high blood pressure in some people because it can cause water retention. This increases your risk of stroke and heart attack. Table salt slows down the human body's production of nitric oxide, a chemical that shuttles blood to the heart, kidneys, brain, and private parts. Very low levels of nitric oxide will squeeze off blood vessels all over your body and cause coronary artery disease. So now you see why blood pressure rises and your risk for stroke and heart attack might increase. Granted, it takes *a lot of salt* to reduce nitric oxide much more than you eat in a day, but there may be a cumulative effect after many years of consumption.

What you may not realize is that low levels of nitric oxide have also been implicated in diabetes and erectile dysfunction. Guys, you heard that right. Viagra—the blockbuster erectile dysfunction drug—works by increasing levels of nitric oxide in your bloodstream. Table salt *reduces* it, to some degree.

Now one more thing before we leave the subject of salt. Many menopause-aged women suffer from low blood pressure, brain fog, and extreme fatigue. They also crave carbs, sugar, and salty foods. Medical research has found that a diet high in sugar and refined carbs can cause high blood pressure and also chronically high insulin levels, which makes the blood vessels saggy. Blood pressure needs to go up in order to keep the blood flowing properly. So it's a vicious cycle.

Granted, those who live on processed food get way too much of the wrong kinds of salt, but those who strictly keep their salt (sodium) intake very low in an effort to be healthy may suffer for it, especially if they take antihypertensive medications to lower blood pressure or diuretics. They may develop fatigue, low blood pressure, and problems with bloodflow or kidney function. We do need some sodium, but not a lot.

When it comes to salt, the middle road is ideal, and real sea salt (not pure sodium chloride) is truly essential for good health. It's high time you switched what's in your saltshaker. So now, let's talk about the kind of salt I want you to eat on a daily basis because it's good for you.

Salt of the Earth

Let's remember that authentic sea salt is an essential nutrient for the body and that in olden days it was traded like money! Sea salt consists of some sodium chloride, just like table salt. The difference between high-quality sea salt and table salt is massive, though.

Healthy brands of gourmet sea salt are pure and unadulterated. They often have a little bit of color to them since they are not bleached white. That's good. You want the color. And remember we agreed back in Chapter 1 that there would be "no more white." The colorful granules you see in unrefined sea salt represent the natural colors of various minerals, such as copper, iodine, potassium, magnesium, chromium, zinc, and iron. Sea salt is derived from water from the sea (or river) that gets evaporated and purified. Dried sea salt retains healthy minerals that you need for normal thyroid, muscle, heart, and pancreatic function.

Where the salt comes from and how it is processed are very important. Great salts are naturally processed—evaporated by the sun and the wind rather than being heated by hot ovens.

Some of the highest-quality salts I've ever tasted—and use in my home—are those that contain a lot of minerals. Natural unrefined sea salt provides your body with healthy natural minerals that make your pancreas and heart very happy.

If you have diabetes, getting minerals is critical to your health and well-being. There is a full discussion of minerals and how they affect your blood sugar in Chapter 14. Good salts that are mineral-rich may help you with leg cramps or the blues. You body craves minerals.

There are two salts that I recommend you use in your home from now on. You can buy them at health food stores or online. Since I'm picky, and I love and crave gourmet salt, I buy mine from a specialty company that insists on purity. They get their salt from mines from all over the world. They are called SaltWorks (www.seasalt.com) and they carry dozens of different types of gourmet salts.

Here are the best two salts that I suggest for people with diabetes.

HIMALAYAN SALT. When it's mined properly from the Himalayan Mountains in Pakistan, it contains about 84 minerals. Good Himalayan salt will look slightly pink because of the extremely high content of iron and other minerals.

FRENCH GREY SEA SALT. This salt does not have quite as many different minerals in it as the Himalayan sort; however, it has the *highest* content (gram for gram) of minerals. So it's a great way to boost levels of healthy minerals in your body. And trust me, your body is hungry for this. Another name this goes by is grey Celtic sea salt.

Experiment with your salts, and use them as a finishing ingredient, meaning at the end of your cooking. This is important, because if you cook with your good sea salt, it may lose flavor, and then you will have to resalt your meal at the dinner table. Remember, sea salt does have some sodium chloride in it, so if you are salting twice, you're getting twice the amount of sodium chloride. Salt *after* the cooking is done. If you need to salt while you're cooking, use a basic sea salt (such as RealSalt) and save the specialty gourmet salts for the final finish.

Many companies manufacturing sea salt bleach their salts or mine them from impure waters. Now that you know how to pick sea salt, you can refer to my resources on page 389 to find genuine salt companies that have your health in mind.

Recipes to Save Your Life and Limbs

CHAPTER
17

It's time to stop making yourself crazy and just enjoy your food again. Of course, you need to track your blood glucose numbers and make sure you're getting enough of the right fat and protein (carbs are easier). But if you choose to follow my suggestions on how to eat and even use some of my recipes, you can focus on the pleasure of food, rather than the business of food, if you know what I mean. I'm guessing that if you have diabetes, or some form of blood sugar issue, you know exactly what I mean.

You can stop the nonsense if you start eating the RIGHT foods. It's true! The right foods are those that sustain and improve your health. The right foods come straight from Mother Earth. They are not adulterated, processed, refined, stripped of their amazing nutritional benefits, boxed, or canned. They are natural, and you will find them to be delicious once your taste buds adjust to real food, instead of food that comes from a box.

These recipes probably won't taste like what you are used to. My goal is to retrain your taste buds so that eventually you find joy in eating these healthful foods, as I do. I want to encourage you to experience different tastes and textures. It may be different at first, but it will be worth the effort and commitment.

After all, eating healthy foods could very well save your limbs, if not your life. All the science points in this direction. There's a new study every day on the dangers of high-sugar, high-salt, and high-fat foods. This science is why states like New York and California banned trans fats—these foods were literally killing people, and the legislators felt so strongly about protecting their people, they outlawed trans fats in restaurants.

Now that's impressive. I wish my state would ban trans fats from restaurants. But you can do it in your home—you can ban all the trans fats and all the high-sugar, empty-calorie food from your diet. And you can start now.

Think about it: You are more likely to become obese, develop heart disease, or lose a limb by eating foods loaded with high-fructose corn syrup and trans fats than by eating fruits and veggies.

WHERE TO BUY THE ALMOND FLOUR

My recipes are incredibly novel. Many are based on almond flour, have practically no carbs, and should not spike blood sugar. Almonds have amazingly impressive health benefits because of their content of vitamin E, magnesium, calcium, potassium, and fiber. Almonds are also a great source of mono-unsaturated fat and healthy protein. Using almond flour is perfect for people who are reversing their type 2 diabetic status.

Almond flour is thicker and heavier than what you are probably used to. That's because it's just ground-up almonds, so the texture is heavier than that of processed white flour. This also means that your baked items are going to be heavier in texture. It's not hard to get used to.

Almond flour gets very expensive if you buy the type sold at health food stores because it comes in little bags for about $5 a bag. I buy my flour in bulk because it's all I use in my house. I buy 25 pounds and I find that the brands I use taste great and have a better texture.

These are the places I recommend that you buy your flour from. If you find other sources for almond flour that is similar to these brands, please drop me an email at info@dearpharmacist.com

www.JustAlmonds.com; 877-287-0233
www.LucysKitchenShop.com; 888-484-2126

In the coming pages, I am going to share with you some of my incredible recipes that substitute bad foods for good ones. Why?

Because people with diabetes have the same nutritional needs as anyone else. You have to eat well-balanced meals to keep your blood glucose levels within the normal healthy range. You can do that without becoming schizo over every meal choice. For example, when baking bread, you can use almond flour instead of regular alloxan-poisoned white or all-purpose bleached flour. Almond flour has 20 carbs per cup, versus over 70 carbs for wheat flour. You can eat delicious cakes and cookies without gluten-containing wheat flour also.

See how easy it is? If you want to eat muffins, bread, and cookies, now you can! I have all sorts of secrets that I will share in the coming pages. These are the exact recipes that I use in my own kitchen and have for many years.

Before we get to the recipes, I'd like to share with you a few basic tips and pointers.

FORGET ABOUT ARTIFICIAL SWEETENERS. You will never find a recipe in my book that contains an artificial sweetener. These are not naturally occurring

GREEN BAGS

Evert-Fresh Green Bags help your vegetables stay fresher longer, so you don't have to go to the grocery store every few days. Health food stores and supermarkets often carry these. They are fantastic and save you money because you don't have to toss dying veggies and fruits. For more information see www.evertfresh.com.

in nature, and there is enough documentation to suggest that they can fuel tumors or damage nerve cells and brain cells. So you will only see sweeteners that come from Mother Nature in these recipes.

LEARN TO LOVE SOUP. I love soup myself. When made properly it can act like medicine in your body. You will see I do not use potatoes or gluten-containing thickeners in them. Instead of potatoes, I recommend zucchini or turnips and they turn out perfectly, without the added carbs of potatoes. In my soups, these are virtually tasteless. As a rule, be open to using new veggies and turn all your left-over vegetables into soup.

CHECK YOUR OVEN TEMPERATURE. Not all ovens cook the same, so 30 minutes in my oven might be 60 minutes in yours.

BE ESPECIALLY CAREFUL WITH OILS. You will want to freshen oils periodically so they don't go rancid. Don't use oils that taste sour or have an odor and check expiration dates. I've outlined some of the healthiest oils for you in Chapter 16. Among them are almond oil, grape seed oil, avocado oil, olive oil, and flaxseed oil. I suggest you use Bija brand or other high quality brands, and make sure you have on hand a variety of four or five different oils for different recipes. Each oil provides something different for your body, nutritionally speaking.

PAY ATTENTION TO CHEESE. Some of my recipes contain cheese. If you want to remain casein-free, skip the cheese. In my home, I am casein-free for the most part but when I need a cheese fix, I use goat's cheese because it doesn't seem to spark as many reactions as cow's cheese. If you want to stay dairy-free, that's okay with me too. You might also opt to stay mostly dairy-free, with the exception of one or two meals per week.

AVOID OR STRICTLY LIMIT ALCOHOL. Please pay a few extra dollars to buy extracts of vanilla (or almond) that are alcohol-free. Alcohol damages the pancreas.

BUY A HIGH-PERFORMANCE BLENDER. Since you are ready to make

SUBSTITUTIONS

I recommend against using wheat flour because of the gluten. So here is a list of some substitutions that might work if you want to thicken sauce or gravy. One tablespoon of wheat flour could be substituted with:

1½ teaspoons cornstarch
1½ teaspoons potato starch
5 teaspoons rice flour
5 teaspoons arrowroot starch
2 teaspoons tapioca starch
1 tablespoon sorghum flour

Substitution for Egg

In some biscuits and cookie recipes you may be able to leave out the eggs altogether. Try this handy substitution; it usually works well for me:

To replace 1 egg, blend 2 tablespoons of cornstarch with ¼ cup of water. Note: This works only in some recipes. You'll have to experiment.

healthier choices for yourself and your family, you should consider investing in a high-performance blender. I love to make soup and smoothies, and drink fresh juice in the morning. I got tired of throwing out a blender every year or two. At a convention one year, I watched a demonstration for the incredible Vita-Mix blender and bought one on the spot. I use it almost daily, and it's still perfect after 6 years.

The Vita-Mix company has been improving their product for four generations, and they boast that they have created the "world's most durable, reliable and innovative appliance." If I didn't own one, I would think they were just touting their product, but this thing can honestly grind up your shoes!

Why is that important? Because raw food enthusiasts (and I advocate more raw foods in your diet) actually blend up healthy parts of fruits and veggies. For example, pulverizing the avocado pit to release its anticancer benefits is easy to do with a Vita-Mix 500 or a BlendTec blender, whereas it would destroy a regular blender. I used them to make many of the fresh healthy smoothies, soups, and recipes in the next pages. You can even make ice cream in minutes. Watch videos and learn more about the Vita-Mix at www.vita-mix.com.

Blend Tec is another high-performance blender brand (www.blendtec.com).

YERBA MATÉ LATTE

Yerba maté contains natural compounds that sustain energy, increase alertness, and combat dangerous free radicals. The saponins in yerba maté boost immune function. Yerba maté also appears to help you lose weight by speeding up the way you burn fat. You can drink yerba maté plain, or you can dress it up a little in this almond-flavored latte.

1   yerba maté tea bag
⅛   teaspoon almond extract
1   tablespoon hemp or almond milk

Steep the tea bag in hot water following directions on the package. Add almond extract and milk. You can froth the milk if you like it that way.
Makes 1 serving

PER SERVING: 10 calories, 0 g protein, 1 g carbohydrates, 0.2 g total fat, 0 g saturated fat, 0.1 g fiber, 8 mg sodium

HOMEMADE ALMOND MILK

You can buy commercial brands at the store, but the homemade kind is delicious. Almonds contain lots of calcium, vitamin E, and magnesium, plus they are dairy-free. One ounce of almonds contains about as much calcium as ¼ cup of dairy milk.

2   cups organic raw unblanched almonds
3½   cups filtered water
½   teaspoon vanilla or almond extract
1   or 2 teaspoons agave syrup or organic honey, to taste
       Pinch of sea salt

In a medium bowl, soak the almonds in water to cover for about 6 hours. Drain and rinse. Put the almonds in a Vita-Mix blender or BlendTec with the filtered water. Add the vanilla or almond extract, agave syrup, and salt, and grind on high for a minute. Pour the mixture into a cheesecloth bag and squeeze it over a bowl or pitcher. It keeps for about a day or two in the refrigerator. You also have the option of peeling the almonds (after you soak them for 6 hours). The skin will slide right off. The advantage to peeling the almonds before blending them is that the milk produced will stay fresher for longer (3 to 5 days).

Makes 4½ cups

PER ½ CUP: 24 calories, 1 g protein, 2 g carbohydrates, 1.5 g total fat, 0 g saturated fat, 0.5 g fiber, 93 mg sodium

ALMOND-PAPAYA SMOOTHIE

The papaya puree in this recipe offers your body vitamin C, folate, and potassium. The green tea drink mix used in this smoothie contains barley and wheatgrass, making it a delicious superfood. Talk about a jump-start to cleaning up cells and nourishing your body.

1½	cups almond milk
½	cup coconut water or filtered water
½	cup papaya puree (we use Dynamic Health brand)
2	tablespoons aloe vera juice
1	teaspoon agave syrup (optional)
1	scoop protein powder (we use NanoPro French Vanilla)
1	tablespoon Kyo-Green Green Tea powdered drink mix
2	cups ice cubes

Combine the ingredients in a blender and blend on high for 30 seconds.

Makes 1 serving

PER SERVING: 259 calories, 21 g protein, 29 g carbohydrates, 6.6 g total fat, 1.3 g saturated fat, 4.9 g fiber, 450 mg sodium

MATCHA MINT SMOOTHIE

Matcha tea contains antioxidants that sweep away free radicals. One cup of matcha tea contains the antioxidant equivalent of 8 to 10 cups of regular green tea.

1½   cups almond milk

1   tablespoon matcha green tea powder

Fresh mint leaves (6 to 8)

2   cups ice cubes

1   tablespoon honey, or to taste

Place all ingredients in a blender and blend on high for 30 seconds.

PER SERVING: 140 calories, 3 g protein, 23 g carbohydrates, 4.8 g total fat, 0 g saturated fat, 2.3 g fiber, 276 mg sodium

EVERYTHING-BUT-THE-KITCHEN-SINK SMOOTHIE

This makes a very sweet and filling smoothie. It's perfect for breakfast or a midday snack. If you don't have blueberries, use raspberries or blackberries. The point of this smoothie is that you are getting nutrition in a cup. It's fresh and packed with life-sustaining nutrients, including from the cacao powder, which is pure ground cacao beans, not commercial cocoa powder.

1   banana

1   cup blueberries (I keep mine frozen)

1   cup coconut water or filtered water

1   tablespoon ground flaxseeds

1   tablespoon hulled hemp seeds

1   tablespoon Kyo-Green Green Tea powdered drink mix

1   tablespoon vanilla whey protein powder

1   teaspoon cacao powder

½   teaspoon ground cinnamon

2   cups ice cubes

Combine the ingredients in a blender and blend on high for 30 seconds.

Makes 1 serving

PER SERVING: 405 calories, 20 g protein, 68 g carbohydrates, 8.8 g total fat, 1.5 g saturated fat, 12 g fiber, 280 mg sodium

THANKSGIVING SMOOTHIE

Cinnamon is thought to help regulate blood sugar. The sweet potato contains a lot of nutrients, including beta-carotene, which protects your vision and your skin. (I'm thinking especially about the skin on your feet.) Sweet potato also contains a lot of vitamin C, which helps squash free radicals. Flaxseeds are a source of healthful essential fatty acids, and they're also a great way to suppress the formation of bad estrogen in your body.

1	medium sweet potato, baked and peeled
1	cup almond milk
2	teaspoons ground flaxseeds
½	cup plain So Delicious coconut yogurt (optional)
2	cups ice cubes
1	teaspoon ground cinnamon
½	teaspoon vanilla extract
1	teaspoon agave syrup
	Pinch of nutmeg

Combine the ingredients in a blender and blend on high for 30 seconds.

Makes 1 serving

PER SERVING: 282 calories, 5 g protein, 45 g carbohydrates, 9.4 g total fat, 4.1 g saturated fat, 9.5 g fiber, 228 mg sodium

CHOCOLATE-MINT SMOOTHIE

This smoothie has amazing flavor and is packed with impressive antioxidants and phytochemicals. The ground cacao contains compounds that enhance physical and mental well-being. It also has magnesium, lysine, and neurotransmitters, such as dopamine and anandamide. The spearmint soothes the gastrointestinal tract. The aloe vera juice is the other star in this recipe. It contains over 100 health-promoting chemicals.

1	cup almond milk
2	teaspoons ground flaxseeds
1	tablespoon aloe vera juice
1	container (6 ounces) So Delicious coconut yogurt

1   tablespoon cacao powder

½   teaspoon vanilla extract

2   teaspoons agave syrup

8   to 10 fresh mint leaves

2   cups ice cubes

Combine the ingredients in a blender and blend on high for 30 seconds.

Makes 1 serving

PER SERVING: 222 calories, 3 g protein, 33 g carbohydrates, 9 g total fat, 6 g saturated fat, 5.4 g fiber, 14 mg sodium

GINGER-MINT MATCHA TEA

Ginger is a powerful anti-inflammatory and antimicrobial. It can reduce pain in the joints and soothe some of your digestive woes. It works best when grated fresh (don't use powdered ginger in this recipe). Ginger also may freshen your breath and fight candida. Matcha tea is one of the strongest natural antioxidants on the planet. It's 8 to 10 times stronger than plain green tea in the antioxidant department.

2   tablespoons grated fresh ginger

½   bunch fresh mint (about 1 cup)

1   teaspoon matcha green tea powder

1   teaspoon agave syrup

In a small saucepan, combine the ginger in 2 cups water and heat to boiling. Simmer gently for about 10 minutes. Take off the heat and add the mint leaves and matcha powder. Let steep for about 5 minutes. When you serve the tea, put it through a handheld filter so that you only get liquid. Sweeten with agave syrup. (You may sweeten with natural raw honey or stevia if you prefer.)

Makes 1 serving

PER SERVING: 49 calories, 1 g protein, 11 g carbohydrates, 0.4 g total fat, 0.1 g saturated fat, 0 g fiber, 10 mg sodium

SUPER GREEN PROTEIN SMOOTHIE

The whey provides a source of protein and also provides a source of amino acids that improve mood. The green powder skyrockets the amount of antioxidant protection you get. The coconut yogurt adds a nice texture without having to add more milk.

1   container (6 ounces) So Delicious plain or flavored coconut yogurt

½   cup coconut water or filtered water

1   teaspoon Kyo-Green green powdered drink mix

1   scoop vanilla whey protein powder

1   cup ice cubes

Combine the ingredients in a blender and blend on high for 30 seconds.

Makes 1 serving

PER SERVING: 263 calories, 19 g protein, 27 g carbohydrates, 8.7 g total fat, 7.2 g saturated fat, 4.3 g fiber, 176 mg sodium

SUZY'S NATURAL SODA

This soda can break you of the traditional store-bought soda habit. Pomegranate is known for its heart-health benefits. It is loaded with antioxidants, and preliminary studies show it can improve bloodflow to the heart and to the reproductive organs. (Seriously, pomegranate helps improve erectile dysfunction over time by improving prostate function.)

1   cup plain seltzer

¼   cup POM pomegranate juice

Mix together and serve over ice.

Variations: If you don't like the flavor of pomegranate juice, make this with grape juice (100% juice, not the sweetened kind). Or for "root beer," mix the seltzer with root beer–flavored liquid stevia. It tastes just like root beer, for real! Experiment. You can't mess this up.

Makes 1 serving

PER SERVING: 35 calories, 0 g protein, 9 g carbohydrates, 0 g total fat, 0 g saturated fat, 0 g fiber, 8 mg sodium

VEGETABLE BROTH

When one of my soup recipes calls for water, you can easily substitute this vegetable broth if you want added health benefits. It's also great for cooking brown rice. It will keep in the freezer nicely for 3 months.

2	celery ribs
2	onions
2	carrots, sliced
2	tomatoes
1	leek (white and green parts), well washed
1	zucchini or yellow summer squash
3	garlic cloves
6	cups water
1	bunch parsley
1	or 2 teaspoons Celtic or French grey sea salt

In a large saucepan, combine the celery, onions, carrots, tomatoes, leek, zucchini or squash, garlic, and water. Bring to a boil and cook until the vegetables are tender but the colors are still bright and vivid, about 10 minutes. Add the parsley and sea salt to taste. Cover for 5 minutes. Strain the broth and discard the solids. Refrigerate or freeze.

Makes 6 cups

PER CUP: 20 calories, 0 g protein, 3 g carbohydrates, 0 g total fat, 0 g saturated fat, 0 g fiber, 140 mg sodium

WATERCRESS SOUP

Watercress protects the kidneys and contains a lot of healthful phytochemicals, including carotenes. Fresh onions and garlic are known for their immune-enhancing benefits. You can also make this soup with broccoli instead of watercress.

2	teaspoons flaxseed oil
2	or 3 turnips, peeled and chopped
1	large zucchini, cut into chunks
1	leek (white and green parts), well washed and cut into chunks
1	small onion, cut into chunks
2	garlic cloves, chopped
4	cups water or vegetable broth
1	bunch (or 7-ounce bag) watercress
½	bunch parsley
	Sea salt

In a medium saucepan, warm the flaxseed oil over medium heat. Add the turnips, zucchini, leek, onion, and garlic. Cook, stirring, until they soften slightly. Add the water and simmer for 15 minutes.

Stir in the watercress and parsley, and remove from the heat. Uncover and let cool for about 10 minutes. Pour into a blender and blend on high for 2 minutes. Add more water if you want a thinner soup. Season to taste with sea salt. Serve hot.

Makes 4 servings

PER SERVING: 88 calories, 4 g protein, 15 g carbohydrates, 2.8 g total fat, 0.3 g saturated fat, 3.7 g fiber, 384 mg sodium

PUMPKIN AND MACADAMIA NUT SOUP

This soup has an interesting, delicious, warming taste. In this recipe I used butternut squash, which—just like pumpkin—has potassium, calcium, folate, and loads of beta-carotene. The pumpkin seed oil I use is 100 percent pure, made by Bija Culinary Oils. It has a green color to it because of the high chlorophyll content (in Chapter 12 you'll find that greens and chlorophyll are powerful detoxifiers in the body). The oil is expensive, but I feel it is worth it. Macadamia nuts add fiber and are an excellent source of protein, monounsaturated fats, omega-6 fatty acids, thiamine, and potassium.

1	medium (2 pounds) butternut squash, cooked and scooped out
1	cup peeled and diced apples (Granny Smith)
1	onion, quartered
1	celery rib, chopped
3	small garlic cloves
2	teaspoons grated fresh ginger
½	teaspoon ground cardamom
½	teaspoon ground turmeric
2½	cups water
¾	cup macadamia nuts (3½ ounces), coarsely chopped
2	tablespoons pumpkin seed oil

In a large saucepan, combine the squash, apples, onion, celery, garlic, ginger, cardamom, turmeric, and water. Bring to a simmer and cook until squash is tender, about 15 minutes. Transfer the mixture to a blender. Add the macadamias and pumpkin seed oil. Blend on high for a minute or two.

Makes 4 servings

PER SERVING: 352 calories, 4 g protein, 32 g carbohydrates, 26 g total fat, 4.6 g saturated fat, 9.1 g fiber, 19 mg sodium

Makes 6 servings

PER SERVING: 235 calories, 3 g protein, 21 g carbohydrates, 18 g total fat, 3.1 g saturated fat, 6.1 g fiber, 13 mg sodium

SPINACH SOUP

As children, we all loved Popeye and his impressive transformation from eating spinach. There's a reason for this. The leafy green vegetable is an incredible source of beta-carotene, as well as vitamin C, calcium, and phosphorus. By combining spinach with garlic, onions, and zucchini, you get a soup that contains strong antioxidants, phytochemicals, and anticancer nutrients. The key with this soup (and all of them) is to make sure the greens are put in last, and that they are only just heated through. Don't let them turn an olive color or get wilty.

1	tablespoon grape seed oil
2	small turnips, peeled and chopped
1	large onion, chopped
1	large zucchini, cubed
3	garlic cloves, chopped
1	tablespoon wheat-free tamari
½	teaspoon ground nutmeg
4	cups water
1	bunch (or 10-ounce bag) spinach

In a medium saucepan, warm the oil over medium heat. Add the turnips, onion, zucchini, garlic, tamari, and salt. Cook until the vegetables begin to soften. Add the water and simmer for 15 minutes. Stir in the spinach and remove from the heat. Uncover and let cool for about 10 minutes. Transfer to a blender and blend on high for 2 minutes. Add more water if you want a thinner soup. Adjust seasoning to taste. Serve hot.

This is a great soup to make in the high-speed blender as you can save nutrients by increasing the blend time and eliminating the heating in saucepan step.

Makes 4 servings

PER SERVING: 90 calories, 4 g protein, 12 g carbohydrates, 4 g total fat, 0.5 g saturated fat, 3.8 g fiber, 338 mg sodium

Even though I don't recommend that you eat a lot of meat (or any for that matter), I realize that there's a good chance that you do indulge. I respect your choice, and I have included some delicious recipes that include meat. I have tried all these at home and they are virtually foolproof. The key is in the almond flour. It has a thicker texture, and it adds a hearty flavor to anything you put it on. If you are a meat eater, I'd stick primarily to fish as much as you can, preferably wild caught, from cold oceans. These include salmon, Arctic char, cod, mackerel, tuna, and haddock. If you are going to enjoy some beef, I'd prefer that it be grass fed (as opposed to grain fed) and that it be designated as free range.

ALMOND CHICKEN

The turmeric and rosemary are the stars in this recipe. When you put these anti-inflammatory and anticancer spices into the breading mixture for the chicken, it loads the dish with good nutrients—especially when you compare it to typical store-bought fried chicken. The ground flaxseed won't be detectable to your taste buds, but it adds fiber and essential fatty acids to your plate (and you can add any other herbs or spices you like). This recipe passes any kid's fuss factor too.

1	sprig fresh rosemary
1	cup almond flour
½	cup chopped parsley
1	tablespoon ground flaxseeds
1	teaspoon salt
1	teaspoon ground turmeric
8	bone-in chicken thighs or 4 bone-in breast halves, skin removed

Preheat the oven to 350°F.

Strip the leaves from the rosemary sprig and coarsely chop. In a shallow bowl or pie plate, combine the rosemary, almond flour, parsley, ground flaxseeds, salt, and turmeric. Rinse the chicken and dip it into the breading. Place it in a glass baking dish (or stone baking dish) and bake for 20 to 30 minutes, or until cooked through but still juicy.

Makes 4 servings

PER SERVING: 386 calories, 33 g protein, 7 g carbohydrates, 26 g total fat, 4.2 g saturated fat, 3.6 g fiber, 397 mg sodium

BREADED ORANGE ROUGHY

Orange roughy has a mild flavor and a texture that is similar to (but softer than) lobster. It will take on the taste of any seasoning you put on it. I use hemp seeds in this recipe to pull in an extraordinary amount of healthy essential fatty acids—omega-3s, omega-6s, and gamma linolenic acid. The fish can be baked, or you can pan-fry it lightly in unrefined grape seed oil or ghee. If you'd like, make this with 1 teaspoon fresh thyme instead of dill.

2	cups almond flour
½	cup chopped parsley
2	tablespoons chopped fresh dill
1	tablespoon hulled hemp seeds
1	tablespoon ground flaxseeds
1	garlic clove, crushed
1	teaspoon salt
½	teaspoon grated lemon zest
4	large orange roughy fillets (about 6 ounces each)
	Lemon, lime, or orange slices (or mix them up to make it pretty)
	Grape seed oil, for the baking dish

Preheat the oven to 325°F. Grease a baking dish with grape seed oil.

In a shallow bowl or pie plate, combine the almond flour, parsley, dill, hemp seeds, ground flaxseeds, garlic, salt, and lemon zest. Wash the fish but don't dry it. Dip the moist fish into the breading to coat it and lay it in the baking dish. Put the citrus slices on top of the fish and bake for 25 to 30 minutes, or until the fish is cooked through but still moist.

Makes 4 servings

PER SERVING: 324 calories, 35 g protein, 7 g carbohydrates, 18 g total fat, 1.3 g saturated fat, 3.6 g fiber, 428 mg sodium

QUINOA PASTA WITH SCALLOPS AND ARTICHOKES

I use angel hair quinoa pasta in this recipe. But you can try spaghetti squash, rice pasta, or glass noodles, if you prefer. I cook the scallops along with the vegetables, but if you want them browned, broil them separately.

8	ounces angel hair quinoa pasta
2	tablespoons olive oil or grape seed oil
12	large sea scallops
1	bag (9 ounces) frozen artichoke hearts, thawed and drained (dry them as much as possible before cooking)
1	large zucchini or Japanese eggplant, peeled and chopped
2	shallots or 1 medium onion, chopped
½	leek (green and white parts), washed and chopped
¼	cup chopped red bell pepper or ¼ cup sun-dried tomatoes
1	or 2 garlic cloves, minced
12	grape or cherry tomatoes, halved
	Himalayan sea salt or Herbamare
	Pepper (optional)
	Handful parsley and basil leaves, chopped

Cook pasta according to package directions.

In a large skillet, heat the oil over medium heat. Add the scallops, artichokes, zucchini, shallots, leek, bell pepper or sun-dried tomatoes, and garlic. Cook until scallops are opaque throughout (turning them as they cook), about 10 minutes. Add grape or cherry tomatoes for the last 2 minutes. Season with salt and pepper to taste. Serve over the hot pasta, sprinkled with parsley and basil.

Makes 4 servings

PER SERVING: 359 calories, 16 g protein, 52 g carbohydrates, 10 g total fat, 1 g saturated fat, 8.5 g fiber, 278 mg sodium

LAMB CUTLETS

1   tablespoon avocado oil

6   lamb cutlets (about 3 ounces each), preferably grass fed and free range

1   teaspoon sea salt (I use flavored Fusion's Spanish Rosemary)
     Chopped fresh mint leaves
     Lime wedges

In a large skillet, in batches if necessary, heat the oil over medium-low heat. Season the lamb with the salt. Add to the pan and cook for about 5 minutes on each side for medium. Serve garnished with fresh mint and a squeeze of lime.

Makes 6 servings

PER SERVING: 262 calories, 21 g protein, 0 g carbohydrates, 19 g total fat, 7.3 g saturated fat, 0 g fiber, 445 mg sodium

RICE PAPER WRAPS

This is more of a general guideline than an actual recipe. Serve it with the sauce that follows. If you're vegan, leave out the shrimp.

Glass noodles

Chives

Avocado, sliced thin

Zucchini, peeled and sliced

Carrots, shredded

Bean sprouts (optional)

Cooked shrimp (optional)

Rice paper wraps

Cook the glass noodles according to package directions. Prepare the veggies and shrimp. Place room-temperature water in a shallow bowl or pan. Submerge a rice paper wrapper in the water until it is pliable. Spread the softened rice paper on a work surface and add fillings to taste and in any ratio.

DIPPING SAUCE FOR RICE PAPER WRAPS

¼ cup red wine vinegar

¼ cup wheat-free tamari

2 teaspoons honey

1 tablespoon sesame oil

1 scallion, thinly sliced

1 teaspoon fresh lime or lemon juice

2 teaspoons grated fresh ginger

   Dash of cayenne pepper

Whisk all these ingredients together in a small bowl. Let chill in the fridge while you are preparing the wraps.

Makes ⅔ cup

PER TABLESPOON: 22 calories, 1 g protein, 2 g carbohydrates, 1.4 g total fat, 0.2 g saturated fat, 0.1 g fiber, 403 mg sodium

BURGERS NOT MADE WITH MEAT

You can cook the patties in a skillet in some grape seed oil, or you can bake them. These will freeze well too.

1 can (15.5 ounces) red kidney beans, drained and rinsed

1 cup hulled sunflower or pumpkin seeds

½ cup grated carrot

¼ cup chopped onion

¼ cup chopped leek

1 tablespoon minced parsley

1 tablespoon minced fresh basil

   A few leaves of fresh rosemary (thin little leaves, not sprigs; it's strong!)

   Celtic or French grey sea salt

4 eggs

Combine the beans, seeds, carrot, onion, leek, parsley, basil, rosemary, salt to taste, and eggs in a blender or food processor. Process until ground. Form into patties.

Makes 4 servings

PER SERVING: 338 calories, 19 g protein, 25 g carbohydrates, 20 g total fat, 3.1 g saturated fat, 10 g fiber, 227 mg sodium

CRAB CAKES

These are great served with my Rainbow Salad.

1	container (8 ounces) crabmeat (I prefer claw meat)
1	celery rib, thinly sliced
¼	cup minced red or green bell pepper
¼	cup chopped onion
¼	cup hulled hemp seeds
2	tablespoons minced parsley
1	tablespoon ground flaxseeds
2	tablespoons mayonnaise
1	teaspoon Dijon mustard
½	teaspoon Worcestershire sauce
½	teaspoon salt
¼	teaspoon cayenne pepper
½	cup almond flour
1	tablespoon grape seed oil

In a medium bowl, combine crabmeat, celery, bell pepper, onion, hemp seed, parsley, ground flaxseeds, mayonnaise, mustard, Worcestershire, salt, and cayenne. Mash together and form into crab cakes about 3 inches in diameter. Dip the cakes into the almond flour, coating them well.

In a skillet, heat a small amount of oil over medium heat. Add and cook until browned on both sides.

Makes 4 servings

PER SERVING: 289 calories, 19 g protein, 8 g carbohydrates, 21 g total fat, 1.9 g saturated fat, 2.6 g fiber, 595 mg sodium

TURKEY AVOCADO BOATS

Here's something new to do with leftover turkey. Serve it with a fresh salad or warm onion rolls. If you are vegetarian, substitute the turkey with warm brown rice and leave the mayo out.

1   cup chopped cooked turkey meat (dark and light)

½   cup chopped red onion (optional)

¼   cup mayonnaise (no substitute mayos; they're worse than genuine mayonnaise)

1   tablespoon dried cranberries

½   teaspoon salt (I use Fusion's Ginger Salt)

1   avocado, halved and pitted (but not peeled)

In a medium bowl, combine the turkey, onion, mayonnaise, cranberries, and salt. Mound the turkey mixture in the avocado halves.

Makes 2 servings

PER SERVING: 435 calories, 22 g protein, 9 g carbohydrates, 35 g total fat, 5.2 g saturated fat, 4.8 g fiber, 812 mg sodium

ZUCCHINI "PIZZA"

Be sure to use a brand of pasta sauce that does not have any high-fructose corn syrup in it.

2   large zucchinis, peeled and cut crosswise into ¼-inch-thick rounds

1   cup bottled marinara sauce

½   cup grated cheese (Parmesan, mozzarella, Asiago, or goat cheese)

2   teaspoons chopped fresh oregano

½   cup chopped flat-leaf parsley

Preheat the oven to 350°F. Spread the zucchini on a baking sheet and bake for 20 to 30 minutes, or until somewhat dry. Remove from the oven and put a spoonful of marinara sauce on each slice. Sprinkle with some cheese, oregano, and flat-leaf parsley. Return to the oven and bake for 5 more minutes to melt the cheese.

Makes 4 servings

PER SERVING: 97 calories, 7 g protein, 12 g carbohydrates, 3.5 g total fat, 1.8 g saturated fat, 2 g fiber, 338 mg sodium

RAINBOW SALAD

You'll notice that this salad contains all the colors of the rainbow. There are no amounts listed. Simply toss in as much as you want of as many ingredients as you choose. Use your favorite dressing, or try my Lime Vinaigrette (page 367). The blue vegetables give us powerful antioxidants known as anthocyanins. According to one study, those who consumed purple/blue fruits and vegetables had significantly reduced risk of hypertension, better cholesterol ratios, and smaller waistlines compared to those who did not. The analysis found that adults who consumed purple/blue fruits and vegetables had reduced risk for metabolic syndrome. The other colors contain equally potent nutrients.

Red leaf lettuce

Red beets, peeled and shredded

Red bell peppers

Orange tomatoes

Yellow squash or yellow bell peppers

Broccoli florets or cucumbers or avocado or kiwis

Blueberries (yes, try it!) or blackberries or chopped figs

Red cabbage shreds or raisins

EVERYDAY DELICIOUS SALAD

I make this salad almost every day and love it. You can include whatever you have in the house in this salad. I am one of those cooks that hardly ever repeat the same meal twice because the meal consists of whatever I have in my kitchen. I share this little secret because I want you to have the confidence to follow your taste buds and try new things. Just because you are out of cucumbers, don't sweat it. Throw in sliced zucchini instead. If you don't have cranberries, throw in goji berries or fresh blueberries. Here's my basic template for an everyday delicious salad. Use whatever salad dressing you prefer. It can be as simple as a tablespoon of vinegar and a sprinkling of oil and dried herbs. Try to put in as many superfoods as you can, and experiment with the optional items listed below.

1	head of red leaf lettuce (or romaine), torn into bite-size pieces
1	tomato (I like Roma but you can use what you have), cut into wedges
½	zucchini, chopped
¼	cup chopped red onion (or scallions)
1	teaspoon ground flaxseeds
1	tablespoon hulled hemp seeds
1	tablespoon chia seeds
½	cup warm cooked brown rice
	Sea salt, to taste

OPTIONAL ITEMS:

¼	cup goat feta cheese (not cow's milk), crumbled
½	cup chopped strawberries (they contain fesitin, a powerful antioxidant compound)
½	cup blueberries or cantaloupe

¼   cup shredded beets (peeled, raw)

¼   cup cooked black beans or adzuki beans

Place all ingredients together in a salad bowl and toss with your favorite dressing.

Makes 1 serving

PER SERVING (with no optional ingredients or dressing): 317 calories, 15 g protein, 47 g carbohydrates, 9.2 g total fat, 0.9 g saturated fat, 11 g fiber, 105 mg sodium

Makes 2 servings

PER SERVING (with no optional ingredients or dressing): 158 calories, 7 g protein, 23 g carbohydrates, 4.6 g total fat, 0.4 g saturated fat, 5.7 g fiber, 52 mg sodium

WALNUT-CRUSTED GOAT CHEESE ON A BED OF ORGANIC GREENS

Bake these goat cheese rounds just until the cheese starts to bubble out of the breading.

Mild goat cheese (11-ounce log)

½   cup finely chopped walnuts

½   cup almond flour

1   tablespoon minced fresh herbs (your choice)

Sea salt and pepper

5   ounces mixed organic greens, spinach, or romaine lettuce

2   tomatoes, chopped

¼   cup pitted kalamata olives, chopped

2   tablespoons salad dressing: your choice or try my Lime Vinaigrette (page 367)

Wrap the goat cheese in plastic wrap and put it in the freezer for about 10 minutes. This makes it firm and easier to cut.

Meanwhile in a shallow bowl or pie plate, combine the walnuts, almond flour, herbs, and salt and pepper to taste.

Unwrap the cheese and slice it with some dental floss or a wet knife. The goal is to make clean, neat slices. Dampen each slice with a little water and then dip it into the breading.

Preheat the oven to 350°F.

Place the goat cheese on a parchment-lined baking sheet and bake for about 10 minutes, or until the cheese starts to bubble out of the breading. Serve them on a bed of greens. Add the chopped tomatoes and olives, and drizzle with a little salad dressing.

Makes 6 servings

PER SERVING (with Lime Vinaigrette): 304 calories, 14 g protein, 8 g carbohydrates, 25 g total fat, 8.8 g saturated fat, 3 g fiber, 374 mg sodium

GUACAMOLE

Cilantro is a strong chelator, so it's a natural way to pull heavy metals and other toxins out of your bloodstream. Detoxification is one way to help support general health and reduce risk of cardiovascular damage. The avocados contain healthy essential fats as well as glutathione, a strong antioxidant that sweeps away free radicals. For your dipping pleasure, I recommend gluten-free chips. So make sure you buy 100 percent corn chips or rice chips. It should say gluten-free on the label.

 4 avocados, scooped out
 5 or 6 Roma tomatoes, chopped
 ½ bunch cilantro, chopped
 ¼ cup chopped red onion
 Juice of ½ small lemon (also grate a little of the zest into the bowl)
 Fresh jalapeño or cayenne pepper, minced (optional)
 Sea salt and black pepper

In a large bowl, combine the avocados, tomatoes, cilantro, onion, lemon juice, jalapeño (if using), and salt and black pepper to taste. I like my guacamole kind of chunky, so I mash it together with a fork. If you like yours smooth, then blend it instead.

Makes 8 servings

PER SERVING: 125 calories, 2 g protein, 9 g carbohydrates, 11 g total fat, 1.5 g saturated fat, 5.4 g fiber, 155 mg sodium

CRAVEABLE SALAD

This salad is packed with living nutrition, and it's pretty to look at. I eat this frequently for breakfast. Hard to believe, isn't it? But once your palate changes, you will see what I mean about craving this dish. And it's a million times better for you than the typical American breakfast. Make extra and keep it in the fridge (without the dressing) so you can snack throughout the day.

1	avocado, sliced
1	large tomato, sliced
½	cucumber, peeled and sliced
	Optional: Smoked salmon (nova or lox) or herring (rinse off the marinade, which has high-fructose corn syrup in it)
	Sea salt (preferably Celtic or French grey, any flavor)
	Capers
1	tablespoon hulled hemp seeds
1	tablespoon olive or coconut oil
	Sprinkle of red wine vinegar or apple cider vinegar

Divide the avocado, tomato, and cucumber between 2 salad plates. If you want protein, include the seafood. Sprinkle the salad with salt and capers to taste, the hemp seeds, oil, and vinegar. It is now ready to devour.

Makes 2 servings

PER SERVING (without seafood): 225 calories, 4 g protein, 12 g carbohydrates, 20 g total fat, 2.6 g saturated fat, 6.2 g fiber, 429 mg sodium

QUINOA THAI STYLE

Be sure that you do not skip the rinsing and draining step for the quinoa, or there will be a bitter residue.

1½	cups dry quinoa, rinsed (3 times) and well drained
3	cups water
2	tablespoons unsweetened coconut milk (canned is okay)
8	fresh basil leaves, chopped
4	sprigs cilantro, chopped

¼   cup chopped red onion

¼   fresh jalapeño pepper, seeded and minced

2   tablespoons grape seed oil

2   tablespoons plus 1 teaspoon fresh lime juice

Fine sea salt (I use Fusion's Thai Ginger Salt)

Put the drained quinoa into a saucepan and add the water and coconut milk. Bring to a boil over high heat, then reduce to a simmer and cook until the water is absorbed, 10 to 15 minutes (the grains will be translucent or the outer layer will have come off). Drain well.

Meanwhile, in a medium bowl, combine the basil, cilantro, onion, and jalapeño. Drizzle in the oil and lime juice. Add ½ teaspoon sea salt and stir to combine.

Add the drained quinoa and toss to combine. Season with more salt to taste. Serve warm or at room temperature.

Makes 4 servings

PER SERVING: 316 calories, 9 g protein, 43 g carbohydrates, 12 g total fat, 2.4 g saturated fat, 4.9 g fiber, 304 mg sodium

QUINOA SALAD

You can make this with cut-up asparagus instead of broccoli. To dress up the quinoa a bit, garnish with a sprig of parsley (and yes, it's fine to eat!). You also might want to sprinkle it with some goat cheese or grated sheep cheese (which tastes like Parmesan). This is great served with any green soup.

2   cups dry red quinoa, rinsed (3 times) and well drained

3½   cups water

Pinch of salt

1   tablespoon olive oil

½   large broccoli stalk, broken into small florets

¼   cup chopped red bell pepper

2   scallions, chopped

1   garlic clove, minced

3   fresh basil leaves, slivered

Place the drained quinoa in a saucepan with the water and salt. Bring to a boil, reduce to a simmer, cover tightly, and cook until tender, about 25 minutes (the grains will be translucent or the outer layer will have come off). Set aside.

Meanwhile, in a skillet, heat the oil over medium-low heat. Add the broccoli, bell pepper, scallions, and garlic. You want this to cook for only a few minutes so it stays bright colored and somewhat crisp. If you overcook, you've lost the vital nutrients. Remove from the heat and stir in the basil.

Combine with the quinoa and toss.

Makes 4 servings

PER SERVING: 355 calories, 13 g protein, 57 g carbohydrates, 8.7 g total fat, 1.1 g saturated fat, 6.7 g fiber, 23 mg sodium

PESTO SAUCE

Use this sauce over brown rice, or over artichokes or pasta. It's delicious and loaded with healthy nutrients. Pesto will keep well in the refrigerator for a week or more. This recipe (which makes about 3½ cups) can be easily halved.

2	cups packed basil leaves
2	garlic cloves, peeled and lightly crushed
½	cup pine nuts or walnuts (or a combination of the two)
½	cup grated Parmesan or Asagio cheese
¼	cup grape seed oil
1	tablespoon aloe vera juice
	Lemon juice (optional)
¼	cup filtered water
	Salt and pepper

Combine basil and garlic in a food processor or blender. Process until the basil is finely chopped. Add the nuts and process until they are finely chopped. Add the cheese and process until combined. With the machine running, add the oil in a slow, steady stream. Blend in the aloe vera juice and lemon juice (if using). If you want a thinner sauce, add the water. Add salt and pepper to taste. If not using immediately, store in an airtight container with a thin coating of oil on top to keep the sauce from turning dark.

Makes 3½ cups

PER TABLESPOON: 19 calories, 1 g protein, 0 g carbohydrates, 1.8 g total fat, 0.4 g saturated fat, 0.1 g fiber, 22 mg sodium

BROCCOLI PESTO SAUCE

I have poured this sauce over rice, fresh sliced tomatoes, cooked seafood (like salmon), or noodles. I've also used it as salad dressing.

2	cups chopped broccoli florets
½	cup chopped parsley
½	cup shredded Parmesan cheese
½	cup part-skim ricotta cheese (I use goat ricotta cheese)
½	cup extra-virgin olive oil
¼	cup pine nuts (toasted if you have time)
2	garlic cloves, peeled
1	tablespoon ground flaxseeds
	Sea salt and pepper
¼	cup water (optional)

In a steamer, cook the broccoli until just slightly tender, 3 to 4 minutes. It should retain its bright green color. Combine the cooked broccoli, parsley, Parmesan, ricotta, oil, pine nuts, garlic, ground flaxseeds, and salt and pepper to taste in a food processor or blender. Process or blend until smooth. Add the water if you want a thinner sauce.

Makes 4 cups

PER ¼ CUP: 99 calories, 3 g protein, 2 g carbohydrates, 9.4 g total fat, 2 g saturated fat, 0.6 g fiber, 93 mg sodium

ARTICHOKE-SPINACH DIP

1	tablespoon flaxseed oil
2	packages (9 ounces each) frozen artichoke hearts, thawed and well drained
2	garlic cloves, grated
1	teaspoon Herbamare or other herb-flavored sea salt
¼	teaspoon cayenne pepper
5	ounces baby spinach
1	cup chopped Roma tomatoes
8	ounces cream cheese
½	cup grated Parmesan cheese

In a medium saucepan, heat the oil over medium heat. Add the artichokes, garlic, Herbamare, and cayenne. Cook, stirring often, for 5 minutes. Stir in the spinach, tomatoes, and cream cheese. When the spinach is wilted but still bright green, add the Parmesan. Serve warm.

Makes 6 cups

PER ¼ CUP: 60 calories, 2 g protein, 3 g carbohydrates, 4.5 g total fat, 2.4 g saturated fat, 1.6 g fiber, 174 mg sodium

SHIITAKE-SPINACH SAUTÉ

I like to use Italian cipolline onions here, but use whatever you like.

- 1   tablespoon grape seed oil
- 1   small onion, thinly sliced
- 8   ounces shiitake mushrooms, stems discarded and caps sliced crosswise
- 10   ounces fresh spinach
-     Juice of 1 lemon
- 1   tablespoon cornstarch
-     Sea salt

In a large skillet, heat the oil over medium-low heat. Add the onion and mushrooms and cook until beginning to soften, about 2 minutes. Add the spinach and cover. Stir occasionally until the spinach is wilted but still bright green.

In a small bowl, whisk the lemon juice into the cornstarch. Pour the cornstarch mixture into the pan and cook, stirring, until the sauce thickens, about 1 minute. Season with salt to taste. Serve hot.

Makes 4 servings

PER SERVING: 89 calories, 3 g protein, 14 g carbohydrates, 3.8 g total fat, 0.4 g saturated fat, 2.8 g fiber, 349 mg sodium

ACORN SQUASH DELIGHT

This dish is so easy and delicious. Serve with a fresh salad or just on its own. Sometimes this is my breakfast! Acorn squash contains beta-carotene and vitamin C.

> 1   acorn squash
> ½   teaspoon ground cinnamon
>   Sea salt
>   Black strap molasses

Preheat the oven to 350°F. Line a rimmed baking sheet with foil.

Halve the squash lengthwise and place it cut-side down on the baking sheet. Bake for 30 to 40 minutes, or until fork-tender.

When cool enough to handle, scoop out the seeds. Sprinkle the squash with the cinnamon and salt to taste. Drizzle with agave syrup, if desired.

Makes 2 servings

PER SERVING: 88 calories, 2 g protein, 23 g carbohydrates, 0.2 g total fat, 0 g saturated fat, 3.6 g fiber, 297 mg sodium

ARTICHOKE SAUTÉ

This recipe works well for any frozen vegetable.

> 2   packages (9 ounces each) frozen artichokes
> 1   tablespoon extra-virgin olive oil
> 1   garlic clove, minced
>   Sea salt (I use Fusion's Black Truffle Sea Salt)

In a saucepan of boiling water, cook the artichokes according to package directions. Drain them well so they are not soggy. Return them to the pan, along with the oil and garlic. Warm for a minute. Season with salt to taste and serve.

Makes 4 servings

PER SERVING: 93 calories, 3 g protein, 11 g carbohydrates, 4.1 g total fat, 0.5 g saturated fat, 7.6 g fiber, 375 mg sodium

LIME VINAIGRETTE

The dressing will keep a week refrigerated.

¾　cup grape seed oil

½　cup flaxseed oil

½　cup cider vinegar or balsamic vinegar

¼　cup filtered water

½　cup packed chopped mixed green herbs: fresh basil, cilantro, and parsley

1　garlic clove, minced

½　teaspoon grated lime zest

　　Juice of 1 large lime

½　teaspoon salt

In a screw-top jar, combine all the ingredients and shake well. Store in the refrigerator.

Makes 2½ cups

PER TABLESPOON: 64 calories, 0 g protein, 0 g carbohydrates, 6.9 g total fat, 0.6 g saturated fat, 0 g fiber, 29 mg sodium

ROASTED GARLIC

Garlic contains allicin, a powerful antioxidant that, along with flavonoids, has been shown to reduce heart disease, lower cholesterol, prevent complications of diabetes, and raise serum insulin (thereby lowering blood sugar).

2　whole heads of garlic

1　tablespoon almond oil

　　Grated Parmesan or Asiago cheese (optional)

　　Salt (optional)

Preheat the oven to 350°F.

Peel off the papery outer layers of the garlic heads. Slice about ½ inch off the tops, exposing the garlic cloves. Place the garlic heads on a piece of foil. Pour the almond oil onto the tops and enclose the heads with foil. Bake for 30 to 35 minutes, or until the garlic is quite soft.

When cool enough to handle, squeeze the roasted garlic cloves out of their skins. Sprinkle with Parmesan or salt if desired. You can eat it straight or spread it on a cracker or some bread.

Makes 16 servings

PER SERVING: 41 calories, 2 g protein, 7 g carbohydrates, 1 g total fat, 0.2 g saturated fat, 2.8 g fiber, 3 mg sodium

FETA GREENS DELIGHT

1	pound turnip or mustard greens, well washed and chopped
1	tablespoon extra-virgin olive oil
¼	cup goat feta cheese, crumbled (not cow's milk; be careful)
1	garlic clove, minced
¼	teaspoon ground chia seeds

In a steamer, cook the greens for 15 minutes or until bright green. Don't overcook. Drain well. Pat dry with paper towels.

Place the cooked greens in a saucepan and drizzle with oil. Heat gently over low heat. Add the goat cheese and garlic. Remove from the heat, cover, and let sit for a minute or two. Serve warm.

Makes 4 servings

PER SERVING: 94 calories, 3 g protein, 9 g carbohydrates, 5.8 g total fat, 2 g saturated fat, 3.8 g fiber, 150 mg sodium

SUN-DRIED TOMATO KALE

1 bunch (about 1 pound) fresh kale, well washed

2 garlic cloves, minced

½ cup oil-packed sun-dried tomatoes, chopped

1 tablespoon avocado oil

In a steamer, cook the kale until tender but still bright green, about 10 minutes. Don't overcook. Drain well. Pat dry with paper towels. In a bowl (or the pan where you steamed the kale if you didn't use an electric steamer), toss the kale with the garlic, sun-dried tomatoes, and avocado oil.

Makes 4 servings

PER SERVING: 119 calories, 5 g protein, 15 g carbohydrates, 6.2 g total fat, 0.8 g saturated fat, 3.1 g fiber, 86 mg sodium

ALMOND FLOUR BREAD

This is a good, basic bread. Play around with it. If you are craving something sweet, throw in some cranberries or dried blueberries and cinnamon. If you are craving salt, throw in about 1 teaspoon sesame or poppy seeds and ¼ cup grated aged sheep cheese (similar to Parmesan).

2½	cups almond flour
¼	cup olive, hemp seed, or sunflower oil
1	package (7 ounces) dry-curd cottage cheese (also called farmer's cheese)
1	teaspoon baking soda
1	tablespoon hulled hemp seeds
1	teaspoon ground flaxseeds (or ground chia seeds)
¼	teaspoon sea salt
3	eggs

Preheat the oven to 350°F. Lightly grease a stoneware loaf pan.

In a large bowl, mix together the flour, oil, cheese, baking soda, hemp seeds, ground flaxseeds, sea salt, and eggs. Transfer batter to the loaf pan. Bake for 1 hour, or until a toothpick inserted in the center comes out clean. If it's still uncooked in the center, reduce the temperature to 300°F and continue baking until done.

Makes 1 loaf (16 slices)

PER SLICE: 169 calories, 7 g protein, 4 g carbohydrates, 15 g total fat, 2.1 g saturated fat, 1.9 g fiber, 134 mg sodium

CRUSTY ONION-CHEDDAR BISCUITS

These biscuits are hearty, so one can really fill you up, and they are low on the glycemic index. I also make these without the onions, or I'll switch the cumin with curry just for fun. Play around with the recipe. Serve these with a salad or soup.

3	cups almond flour
1	cup shredded Cheddar or Gouda cheese
⅓	cup chopped onion
1	tablespoon ground flaxseeds
1	teaspoon baking soda
1	teaspoon sea salt
½	teaspoon ground cumin
¼	cup hemp seed or grape seed oil
1	tablespoon brown rice syrup or honey
2	eggs

Preheat the oven to 350°F. Grease a 13" × 9" glass baking dish or use a stoneware baking sheet.

In a large bowl, combine the flour, cheese, onion, ground flaxseeds, baking soda, salt, cumin, oil, rice syrup, and eggs. Stir just to blend. Do not overbeat. Form into 2-inch round biscuits and place in the baking dish. Bake for 30 minutes, then reduce the temperature to 300°F and continue baking for about 20 minutes, until the biscuits are browned.

Makes 12 biscuits

PER SERVING: 263 calories, 9 g protein, 8 g carbohydrates, 23 g total fat, 4.2 g saturated fat, 3.3 g fiber, 384 mg sodium

Makes 24 biscuits

PER SERVING: 132 calories, 5 g protein, 4 g carbohydrates, 12 g total fat, 2.1 g saturated fat, 1.6 g fiber, 192 mg sodium

BLUEBERRY CINNAMON CAKE

2½   cups almond flour

1   teaspoon ground cinnamon

1   teaspoon baking soda

¼   teaspoon salt

½   cup maple syrup

½   cup grape seed oil

1   teaspoon vanilla extract

1   egg

¾   cup fresh blueberries

½   cup dried cranberries

¼   teaspoon ground chia seeds

Preheat the oven to 350°F. Grease a 6" × 9" glass baking dish. AU: Confirm size.

In a large bowl, combine the flour, cinnamon, baking soda, and salt and blend well. Stir in the maple syrup, oil, vanilla, and egg. Fold in the blueberries and cranberries.

Pour the batter into the baking dish. Bake for 25 minutes. Reduce the oven temperature to 300°F and bake for 30 minutes, or until a toothpick inserted in the center comes out clean.

Makes 12 servings

PER SERVING: 268 calories, 6 g protein, 17 g carbohydrates, 21 g total fat, 1.8 g saturated fat, 3.1 g fiber, 168 mg sodium

PIÑA COLADA PLEASURE CAKE

3   cups almond flour

½   cup unsweetened coconut flakes

1   teaspoon baking soda

¼   teaspoon ground cinnamon

⅛ teaspoon salt

½ cup maple syrup

½ cup grape seed oil

2 eggs

¼ teaspoon lemon extract or grated lemon zest

1 cup canned juice-packed crushed pineapple, well drained

Preheat the oven to 350°F. Grease a 6" × 9" glass baking dish.

In a large bowl, combine the flour, coconut, baking soda, cinnamon, and salt and blend well. Stir in the maple syrup, oil, eggs, and lemon extract. Fold in the pineapple.

Pour the batter into the baking dish. Bake for 30 minutes. Reduce the oven temperature to 300°F and bake for 10 to 15 minutes, or until a toothpick inserted in the center comes out clean.

Makes 12 servings

PER SERVING: 315 calories, 7 g protein, 16 g carbohydrates, 26 g total fat, 4.2 g saturated fat, 3.7 g fiber, 152 mg sodium

BANANA-NUT BREAD

2½ cups almond flour

½ cup chopped walnuts

1 tablespoon ground flaxseeds (or ground chia seeds)

1 teaspoon baking soda

1 teaspoon ground cinnamon

⅛ teaspoon salt

2 very ripe large bananas, mashed

½ cup agave syrup or honey

½ cup grape seed oil

1 teaspoon vanilla extract

2 eggs

Preheat the oven to 350°F. Grease a 6" × 9" glass baking dish.

In a large bowl, combine the flour, walnuts, ground flaxseeds, baking soda, cinnamon, and salt and blend well. In a medium bowl, combine the bananas, agave syrup, oil, vanilla, and eggs. Stir the banana mixture into the flour mixture. Pour the batter into the baking dish.

Bake for 30 minutes. Reduce the oven temperature to 300°F and bake for 12 to 15 minutes, or until the top is brown and a toothpick inserted in the center comes out clean.

Makes 12 servings

PER SERVING: 322 calories, 7 g protein, 22 g carbohydrates, 25 g total fat, 2.3 g saturated fat, 3.7 g fiber, 150 mg sodium

LIGHT ALMOND BREAD

2½ cups almond flour

1 teaspoon baking soda

¼ teaspoon sea salt

1 tablespoon ground chia seed or flaxseeds

3 eggs, separated

1 cup yogurt

1 tablespoon honey

Preheat the oven to 300°F. Grease and flour (use almond flour) a loaf pan.

In a small bowl, combine the flour, baking soda, sea salt, and chia seeds in a small bowl. Set aside.

In a large bowl, whisk the egg yolks, yogurt, and honey until light and fluffy. Stir in the flour mixture.

In a small bowl, beat the egg whites until stiff peaks form. Fold the egg whites into the batter.

Pour into the loaf pan. Bake for 45 to 50 minutes, or until a toothpick inserted in the center comes out clean.

Makes 16 slices

PER SERVING: 133 calories, 5 g protein, 7 g carbohydrates, 11 g total fat, 1.4 g saturated fat, 2.5 g fiber, 135 mg sodium

PUMPKIN AND ALMOND BREAD

Serve sliced with fresh raspberries and blackberries and a drizzle of honey.

4	cups almond flour
1	teaspoon baking soda
½	teaspoon salt
½	teaspoon ground cinnamon
½	teaspoon pumpkin pie spice
1	tablespoon hulled hemp seeds
3	eggs
¼	cup hempseed oil
1	cup cooked, pureed pumpkin or butternut squash (canned can be substituted)
½	cup chopped walnuts
1	tablespoon grated orange zest

Preheat the oven to 300°F. Grease and flour (use almond flour) a loaf pan.

In a large bowl, combine the flour, baking soda, salt, cinnamon, pumpkin spice, and hemp seeds. Set aside.

In another large bowl, whisk the eggs with the oil. Add the pumpkin puree, walnuts, and orange zest and stir. Add the flour mixture and stir to combine. Pour the batter into the loaf pan. Bake for 45 minutes or until lightly browned and a toothpick inserted in the center comes out clean.

Makes 16 slices

PER SERVING: 237 calories, 8 g protein, 8 g carbohydrates, 21 g total fat, 1.9 g saturated fat, 4 g fiber, 175 mg sodium

AMAZINGLY MOIST CARROT CAKE

1½	cups almond flour
1½	cups finely shredded carrots
½	cup maple syrup
½	cup dried cranberries
½	cup grape seed oil

1   teaspoon baking soda

2   eggs

1   teaspoon ground cinnamon

1   teaspoon vanilla extract

    Pinch of salt

Preheat the oven to 350°F. Grease a 6" × 9" glass baking dish.

In a large bowl, combine the flour, carrots, maple syrup, cranberries, oil, baking soda, eggs, cinnamon, vanilla, and salt. Pour the batter into the baking dish and bake for 30 minutes, or until a toothpick inserted in the center comes out clean. It will not rise like a traditional cake, and it may or may not brown on top.

Makes 12 servings

PER SERVING: 221 calories, 4 g protein, 15 g carbohydrates, 17 g total fat, 1.6 g saturated fat, 2.3 g fiber, 134 mg sodium

CRANBERRY-NUT BREAD

2½   cups almond flour

½   cup turbinado sugar

2½   teaspoons baking powder

¾   teaspoon sea salt

¾   cup water

½   cup walnut or almond oil

⅓   cup egg whites

3   eggs

2   cups frozen cranberries

½   cup chopped walnuts or pecans

Preheat the oven to 350°F. Grease a loaf pan.

In a large bowl, combine the flour, sugar, baking powder, and salt and blend well. Stir in the water, oil, egg whites, and whole eggs. Mix just until evenly moist. Fold in the cranberries and nuts.

Pour the batter into the loaf pan. Bake for 30 minutes, until lightly browned on top and a toothpick inserted in the center comes out clean.

Makes 16 slices

PER SERVING: 231 calories, 6 g protein, 13 g carbohydrates, 19 g total fat, 1.8 g saturated fat, 2.6 g fiber, 223 mg sodium

CHOCOLATE CHIP COOKIES

These are really good, fresh, healthy, warm, and free of allergy-causing ingredients. My teenagers love these cookies. The cornstarch mixture is used as an egg substitute. You can also use ¾ cup almond flour and ¾ cup rice flour. This lightens the texture somewhat. Everything else remains the same.

1½	cups almond flour
½	cup turbinado sugar
¼	teaspoon ground cinnamon
⅛	teaspoon sea salt
½	ripe banana, mashed
2	tablespoons cornstarch blended with ¼ cup water
2½	tablespoons sunflower or almond oil (or a combination)
1	teaspoon vanilla extract
½	teaspoon almond extract
½	cup semisweet chocolate chips
¼	cup hulled hemp seeds
¼	cup chopped walnuts

Preheat the oven to 350°F. Grease a stoneware baking sheet.

In a large bowl, combine the flour, sugar, cinnamon, salt, banana, cornstarch mixture, oil, vanilla, almond extract, chocolate chips, hemp seeds, and walnuts. Form 24 cookie balls in your hands, keeping your hands moist. Place the cookies on the baking sheet and flatten them slightly. These cookies will not spread like other cookies, so you do not have to space them far apart. Bake for 20 to 30 minutes, until the tops turn lightly brown. Let cool 5 minutes on the baking sheet.

Makes 24 cookies

PER COOKIE: 107 calories, 2 g protein, 9 g carbohydrates, 7.5 g total fat, 1.2 g saturated fat, 1.1 g fiber, 15 mg sodium

MAMMOTH COOKIES

5	cups almond flour
1	teaspoon baking soda
⅛	teaspoon sea salt

1   cup golden raisins

1   cup chopped walnuts or Brazil nuts

1   cup unsweetened coconut flakes

1   tablespoon hulled hemp seeds

1   cup raw honey, unrefined blue agave syrup, or brown rice syrup

¼   cup grape seed oil

2   eggs, beaten

Preheat the oven to 350°F. Grease a baking sheet.

In a large bowl, combine the flour, baking soda, salt, raisins, nuts, coconut, hemp seeds, honey, oil, and eggs. Blend well. Form into 36 or 48 balls and place on the baking sheet. Bake for 20 minutes, or until the tops are slightly browned.

Makes 36 cookies

PER COOKIE: 191 calories, 5 g protein, 16 g carbohydrates, 14 g total fat, 2.4 g saturated fat, 2.4 g fiber, 54 mg sodium

Makes 48 cookies

PER COOKIE: 143 calories, 3 g protein, 12 g carbohydrates, 10 g total fat, 1.8 g saturated fat, 1.8 g fiber, 40 mg sodium

WANT MORE RECIPES?

Here are the cookbooks that I recommend and refer to in my own home. These are very good choices for anyone with diabetes. The first three cookbooks on this list use almond flour. The rest of the cookbooks are listed in no particular order.

Healing Foods by Sandra Ramacher

The pictures are beautiful (the author happens to be a photographer) and her recipes are foolproof if you follow directions.

Recipes for the Specific Carbohydrate Diet: The Grain-Free, Lactose-Free, Sugar-Free Solution to IBD, Celiac Disease, Autism, Cystic Fibrosis, and Other Health Conditions by Raman Prasad

Eat Well Feel Well: Meals to Help Manage Crohn's Disease, Ulcerative Colitis, IBS, Celiac Disease, Diverticulitis and Other Digestive Conditions by Kendall Conrad

Allergy-Free Recipes

The Whole Life Nutrition Cookbook: Whole Foods Recipes for Personal and Planetary Health by Alissa Segersten and Tom Malterre

Evidence-based information on whole foods and food sensitivities. Many recipes are gluten-free, dairy-free, or egg-free.

The Gluten-Free Gourmet Cooks Comfort Foods by Bette Hagman

Gluten-free cookbook. It does include dairy.

EveryDay Grain-Free Gourmet by Jodi Bager and Jenny Lass

Uses whole foods to create gluten-free, refined sugar–free, low-lactose meals.

Conscious Eating by Gabriel Cousens, MD
(founder of the Tree of Life Rejuvenation Center in Arizona)

This book offers information that links nutrition with spiritual, emotional, and physical vitality. If you are interested in becoming more of a raw foodist or vegan you will love this book. It could be life-changing.

Eating Your Way to Good Health by Doug Kaufmann and Jami Clark, RN

Dr. Kaufmann is the host of the most popular health television show, *Know the Cause*, and Jami is a nurse. This book offers simple recipes that help you to reduce your body's load of fungus (like candida). These are healthy, quick, and delicious recipes.

Resources

Teas

Agape Tea Store
A source for U.S. certified organic hibiscus herbal tea.

www.agapetea.com

Alvita Tea
A source for pau d'arco tea.

800-437-2257
www.alvita.com

Charantea
This is a high-quality resource for bitter melon tea, which is useful in protecting beta cells of the pancreas.

877-347-2290
www.charanteausa.com

Guayaki
A leader in the production of yerba maté tea.

888-482-9254
www.guayaki.com

Matcha Source
A leading supplier for various types of matcha tea, cultivated from some of the world's finest resources. For more information, please read the column I wrote about matcha, which is still posted at my Web site, www.DearPharmacist.com.

877-962-8242
www.matchasource.com

Mountain Rose Herbs
These teas contain herbs certified U.S. organic, and I have about a dozen different flavors in my house. One of their popular teas, Evening Repose, might help you with sleeping problems. It contains chamomile, lavender, lemon verbena, blue malva flowers, rose petals, and peppermint. It's also certified kosher. Infuse 1 teaspoon of the herbs into 1 cup hot water for 5 to 15 minutes.

800-879-3337
www.mountainroseherbs.com

Republic of Tea
One of the leaders in tea cultivating. This brand is sold at many health food stores and bookstores nationwide. I often recommend their rooibos (red) tea. A complete line of teas target various aspect of health and wellness, including Get Heart, Get Relaxed, and Get Happy.

800-298-4832
www.republicoftea.com

Teavana
A source for teas of any sort. I have many of their delicious flavors.

877-832-8262
www.teavana.com

Recommended Reading

The Fungus Link Audio Trilogy
Audiobook by Doug Kaufmann, an expert in fungus.

972-772-0990
www.knowthecause.com

Omega 3 Cuisine by Chef Alan Roettinger
www.omega3cuisine.com

The Omnivore's Dilemma by Michael Pollan (Penguin, 2007)
Available at bookstores nationwide and amazon.com

Recognizing Celiac Disease by Cleo J. Libonati, RN, BSN
215-591-4565
www.recognizingceliacdisease.com

Stop Prediabetes Now by Jack Challem and Ron Hunninghake, MD (Wiley, 2007)
www.thenutritionreporter.com

Superfoods by David Wolfe (North Atlantic Books, 2009)
www.davidwolfe.com

Is Your Cardiologist Killing You? by Sherry Rogers, MD (Prestige Publishing, 2009)

210-614-7246
www.painstresscenter.com

The UV Advantage by Michael Holick

www.uvadvantage.org

The 24-Hour Pharmacist by Suzy Cohen, RPh (Rodale, 2008)

www.DearPharmacist.com and amazon.com

Recommended Movies

Fast Food Nation

Director: Richard Linklater

Available through Netflix, Blockbuster, and certain retailers

Food Matters

Director and producer: James Colquhoun and Laurentine ten Bosch

+61 (07) 3040-7073
www.foodmatters.tv

Simply Raw

Created by Mark Perlmutter

800-419-3886
www.rawfor30days.com

Supplements and Supplement Sources

AstaVita

Source for high-quality astaxanthin

800-507-4011
www.astavita.com

Bioenergy

Source for Corvalen, a high-quality ribose supplement mentioned in Chapter 8.

866-267-8253
www.bioenergy.com

Biopharma Scientific

I recommend their NanoGreens in Chapter 12. You just mix it with water or juice and it provides a lot of powerful antioxidants and phytonutrients.

877-772-4362
www.biopharmasci.com

Biotivia

Source for Transmax Trans Resveratrol. They have other antiaging supplements, too. This company is found primarily through online sources.

800-458-0993
www.biotivia.com

Bluebonnet Vitamins

Source for Buffered Vitamin C Plus Citrus Bioflavonoids

281-240-3332
www.bluebonnetnutrition.com

Boku Superfoods

I recommend their Boku green food supplement in Chapter 12. This is definitely one super superfood because it contains all sorts of antioxidants and phytonutrients, many derived from the sea. I often advocate the use of marine-derived superfoods for good health.

877-265-8366
www.bokusuperfood.com

Cellfood Silica

This supplement was mentioned in Chapters 10 and 12.

800-456-9887
www.toolsforwellness.com

Doctor's Best

800-333-6977
www.drbvitamins.com

Econugenics

I mentioned their MycoPhyto and Organic Ten Mushroom Formula in Chapter 8. This product line was formulated by Isaac Eliaz, MD, who specializes in many other condition-specific formulas that may help you detoxify from heavy metal and plastics.

800-308-5518
www.econugenics.com

Enzymatic Therapy

I recommended their ubiquinol in Chapter 8. They use a high-quality form of ubiquinol (produced by Kaneka QH), so I often recommend this product. I also recommend their Resveratrol Forte because it is 100 percent trans resveratrol, the proper type of resveratrol. (You want "trans," not "cis.")

800-783-2286
www.enzymatictherapy.com

Enzymedica

I recommend their Natto-K in Chapter 8.

888-918-1118
www.enzymedica.com

GNC

Source for fenugreek. Their stores are sprinkled all over the United States.

877-462-4700
www.gnc.com

Good Health Naturally Nutrition

Source for Curcumin 98. This product is strong and free of common allergens. You can see the purity in the bright orange color of the capsules, which is the color of pure curcumin. They combine it with piperine (a black pepper extract) to aid absorption and improve efficacy.

44 (0) 1772 780562

info@goodhealth-naturally.co.uk

Healthy Origins

I recommended their coenzyme Q10 and ubiquinol in Chapter 8.

888-228-6650

www.healthyorigins.com

Jarrow

I recommended their QH-Absorb in Chapter 8. They carry a wide range of excellent vitamins, herbs, and dietary supplements. Their products are easy to find and affordable.

310-204-6936

www.jarrow.com

JHS

This is a high-quality supplier for medicinal mushrooms. I have purchased various formulas over the years and experienced well-being as a result. I mentioned their 5 Mushroom Formula in Chapter 8.

888-330-4691

www.jhsnp.com

Kaneka

The world's leading manufacturer of coenzyme Q10 and ubiquinol.

866-888-1723

www.kaneka.com

Lantus

This is a type of injectable insulin that requires a prescription. It is discussed in Chapter 5. You can visit the site to learn about basal insulin and keep up to date with usage, dosage, and warnings.

800-981-2491

www.lantus.com

Latisse

I mentioned this product in Chapter 7 because it was derived from a glaucoma medication when users experienced a lash-growing side effect from the drops. The makers (Allergan) decided to market a product that lengthens lashes.

800-433-8871

www.latisse.com

Life Extension

This company has high-quality dietary supplements, and you don't need to be a member to buy from them.

Order: 800-544-4440; customer care: 800-678-8989; health advisor: 800-226-2370

www.lef.org

Lily of the Desert

They make one of the best brands of aloe vera juice I've tried. It is virtually tasteless. I used this brand in all of my smoothie recipes in Chapter 17. Their products are sold widely at health food stores nationwide.

800-229-5459

www.lilyofthedesert.com

Metagenics

This company produces high-quality vitamins, minerals, and dietary supplements, and I have recommended them for many years in all of my books. This is the company that Dr. Jeffrey Bland founded, based on functional medicine. I think they are among the best you can buy; however, they sell only through licensed practitioners and online. Because I am one of their practitioners, you can find some of their supplements sold at my Web site, too, if this is easier for you. Hopefully, though, your physician won't mind becoming one of their practitioners and faxing in his or her license so he can buy for you, whatever you want. See their products online.

800-692-9400

www.metagenics.com

New Chapter

Source for Zyflamend, Supercritical Holy Basil, Aloe Vera Force, and E Food Complex. This company is a high-quality dietary supplement maker that has unique multitasking formulas to support good health.

800-543-7279

www.newchapter.com

Nordic Naturals

Source for high-quality essential fatty acid supplements, such as omega-3 fish oils and cod liver oil. Many of their newer products contain other ingredients that support vision, immune, and metabolic functions.

800-662-2544

www.nordicnaturals.com

NSI (Nutraceutical Sciences Institute)

Source for curcumin supplement, Turmeric Extract Curcumin C3 Complex. It also contains bioperine, the black pepper extract that helps improve bioavailablity. They have many other high-quality, affordable supplements that are sold direct-to-consumer.

800-381-0759

www.vitacost.com

Nutrex Hawaii

Source for astaxanthin and high-quality Hawaiian spirulina.

800-453-1187

www.nutrex-hawaii.com

Nutricology

I mention their NattoZyme nattokinase, 100 mg, in Chapter 8.

800-545-9960

www.nutricology.com

Origin Biomed

I mentioned their topical nerve pain product in Chapter 11.

888-234-7256

www.neuragen.com

Puritan's Pride

I recommended their ubiquinol in Chapter 8.

800-645-1030

www.puritan.com

Solgar

Good source for citrus bioflavonoid complex. A leader in the dietary supplement field, their products are sold widely at health food stores nationwide.

201-944-2311

www.solgar.com

Source Naturals

I mentioned their high-quality Nattokinase in Chapter 8. This company is one of many leaders in the nutriceutical industry, and they offer many fine products that are sold online and at health food stores nationwide.

800-815-2333

www.sourcenaturals.com

Stages of Life

Good source for Magic Minerals, mentioned in Chapter 10. Pain specialist Dr. David Klein founded this company to create high-quality supplements that, unlike many other brands, are not physician-exclusive. This brand offers a wide range of dietary supplements.

407-679-3337

www.stages-of-life.com

Standard Process

800-558-8740

www.standardprocess.com

Swanson

Source for Full Spectrum E with tocotrienols.

800-824-4491

www.swansonvitamins.com

Thorne Research

Good source for Perfusia SR, Polyresveratrol, and Meriva. This company produces high-quality vitamins, minerals, and dietary supplements, and I have recommended them for many years in all of my books. I think they are among the best you can get because they are bent on purity, refusing to add any fillers whatsoever—not even magnesium stearate, which some people consider an unnecessary additive. They also offer most vitamins in their active body-ready form. While many other products are sold direct-to-consumer, a few of their products are physician-exclusive, so your doctor/practitioner must fax in a license to order it for you. Because I am one of their practitioners, you can find some of their supplements sold at my Web site.

800-228-1966

www.merivaonline.com (to buy Meriva), www.thorne.com (to purchase other supplements)

Twinlab

I mentione their L-arginine in Chapter 8. This is another popular brand name that is easy to find and very affordable.

800-645-5626

www.twinlab.com

Xymogen

They make ALAMax and Resveratin, mentioned in Chapter 13.

800-647-6100

www.xymogen.com

Organizations

ADA (American Diabetes Association)

800-342-2383

www.diabetes.org

Broda Barnes Foundation

This is an excellent resource to learn about thyroid disease. This nonprofit organization can help educate you and provide research and training in the field of metabolic disorders.

203-261-2101

www.brodabarnes.org

CDC (Centers for Disease Control and Prevention)

800-232-4636
www.cdc.gov

Celiac Disease Foundation

This comprehensive site can help you understand the disorder and learn about the best resources, diets, and lifestyles.

818-990-2354
www.celiac.org

Clinical Trials

This is a service by the U.S. National Institutes of Health. If you want to participate in a clinical trial, here is a resource for you.

www.clinicaltrials.gov

Clinical Trials

This company is not part of the National Institutes of Health, but it is another source of information for you.

www.clinicaltrials.com

EPA (Environmental Protection Agency)

202-272-0167
www.epa.gov

FDA (Food and Drug Administration)

888-463-6332
www.fda.gov

Glycemic Index

This site allows you to find information on the glycemic index and how foods rank according to their system. I like some of the links and articles on this site.

www.glycemicindex.com

IFM (Institute of Functional Medicine)

800-228-0622
www.functionalmedicine.org

Juvenile Diabetes Research Foundation International

This Web site offers parents and people with type 1 diabetes a wealth of resources, including fact sheets, publications, and research. It features an area for scientists and consumers.

800-533-2873
www.jdrf.org

LADA (Latent Autoimmune Diabetes in Adults)

44 207 601 7450
www.actionlada.org
r.d.g.leslie@qmul.ac.uk

Matthias Rath Research

This Web site is home to Dr. Matthias Rath, a researcher and author. The site will help you understand the benefit of vitamin C for heart and cholesterol health.

800-624-2442
www.drrathresearch.org

MedWatch Side Effect Reporting

Offers information and online submission for people to report side effects associated with medication.

800-332-1088
www.fda.gov/safety/medwatch

National Dairy Council

www.nationaldairycouncil.org
ndc@dairyinformation.com

National Kidney Foundation

800-622-9010
www.kidney.org

National Institute of Diabetes and Digestive and Kidney Diseases

www2.niddk.nih.gov

Not Milk Web Site

You can spend hours on this eye-popping Web site, which will convince you that milk is not good for you. There are some scientific data (and links) that show milk to contain all sorts of dangerous ingredients, including growth hormones, fat, cholesterol, allergenic proteins, blood, pus, and infectious organisms. There are links that provide information or clinical studies regarding milk (dairy) and its association with many diseases, including osteoporosis, diabetes, allergies, asthma, and autism, among many others.

201-967-7001
www.notmilk.com

No Milk Web Site

This is similar to the site listed above. There are hundreds of links that tie dairy to disease and various areas where you can see the literature, the research studies, books, magazine articles, and so forth.

www.nomilk.com
donwiss@panix.com

WHO (World Health Organization)

+ 41 22 791 2111
www.who.int/en
info@who.int

Products

Diapedic Foot Cream

800-542-7546
www.amlab.com

DiabetiDerm Heel and Toe Cream

I mentioned this in Chapter 11. I've found it on amazon.com and also at various online sellers. Here are two of them.

877-241-9002
www.americandiabeteswholesale.com
800-633-7167
www.diabeticcareservices.com

Green Produce Bags

This is an impressive invention. It's a green plastic bag that you can put your fruits and veggies in. The bags will keep your fresh produce from spoiling for many days, extending the lifespan of your food. After throwing away hundreds of dollars in spoiled produce, I really appreciate these bags. They really work!

800-822-8141
www.evertfresh.com

Kerasal's Moisturizing Foot Ointment

This product contains a form of aspirin along with urea. On their Web site they offer a coupon and a link where you can get a free sample.

877-674-3475
www.kerasal.com

Life Solution Telescoping Mirror

Mentioned in Chapter 11, this mirror is useful to view your feet.

877-785-8326
www.lifesolutionsplus.com

Medical ID Bracelet

I mentioned this in Chapter 5.

318-397-8441
www.medids.com

Labs and Testing

Appraise

I mentioned their hemoglobin A1c test in Chapter 6.

888-764-2384
www.appraisetests.com

Coastal Carolina Eye Clinic

Mentioned in Chapter 7.

910-763-7316, 910-686-8509
www.coastalcarolinaeye.com

Enterolab

I mentioned their gluten antibody test in Chapter 4.

972-686-6869
www.enterolab.com/Home.htm

Immunosciences Lab

www.immuno-sci-lab.com

SpectraCell Laboratories

One of the nation's leaders in nutritional testing, they can check your levels of micronutrients and minerals so you can actually see what you are deficient in. Physicians who are holistic or trained in functional medicine often use SpectraCell testing. Some tests require stool or blood. The laboratory is a CLIA (Clinical Laboratory Improvement Amendments)-accredited lab, so you can trust their results and assessments. I have personally taken many of their tests with success.

800-227-5227
www.spectracell.com

ZRT

I mentioned their CardioMetabolic Profile in Chapter 6.

866-600-1636
www.zrtlab.com

Food and Food Products

Barlean's Oils

800-445-3529
www.barleans.com

Bija oils

I love this brand because the products are of high quality and feature some hard-to-find oils, such as almond oil and pumpkin seed oil. I have all their oils and use them interchangeably to give my family a healthy ratio of all the different essential fatty acids that are found in various oils.

800-446-2110
www.florahealth.com/flora/home/usa/products/TGU11.htm

Boomi Bar Snacks

800-440-6476
www.boomibar.com

Coconut information

This Web site has some links to peer-reviewed research articles.
www.coconutoil.com

Just Almonds

A great source to purchase almond flour, especially in bulk. They provide a good deal of nutritional information on almond flour, pasteurization processes, and other important details on almond flour.

877-287-0233

www.justalmonds.com

Larabar Snacks

720-945-1155

www.larabar.com

Lucy's Kitchen

This is where I've purchased my almond flour for many years because it is fresh and the consistency is nice. I buy it in bulk, usually 10 or 25 pounds at a time. It stores well in the refrigerator and makes excellent bread. The site also offers cookbooks and yogurt makers.

888-484-2126

www.lucyskitchenshop.com

Mrs. Mays Snacks

877-677-6297

www.mrsmays.com

Nutiva Oils

This company sells 100 percent raw, organic, unrefined, cold-pressed extra-virgin coconut oil. I found this product at my local health food store and online at vitacost.com. Their company Web site has lots of information.

800-993-4367

www.nutiva.com

Real Salt

I mentioned their brand of salt in Chapter 9.

800-367-7258

www.realsalt.com

SaltWorks

I often recommend their flavored, pure Fusion salt, which I consider gourmet.

800-353-7258

www.seasalt.com

So Delicious Coconut Yogurt and Milk

866-388-7853

www.turtlemountain.com

Spectrum Naturals Oils

They make a full line of healthy oils, including coconut oil.

800-434-4246

www.spectrumorganics.com

Udo Oils

This is a very good Web site to help you understand fats and how to pick healthy oils. You can spend hours there. The founder, Dr. Udo Erasmus, is the same man who formulated all those high-quality oils that you can buy at health food stores nationwide.

www.udoerasmus.com

Sweeteners

Coconut Sugar

www.LiveSuperfoods.com

63075 Crusher Avenue

Unit 101

Bend, OR 97701

800-481-5074

support@livesuperfoods.com

LifeMel Honey

This honey from Israel has some science—about three decades of research—behind its benefits. The honey hasn't been processed, so it contains significant phytonutrients and antioxidants.

888-543-3635

www.lifemelusa.com

Manuka Honey

This honey from New Zealand is one of the most biologically active types of honey. Many store-bought brands have been processed or heated and lose their benefits. This brand is delicious and healthy.

877-919-9992

www.manukahoneyus.com

NuNaturals White Stevia

This is a brand found in health food stores. It is pure stevia.

800-753-4372

www.nunaturals.com

SweetLeaf

This is the brand name for a stevia-based sweetener. SweetLeaf sweetener became the first stevia-based product to achieve GRAS status (GRAS means "generally recognized as safe.") It remains the only stevia-based product with zero calories, zero carbs, and zero glycemic index.

800-899-9908

www.sweetleaf.com

Stevia Plus

This brand of stevia comes in packets. The stevia is combined with a fiber called inulin, not to be confused with insulin, and these sweeteners are sold at Vitamin Shoppes and online.

Diabetes Resources and Organizations

American Diabetes Association

800-342-2383
www.diabetes.org

American Dietetic Association

800-877-1600
www.eatright.org

National Center for Complementary and Alternative Medicine

888-644-6226
www.nccam.nih.gov

National Institutes of Health Office of Dietary Supplements

301-435-2920
www.ods.od.nih.gov

Other

Natural Pedia

An online resource (encyclopedia) to find terrific health books and information on diseases and dietary supplements. This resource is one of the best I've ever seen.
www.naturalpedia.com

Natural News

This Web site offers breaking natural news and citizen journalism founded by Mike Adams. I receive his informative newsletter.
www.naturalnews.com

Needle Disposal

I mentioned that insulin needles need to be disposed of properly in Chapter 6. You can stay up to date by visiting these Web sites to learn about the safest way to dispose of your needles.

800-643-1643
www.safeneedledisposal.org
800-232-4636
www.cdc.gov/needledisposal

Vitamin D Council

info@vitamindcouncil.org

References

PART 1: UNDERSTANDING DIABETES

Chapter 1: It's Not Science Fiction; It's on Your Plate

American Public Health Association. www.apha.org

Associated Press. Life Expectancy in U.S. Rises to Nearly 78 Years. September 12, 2007. www.foxnews.com/story/0,2933,296534,00.html

Djoussé, L., Gaziano, J.M., Buring, J.E., Lee, I.M. Egg Consumption and Risk of Type 2 Diabetes in Men and Women. *Diabetes Care.* 2009, volume 32, pages 295–300.

Gottlieb, D.J., Punjabi, N.M., Newman, A.B., et al. Association of Sleep Time with Diabetes Mellitus and Impaired Glucose Tolerance. *Archives of Internal Medicine.* 2005, volume 165, pages 863–867.

Environmental Literacy Council. Deicing. www.enviroliteracy.org/article.php/709.html

McGill Office for Science and Society. www.oss.mcgill.ca/schwarcz.php

National Library for Health. Incidence and prevalence of diabetes. www.library.nhs.uk/diabetes/viewResource.aspx?resID=82774

New World Order 101. www.nwo101.com/2008/03/life-expectancy-in-america-now-at-693.html

ThaiIndian News. Diets that could make kids die a decade younger than their parents, December 30, 2007. www.thaindian.com/newsportal/india-news/diets-that-could-make-kids-die-a-decade-younger-than-their-parents_10010738.html

Chapter 2: The Many Faces of Diabetes: Know Your Risk Factors

Centers for Disease Control and Prevention. Healthy weight—it's not a diet, it's a lifestyle! www.cdc.gov/healthyweight/assessing/bmi/adult_bmi/index.html

Centers for Disease Control and Prevention. Obesity: Halting the epidemic by making health easier. www.cdc.gov/NCCDPHP/publications/AAG/obesity.htm

Diabetes.co.uk. Type 3 diabetes. www.diabetes.co.uk/type3-diabetes.html

Juvenile Diabetes Research Foundation International. www.jdrf.org/

Kash, P.M., Lombard, J., Monte, T. Freedom from *Disease: The Breakthrough Approach to Preventing Cancer, Heart Disease, Alzheimer's, and Depression* by Controlling Insulin. St Martin's Press, 2008.

National Institute of Diabetes and Digestive and Kidney Diseases. www2.niddk.nih.gov

The National Obesity Forum. www.nationalobesityforum.org.uk/

Reger, M.A., Watson, G.S., Green, P.S., et al. Intranasal Insulin Improves Cognition and Modulates Beta-Amyloid in Early AD. Neurology. February 5, 2008, volume 70, number 6, pages 440–448.

Russo, M.W., Wei, J.T., Thiny, M.T., et al. Digestive and Liver Disease Statistics, 2004. *Gastroenterology.* 2004, volume 126, pages 1448–1453.

World Health Organization. Obesity and overweight. www.who.int/dietphysicalactivity/publications/facts/obesity/en

Chapter 3: Protecting Your Pancreas from Free-Radical Damage

Barkoukis, H., Marchetti, C.M., Nolan, B., et al. A High Glycemic Meal Suppresses the Postprandial Leptin Response in Normal Healthy Adults. *Annals of Nutrition and Metabolism.* 2007, volume 51, number 6, pages 512–518.

Bhardwaj, P., Garg, P.K., Maulik S.K., et al. A Randomized Controlled Trial of Antioxidant Supplementation for Pain Relief in Patients with Chronic Pancreatitis. *Gastroenterology.* January 2009, volume 136, number 1, pages 149–159.e2.

Canto, C., Auwerx, J. PGC-1 alpha, SIRT1 and AMPK, an Energy Sensing Network That Controls Energy Expenditure. *Current Opinion in Lipidology.* 2009, volume 20, pages 98–105.

Carro, E., Torres-Aleman, I. Serum Insulin-Like Growth Factor I in Brain Function. Keio *Journal of Medicine*. June 2006, volume 55, number 2, pages 59–63.

Corton, J.C., Brown-Borg, H.M. Peroxisome Proliferator-Activated Receptor Gamma Coactivator 1 in Caloric Restriction and Other Models of Longevity. Journals of Gerontology. Series A, *Biological Sciences and Medical Sciences*. December 2005, volume 60, number 12, pages 1494–1509.

Dor, Y., Brown, J., Martinez, O.I., Melton, D.M. Adult Pancreatic Bold Beta-Cells Are Formed by Self-Duplication Rather Than Stem-Cell Differentiation. *Nature*. May 6, 2004, volume 429, pages 41–46.

Farshchi, H.R., Taylor, M.A., Macdonald, I.A. Regular Meal Frequency Creates More Appropriate Insulin Sensitivity and Lipid Profiles Compared with Irregular Meal Frequency in Healthy Lean Women. *European Journal of Clinical Nutrition*. July 2004, volume 58, pages 1071–1077.

Fischer, S., Hanefeld, M., Haffner, S.M., et al. Insulin-Resistant Patients with Type 2 Diabetes Mellitus Have Higher Serum Leptin Levels Independently of Body Fat Mass. *Acta Diabetologia*. 2002, volume 39, pages 105–110.

Hamer, M., Chida, Y. Intake of Fruit, Vegetables, and Antioxidants and Risk of Type 2 Diabetes: Systematic Review and Meta-Analysis. *Journal of Hypertension*. December 2007, volume 25, number 12, pages 2361–2369.

Irwin, N., Flatt, P.R. Evidence for Beneficial Effects of Compromised Gastric Inhibitory Polypeptide Action in Obesity-Related Diabetes and Possible Therapeutic Implications. *Diabetologia*. June 17, 2009, volume 52, pages 1724–1731.

Kirk, G., White, J., McKie, L., et al. Combined Antioxidant Therapy Reduces Pain and Improves Quality of Life in Chronic Pancreatitis. *Journal of Gastrointestinal Surgery*. April 2006, volume 10, number 4, pages 499–503.

Lagouge, M., Argmann, C., Gerhart-Hines, Z., et al. Reseveratrol Improves Mitochondrial Function and Protects against Metabolic Disease by Activating SIRT1 and PGC-1 alpha. *Cell*. December 15 2006, volume 127, pages 1109–1122.

Lee, J.H., Reed, D.R., Price, R.A. Leptin Resistance Is Associated with Extreme Obesity and Aggregates in Families. *International Journal of Obesity and Related Metabolic Disorders*. 2001, volume 25, pages 1471–1473.

Liang, H., Ward, W.F. PGC-1 [alpha]: A Key Regulator of Energy Metabolism. *Advances in Physiology Education*. 2006, volume 30, pages 145–151.

Lowenfels, A.B., Maisonneuve, P., Lankisch, P.G. Chronic Pancreatitis and Other Risk Factors for Pancreatic Cancer. *Gastroenterology Clinics of North America*. 1999, volume 28, pages 673–685.

Matarese, G. Leptin and the Immune System: How Nutritional Status Influences the Immune Response. European Cytokine Network. 2000, volume 11, pages 7–14.

Meier, U., Gressner, A.M. Endocrine Regulation of Energy Metabolism: Review of Pathobiochemical and Clinical Chemical Aspects of Leptin, Ghrelin, Adiponectin, and Resistin. *Clinical Chemistry*. September 2004, volume 50, number 9, pages 1511–1525.

Poh, Z. A Current Update on the Use of Alpha Lipoic Acid in the Management of Type 2 Diabetes Mellitus. Endocrine, Metabolic, and Immune Disorders Drug Targets. December 1, 2009. [Epub ahead of print]

Puigserver, P., Spiegelman, B.M. Peroxisome Proliferator-Activated Receptor-Gamma Coactivator 1 Alpha (PGC-1 alpha): Transcriptional Coactivator and Metabolic Regulator. *Endocrine Review*. February 2003, volume 24, pages 78–90.

Teichert, J. Plasma Kinetics, Metabolism, and Urinary Excretion of Alpha-Lipoic Acid Following Oral Administration in Healthy Volunteers. *Journal of Clinical Pharmacology*. November 2003, volume 43, number 11, pages 1257–1267.

Teta, J., Teta, K. New Perspectives on Insulin Contributing Influences on Body Fat and Insulin Resistance. *Townsend Letter*. December 2008.

Verlaan, M., Roelofs, H.M.J., van Schaik, A., et al. Assessment of Oxidative Stress in Chronic Pancreatitis Patients. *World Journal of Gastroenterology*. September 21, 2006, volume 12, number 35, pages 5705–5710.

Villareal, D.T., Banks, M.R., Patterson, B.W., Polonsky, K.S., Klein, S. Weight Loss Therapy Improves Pancreatic Endocrine Function in Obese Older Adults. *Obesity*. June 2008, volume 16, number 6, pages 1349–1354.

Wareski, P., Vaarmann, A., Choubey, V., et al. PGC-1[alpha] and PGC-1[beta] Regulate Mitochondrial Density in Neurons. *Journal of Biological Chemistry*. 2009, volume 284, pages 21379–21385.

Chapter 4: Milk and Bread, Cause for Dread

Akerblom, H.K. Diabetes and Cows' Milk. *Lancet*. December 14, 1996, volume 348, number 9042, pages 1656–1657.

Akerblom, H.K., Knip, M. Putative Environmental Factors and Type 1 Diabetes. *Diabetes Metabolism Reviews.* 1998, volume 14, pages 31–67.

Akerblom, H.K., Vaarala, O., Hyoty H., et al. Environmental Factors in the Etiology of Type 1 Diabetes. *American Journal of Medical Genetics:* Seminars in Medical Genetics. 2002, volume 115, pages 18–29.

Archer, S.L., Greenlund, K.J., Valdez, R., et al. Differences in Food Habits and Cardiovascular Disease Risk Factors among Native Americans with and without Diabetes: The Inter-Tribal Heart Project. *Public Health and Nutrition.* December 2004, volume 7, number 8, pages 1025–1032.

Berkey, C.S., Rockett, H.R.H, Willett, W.C., Colditz, G.A. Milk, Dairy Fat, Dietary Calcium, and Weight Gain: A Longitudinal Study of Adolescents. *Archives of Pediatric and Adolescent Medicine.* 2005, volume 159, pages 543–550.

Chamberlain, L. Media and Censorship: A Project Censored Award Is a Dubious Achievement. *The Plain Dealer.* April 12–18, 2000.

Collins, M.T. M Paratuberculosis in Foods and the Public Health Implications. Proceedings of the Fifth International Colloquium on Paratuberculosis. International Association for Paratuberculosis. 1996, page 352.

Dahl-Jorgensen, K., Joner, G., Hanssen, K.F. Relationship Between Cow's Milk Consumption and Incidence of IDDM in Childhood. *Diabetes Care.* 1991, volume 14, pages 1081–1083.

Eagan, M.S., Lyle, R.M., Gunther, C.W., Peacock, M., Teegarden, D. Effect of 1-Year Dairy Product Intervention on Fat Mass in Young Women: 6-Month Follow-up. *Obesity.* 2006, volume 14, pages 2242–2248.

Elliot, R.B., Wasmuth, H., Hill, J., Songini, M., Bottazzo, G.F. Diabetes and Cows' Milk [Letter]. Sardinian IDDM Study Groups. *Lancet.* December 14, 1996, volume 348, number 9042, page 1657.

Fava, D., Leslie, R.D., Pozzilli, P. Relationship Between Dairy Product Consumption and Incidence of IDDM in Childhood in Italy. *Diabetes Care.* December 1994, volume 17, number 12, pages 1488–1490.

Hubbard, R.W., Ono, Y., Sanchez A. Atherogenic Effect of Oxidized Products of Cholesterol. *Progress in Food and Nutrition Science.* 1989, volume 13, pages 17–44.

International Dairy Federation. Per capita milk consumption in the US. Bulletin 423/2007. www.fil-idf.org/docsharenoframe/netservices/documents/viewpaperpublication.aspx?PortalSource=2331&DocID=8980

International Dairy Foods Association. Size of the dairy industry: 2007. www.idfa.org/facts/trends.cfm

Karjalainen, J., Martin, J.M., Knip, M., et al. A Bovine Albumin Peptide as a Possible Trigger of Insulin-Dependent Diabetes Mellitus. *New England Journal of Medicine.* 1992, volume 327, pages 302–307.

Manning, J. Milk May Be Linked to Intestinal Illness. *Milwaukee Journal Sentinel.* September 6, 1996, page 7.

Medical News Today.com. www.medicalnewstoday.com

Montonen, J., Knekt, P., Harkanen, T., et al. Dietary Patterns and the Incidence of Type 2 Diabetes. *American Journal of Epidemiology.* February 1, 2005, volume 161, number 3, pages 219–227.

Murch, S. Diabetes and Cows' Milk. *Lancet.* December 14, 1996, volume 348, number 9042, page 1656.

Naik, R.G., Palmer, J.P. Preservation of Beta Cell Function in Type 1 Diabetes. *Diabetes Review.* 1999, volume 7, pages 154–182.

Paratuberculosis Awareness & Research Association. MAP and Crohn's Disease Research. Scientific findings. www.crohns.org/research/index.htm

Parillo, M., Riccardi, G. Diet Composition and the Risk of Type 2 Diabetes: Epidemiological and Clinical Evidence. *British Journal of Nutrition.* July 2004, volume 92, number 1, pages 7–19.

Pereira, M.A., Jacobs, D.R. Jr, Van Horn, L., et al. Dairy Consumption, Obesity, and the Insulin Resistance Syndrome in Young Adults: the CARDIA Study. *Journal of the American Medical Association.* April 24, 2002, volume 287, number 16, pages 2081–2099.

Rense.com. Pus cell count in CA's 'Happy Cow' milk soars. www.rense.com/general51/pus.htm. (Citing Hoard's Dairyman; www.hoards.com/home.htm)

Scott, F. AAP Recommendations on Cow Milk, Soy, and Early Infant Feeding. Pediatrics. 1995, volume 96, pages 515–517.

Smyth, D.J., Plagnol, V., Walker, N.M., et al. Shared and Distinct Genetic Variants in Type 1 Diabetes and Celiac Disease. *New England Journal of Medicine.* December 25, 2008, volume 359, number 26, pages 2767–2777.

Soltesz, G., Patterson, C.C., Dahlquist, G.; EURODIAB Study Group. Worldwide Childhood Type 1 Diabetes Incidence—What Can We Learn From Epidemiology? *Pediatric Diabetes.* October 2007, volume 8 (supplement), pages 6–14.

Umpierrez, G.E., Latif, K.A., Murphy, M.B., et al. Thyroid Dysfunction in Patients with Type 1 Diabetes. *Diabetes Care.* 2003, volume 26, pages 1181–1185.

U.S. Animal Health Association. Report of the USAHA Committee on Food Safety. October 5, 1998.
The World's Healthiest Foods. www.whfoods.com/

PART 2: DETECTION, TREATMENT, AND MONITORING OF DIABETES

Chapter 5: Medications: What You Need to Know to Stay Safe

Triplitt, C., McGill, J.B., Porte, D. Jr., Conner, C.S. The Changing Landscape of Type 2 Diabetes: The
    Role of Incretin-Based Therapies in Managed Care Outcomes. *Journal of Managed Care Pharmacy.*
    December 2007, volume 13 (supplement), number 9.
Generex Corporation (Toronto, Ontario, Canada). Product: Generex Oral-Lyn. www.generex.com/prod-
    ucts.php?prod_id=Nzk=
InjuryBoard.com. Avandia, Rezulin, and Actos: same chemical family; similar benefits, and unfortunately,
    quite similar risks.
The Medical News. Search results for Carolinas Medical Center. www.news-medical.net/
    ?keyword=Carolinas%20Medical%20Center
Merck and Co. Januvia. www.januvia.com/sitagliptin/januvia/hcp/januvia/efficacy/study_results_54_
    week.jsp?WT.svl=5.1=

Chapter 6: Diagnostic Tests to Monitor Your Progress

Abdul-Ghani, M.A., Lyssenko, V., Tuomi, T., DeFronzo, R.A., Groop, L. Fasting Versus Postload Plasma
    Glucose Concentration and the Risk for Future Type 2 Diabetes: Results from the Botnia Study. *Dia-
    betes Care.* 2009, volume 32, pages 281–286.

PART 3: STAYING WELL ABOVE THE WAIST

Chapter 7: Protecting Your Precious Eyesight

Albert, C.M., Cook, N.R., Gaziano, J.M., et al. Effect of Folic Acid and B Vitamins on Risk of Cardio-
    vascular Events and Total Mortality among Women at High Risk for Cardiovascular Disease: A Ran-
    domized Trial. *Journal of the American Medical Association.* 2008, volume 299, pages 2027–2036.
Bagchi, D., Sen, C.K., Bagchi, M., Atalay, M. Anti-angiogenic, Antioxidant, and Anti-carcinogenic Prop-
    erties of a Novel Anthocyanin-Rich Berry Extract Formula. *Biochemistry* (Moscow). January 2004,
    volume 69, number 1, pages 75–80.
Balazs, E.A. Hyaluronan as an Ophthalmic Viscoelastic Device. *Current Pharmaceutical Biotechnology.*
    August 2008, volume 9, number 4, pages 236–238.
Hepler, R.S., Frank, I.R. Marijuana Smoking and Intraocular Pressure [Letter]. *Journal of the American
    Medical Association.* 1971, volume 217, page 1392.
Hepler, R.S., Petrus, R.J. Experiences with Administration of Marihuana to Glaucoma Patients. In:
    Cohen, S., Stillman, R.C., eds. *The Therapeutic Potential of Marihuana.* New York: Plenum Medical
    Books, 1976, pages 63–75.
Huang, S.Y., Jeng, C., Kao, S.C., Yu, J.J., Liu, D.Z. Improved Haemorrheological Properties by Ginkgo
    biloba Extract in Type 2 Diabetes Mellitus Complicated with Retinopathy. *Clinical Nutrition.* August
    2004, volume 23, number 4, pages 615–621.
Puupponen-Pimiä, R., Nohynek, L., Alakomi, H.L., Oksman-Caldentey, K.M. Bioactive Berry Com-
    pounds—Novel Tools Against Human Pathogens. *Applied Microbiology and Biotechnology.* April
    2005, volume 67, number 1, pages 8–18.
Quaranta, L., Bettelli, S., Uva, M.G., et al. Effect of Ginkgo biloba Extract on Preexisting Visual Field
    Damage in Normal Tension Glaucoma. *Ophthalmology.* February 2003, volume 110, number 2, pages
    359–3644.
Seddon, J.M., Ajani, U.A., Sperduto, R.D., et al. Dietary Carotenoids, Vitamins A, C, and E, and
    Advanced Age-Related Macular Degeneration. Eye Disease Case-Control Study Group. *Journal of the
    American Medical Association.* 1994, volume 272, pages 1455–1456.
Statement by the Board of Directors of the American Academy of Ophthalmology. The Use of Marijuana
    in the Treatment of Glaucoma. June 1992.
Takeuchi, K., Nakazawa, M., Yamazaki, H., et al. Solid Hyaluronic Acid Film and the Prevention of
    Postoperative Fibrous Scar Formation in Experimental Animal Eyes. *Archives of Ophthalmology.* April
    2009, volume 127, number 4, pages 460–464.

Chapter 8: Improving Heart Disease

Alexander, J.H., Reynolds, H.R., Stebbins, A.L., et al. Effect of Tilarginine Acetate in Patients with Acute Myocardial Infarction and Cardiogenic Shock: The TRIUMPH Randomized Controlled Trial. *Journal of the American Medical Association.* April 18, 2007, volume 297, number 15, pages 1657–1666.

Balazs, E.A., Takeuchi, K., Nakazawa, M., et al. Hyaluronan as an Ophthalmic Viscoelastic Device. *Current Pharmaceutical Biotechnology.* August 2008, volume 9, number 4, pages 236–238.

Baur, J.A., Pearson, K.J., Price, N.L., et al. Resveratrol Improves Health and Survival of Mice on a High-Calorie Diet. *Nature.* November 16, 2006, volume 444, pages 337–342.

Böger, R.H., Sullivan, L.M., Schwedhelm, E., et al. Plasma Asymmetric Dimethylarginine and Incidence of Cardiovascular Disease and Death in the Community. *Circulation.* March 31, 2009, volume 119, number 12, pages 1592–1600.

Carter, O., MacCarater, D., Mannebach, S., et al. D-Ribose Improves Peak Exercise Capacity and Ventilatory Efficiency in Heart Failure Patients. Abstract presented at American College of Cardiology Annual Scientific Session, March 2005, Orlando, Florida.

Centers for Disease Control and Prevention. Heart disease facts and statistics. www.cdc.gov/heartDisease/statistics.htm

Dr. Isaac Eliaz. www.dreliaz.org/

Gerstein, H., Yusuf, S., Riddle, M.C., Ryden, L., Bosch, J. Rationale, Design, and Baseline Characteristics for a Large International Trial of Cardiovascular Disease Prevention in People with Dysglycemia: The ORIGIN Trial (Outcome Reduction with an Initial Glargine Intervention). *American Heart Journal.* January 2008, volume 155, number 1, pages 26–32.

Harvard Medical School Family Health Guide. Aspirin for heart attack: chew or swallow? www.health.harvard.edu/fhg/updates/update0505a.shtml

Hsia, C.H., Shen, M.C., Lin, J.S., et al. Nattokinase Decreases Plasma Levels of Fibrinogen, Factor VII, and Factor VIII in Human Subjects. *Nutrition Research.* March 2009, volume 29, number 3, pages 190–196.

Jung, H.J., Seu, Y.B., Lee, D.G. Candicidal Action of Resveratrol Isolated from Grapes on Human Pathogenic Yeast C. albicans. *Journal of Microbiology and Biotechnology.* August 2007, volume 17, number 8, pages 1324–1329.

Kung, H.C., Hoyert, D.L., Xu, J., Murphy, S.L. Deaths: Final Data for 2005. *National Vital Statistics Reports.* 2008, volume 56, number 10.

Langsjoen, P.H., Langsjoen, A.M. Supplemental Ubiquinol in Patients with Advanced Congestive Heart Failure. *Biofactors.* 2008, volume 32, numbers 1–4, pages 119–128.

Linus Pauling Institute at Oregon State University. Micronutrient Information Center. Resveratrol Sources. http://lpi.oregonstate.edu/infocenter/phytochemicals/resveratrol/index.html#sources

Maccarter, D., Vijay, N., Washam, M., et al. D-Ribose Aids Advanced Ischemic Heart Failure Patients. *International Journal of Cardiology.* July 30, 2008, volume 137, pages 79–80.

Nutrition Data. Seeds, chia seeds, dried. www.nutritiondata.com/facts/nut-and-seed-products/3061/2

Omran, H., Illien, S., MacCarter, D., St Cyr, J., Lüderitz, B. D-Ribose Improves Diastolic Function and Quality of Life in Congestive Heart Failure Patients: A Prospective Feasibility Study. *European Journal of Heart Failure.* October 2003, volume 5, number 5, pages 615–619.

Pace-Asciak, C.R., Hahn, S., Diamandis, E.P., Soleas, G., Goldberg, D.M. The Red Wine Phenolics Trans-Resveratrol and Quercetin Block Human Platelet Aggregation and Eicosanoid Synthesis: Implications for Protection Against Coronary Heart Disease. *Clinica Chimica Acta.* March 31, 1995, volume 235, number 2, pages 207–219.

Quettier-Deleu, C., Voiselle, G., Fruchart, J.C., et al. Hawthorn Extracts Inhibit LDL Oxidation. *Pharmazie.* August 2003, volume 58, number 8, pages 577–581.

Ros, E., Pi Sunyer, A. Nuts and Novel Biomarkers of Cardiovascular Disease. *American Journal of Clinical Nutrition.* May 2009, volume 89, number 5, pages 1649S–1656S.

Rosner, M.H. Hyponatremia in Heart Failure: The Role of Arginine Vasopressin and Diuretics. *Cardiovascular Drugs and Therapy.* June 2009, volume 23, pages 307–315.

Shah, M., Adams-Huet, B., Brinkley, L., Grundy, S.M., Garg, A. Lipid, Glycemic, and Insulin Responses to Meals Rich in Saturated, Cis-Monounsaturated, and Polyunsaturated (n-3 and n-6) Fatty Acids in Subjects with Type 2 Diabetes. *Diabetes Care.* December 2007, volume 30, number 12, pages 2993–2998.

Sinatra, S.T. Metabolic Cardiology: An Integrative Strategy in the Treatment of Congestive Heart Failure. *Alternative Therapies in Health and Medicine.* May–June 2009, volume 15, number 3, pages 44–52.

Takeuchi, K., Nakazawa, M., Yamazaki, H., et al. Solid Hyaluronic Acid Film and the Prevention of Postoperative Fibrous Scar Formation in Experimental Animal Eyes. *Archives of Ophthalmology.* April 2009, volume 127, number 4, page 460.

Walle, T. Methylation of Dietary Flavones Greatly Improves Their Hepatic Metabolic Stability and

Intestinal Absorption. *Molecular Pharmacology*. November–December 2007, volume 4, number 6, pages 862–832.

Walle, T., Hsieh, F., DeLegge, M.H., Oatis J.E., Jr., Walle, U.K. High Absorption but Very Low Bioavailability of Oral Resveratrol in Humans. *Drug Metabolism and Disposition*. December 2004, volume 32, number 12, pages 1377–1382.

Wen, X., Walle, T. Methylated Flavonoids Have Greatly Improved Intestinal Absorption and Metabolic Stability. *Drug Metabolism and Disposition*. October 2006, volume 34, number 10, pages 1786–1792.

World Health Organization. The Global Burden of Disease: 2004 Update. Geneva: World Health Organization, 2008.

Zhang, M., Bi, L.F., Fang, J.H., et al. Beneficial Effects of Taurine on Serum Lipids in Overweight or Obese Non-diabetic Subjects. *Amino Acids*. June 2004, volume 26, number 3, pages 267–271.

Zhang, G.Q., Zhang, W. Heart Rate, Lifespan, and Mortality Risk. *Aging Research Review*. January 2009, volume 8, number 1, pages 52–60.

Chapter 9: Kidneys Deserve Good Care

Ahmed, M.S., Hou, S.H., Battaglia, M.C., et al. Treatment of Idiopathic Membranous Nephropathy with the Herb Astragalus membranaceus. *American Journal of Kidney Disease*. December 2007, volume 50, number 6, pages 1028–1032.

About.com. Alternative Medicine. www.altmedicine.about.com

Anderson, M.L. A Preliminary Investigation of the Enzymatic Inhibition of 5-alpha Reduction and Growth of Prostatic Carcinoma Cell Line LNCap-FGC by Natural Astaxanthin and Saw Palmetto Lipid Extract in Vitro. *Journal of Herbal Pharmacotherapy*. 2005, volume 5, number 1, pages 17–26.

Brookler, K.H., Glenn, M.B. Ménière's Syndrome: An Approach to Therapy. *Ear Nose and Throat Journal*. August 1995, volume 74, number 8, pages 534–538, 540, 542.

Comhaire, F.H., El Garem, Y., Mahmoud, A., Eertmans, F., Schoonjans, F. Combined Conventional/Antioxidant Astaxanthin treatment for Male Infertility: A Double-Blind, Randomized Trial. *Asian Journal of Andrology*. September 2005, volume 7, number 3, pages 257–262.

Chen, J., He, J., Hamm, L., et al. Serum Antioxidant Vitamins and Blood Pressure in the United States Population. *Hypertension*. December 2002, volume 40, number 6, pages 810–816.

Chen, J., He, J., Ogden, L.G., Batuman, V., Whelton, P.K. Relationship of Serum Antioxidant Vitamins to Serum Creatinine in the US Population. *American Journal of Kidney Disease*. March 2002, volume 39, number 3, pages 460–468.

Chew, B.P., Park, J.S. Carotenoid Action on the Immune Response. *Journal of Nutrition*. January 2004, volume 134, number 1, pages 257S–261S.

Hix, L.M., Lockwood, S.F., Bertram, J.S. Bioactive Carotenoids: Potent Antioxidants and Regulators of Gene Expression. *Redox Report*. 2004, volume 9, number 4, pages 181–191.

Hussein, G., Nakamura, M., Zhao, Q., et al. Antihypertensive and Neuroprotective Effects of Astaxanthin in Experimental Animals. *Biological and Pharmaceutical Bulletin*. January 2005, volume 28, number 1, pages 47–52.

Kim, J.H., Kim, Y.S., Song, G.G., Park, J.J., Chang, H.I. Protective Effect of Astaxanthin on Naproxen-Induced Gastric Antral Ulceration in Rats. *European Journal of Pharmacology*. May 2005, volume 514, number 1, pages 53–59.

Lagouge, M., Argmann, C., Gerhart-Hines, Z., et al. Resveratrol Improves Mitochondrial Function and Protects Against Metabolic Disease by Activating SIRT1 and PGC-1. *Cell*. 2006, volume 127, number 6, pages 1109–1122.

Lockwood, S.F., Gross, G.J. Disodium Disuccinate Astaxanthin (Cardax): Antioxidant and Anti-Inflammatory Cardioprotection. *Cardiovascular Drug Review*. Fall 2005, volume 23, number 3, pages 199–216.

Markus, M.A., Morris, B.J. Resveratrol in Prevention and Treatment of Common Clinical Conditions of Aging. *Clinical Interventions in Aging*. 2008, volume 3, number 2, pages 331–339.

Mauer, M., Zinman, B., Gardiner, R., et al Renal and Retinal Effects of Enalapril and Losartan in Type 1 Diabetes. *New England Journal of Medicine*. July 2009, volume 361, number 1, pages 40–51.

Naito, Y., Uchiyama, K., Aoi, W., et al. Prevention of Diabetic Nephropathy by Treatment with Astaxanthin in Diabetic db/db Mice. *Biofactors*. 2004, volume 20, number 1, pages 49–59.

Nishikawa, J., Minenaka, Y., Ichimura, M., et al. Effects of Astaxanthin and Vitamin C on the Prevention of Gastric Ulcerations in Stressed Rats. *Journal of Nutritional Science and Vitaminology* (Tokyo). June 2005, volume 51, number 3, pages 135–141.

Pennathur, S., Wagner, J.D., Leeuwenburg, C., et al. A Hydroxyl Radical-Like Species Oxidizes Cynomolgus Monkey Artery Wall Proteins in Early Diabetic Vascular Disease. *Journal of Clinical Investigation*. April 1, 2001, volume 107, number 7, pages 853–860.

Ting, H.H., Timimi, F.K., Boles, K.S., et al. Vitamin C Improves Endothelium-Dependent Vasodilation in Patients with Non-Insulin-Dependent Diabetes Mellitus. *Journal of Clinical Investigation*. 1996, volume 97, pages 22–28.

Thornalley, P.J. The Potential Role of Thiamine (Vitamin B(1)) in Diabetic Complications. *Current Diabetes Review*. 2005, volume 1, number 3, pages 287–298.

Venning, E.H., Dyrenfurth, I., Beck, J.C. Effect of Anxiety Upon Aldosterone Excretion in Man. *Journal of Clinical Endocrinology and Metabolism*. 1957, volume 17, number 8, pages 1005–1008.

Wong, Y.T., Gruber, J., Jenner, A.M., et al. Elevation of Oxidative-Damage Biomarkers During Aging in F2 Hybrid Mice: Protection by Chronic Oral Intake of Resveratrol. *Free Radical Biology and Medicine*. March 15, 2009, volume 46, number 6, pages 799–809.

National Kidney Foundation. Glomerular Filtration Rate (GFR) Chart. www.kidney.org/kidneydisease/ckd/knowGFR.cfm#chart

All Cancers: Lappe, J.M., et al. *American Journal of Clinical Nutrition*. 2007;85:1586-91. Breast: Garland, C.F., Gorham, E.D., Mohr S.B., Grant W.B., Garland F.C. Breast Cancer risk according to serum 25-Hydroxyvitamin D: Meta-analysis of Dose-Response (abstract). American Association for Cancer Research Annual Meeting, 2008. Reference serum 25 (OH)D was 5ng/ml. Garland, C.F., et al. American Association Cancer Research Annual Meeting, April 2008. Colon: Gorham, E.D., et al. *American Journal of Preventive Medicine*. 2007;32:210-6. Diabetes: Hypponen E., et al. *Lancet* 2001;358:1500-3. Endometrium: Mohr, S.B., et al. *Preventive Medicine*. 2007;45:323-4. Falls:Broe, K.E., et al. *Journal of the American Geriatrics Society*. 2007;55:234-9. Fractures: Bischoff-Ferrari, H.A., et al. *Journal of the American Medical Association*. 2005. 2005;293:2257-64. Heart Attack: Giovannucci et al. Archives of Internal Medicine/Vol 168 (No 11) June 9, 2008. Multiple Sclerosis: Munger, K.L., et al. *Journal of the American Medical Association*. 2006; 296:2832-8. Non-Hodgkin's Lymphoma: Purdue, M.P., et al. *Cancer Causes Control*. 2007;18:989-99. Ovary: Tworoger, S.S., et al. *Cancer Epidemiology, Biomarkers & Prevention*. 2007;16:783-8. Renal: Mohr, S.B., et al. *International Journal of Cancer*. 2006;119:2705-9. Rickets: Arnaud, S.B.

PART 4: STAYING WELL BELOW THE WAIST

Chapter 10: Natural Approaches to Relieve Neuropathy

Ametov, A.S., Barinov, A., Dyck, P.J., et al. The Sensory Symptoms of Diabetic Polyneuropathy Are Improved with Alpha-Lipoic Acid: The SYDNEY Trial. *Diabetes Care*. March 2003, volume 26, number 3, pages 770–776.

Anand, P., Thomas, S.G., Kunnumakkara, A.B., et al. Biological Activities of Curcumin and Its Analogues (Congeners) Made by Man and Mother Nature. *Biochemical Pharmacology*. December 1, 2008, volume 76, number 11, pages 1590–1611.

Cremer, L., Herold, A., Avram, D., Szegli, G. A Purified Green Barley Extract with Modulatory Properties upon TNF alpha and ROS Released by Human Specialised Cells Isolated from RA Patients. *Roumanian Archives of Microbiology & Immunology*. 1998, volume 57, numbers 3–4, pages 231–242.

Dance with Shadow. Pfizer sues Sun, Wockhardt, Lupin on Lyrica (pregabalin) patents. May 4, 2009. www.dancewithshadows.com/pillscribe/pfizer-sues-sun-wockhardt-lupin-on-lyrica-pregabalin-patents/, DWS Pill Scribe.

De Grandis, D., Minardi, C. Acetyl-L-Carnitine (Levacecarnine) in the Treatment of Diabetic Neuropathy. A Long-Term, Randomised, Double-Blind, Placebo-Controlled Study. *British Journal of Clinical Pharmacology*. March/April 1994, volume 48, number 2, pages 223–231.

Donaghy, M. Assessing the Risk of Drug-Induced Neurologic Disorders: Statins and Neuropathy. *Neurology*. May 14, 2002, volume 58, number 9, pages 1321–1322.

FIR Heals. Far-Infrared Therapy. www.firheals.com

Gaist, D., Jeppesen, U., Andersen, M., et al. Statins and Risk of Polyneuropathy: A Case-Control Study. *Neurology*. May 2002, volume 58, number 9, pages 1333–1337.

Haak, E., Usadel, K.H., Kusterer, K., et al. Effects of Alpha-Lipoic Acid on Microcirculation in Patients with Peripheral Diabetic Neuropathy. *Experimental and Clinical Endocrinology and Diabetes*. 2000, volume 108, number 3, pages 168–174.

Jacob, S., Henriksen, E.J., Schiemann, A.L., et al. Enhancement of Glucose Disposal in Patients with Type 2 Diabetes by Alpha-Lipoic Acid. *Arzneimittelforschung*. August 1995, volume 45, number 8, pages 872–874.

Midaoui, A.E., Elimadi, A., Wu, L., Haddad, P.S., de Champlain, J. Lipoic Acid Prevents Hypertension, Hyperglycemia, and the Increase in Heart Mitochondrial Superoxide Production. *American Journal of Hypertension*. March 2003, volume 16, number 3, pages 173–179.

Morcos, M., Borcea, V., Isermann, B., et al. Effect of Alpha-Lipoic Acid on the Progression of Endothelial Cell Damage and Albuminuria in Patients with Diabetes Mellitus: An Exploratory Study. *Diabetes Research and Clinical Practice*. June 2001, volume 52, number 3, pages 175–183.

Nagamatsu, M., Nickander, K.K., Schmelzer, J.D., et al. Lipoic Acid Improves Nerve Blood Flow, Reduces Oxidative Stress, and Improves Distal Nerve Conduction in Experimental Diabetic Neuropathy. *Diabetes Care*. August 1995, volume 18, number 8, pages 1160–1167.

Neal, J.M. Diabetic Neuropathic Cachexia: A Rare Manifestation of Diabetic Neuropathy. *Southern Medical Journal*. March 2009, volume 102, number 3, pages 327–329.

Sharmaa, S. Curcumin Attenuates Thermal Hyperalgesia in a Diabetic Mouse Model of Neuropathic Pain. *European Journal of Pharmacology*. May 2006, volume 536, number 3, pages 256–261.

Talaei, A., Siavash, M., Majidi, H., Chehrei, A. Vitamin B(12) May Be More Effective Than Nortriptyline in Improving Painful Diabetic Neuropathy. *International Journal of Food Sciences and Nutrition*. February 2009, volume 12, pages 1–6.

Tesfaye, S. Advances in the Management of Diabetic Peripheral Neuropathy. *Current Opinion in Supportive and Palliative Care*. June 2009, volume 3, number 2, pages 136–143.

Ziegler, D., Ametov, A., Barinov, A., et al. Oral Treatment with Alpha-Lipoic Acid Improves Symptomatic Diabetic Polyneuropathy: The SYDNEY 2 Trial. *Diabetes Care*. November 2006, volume 29, number 11, pages 2365–2370.

Ziegler, D., Schatz, H., Conrad, F., et al. Effects of Treatment with the Antioxidant Alpha-Lipoic Acid on Cardiac Autonomic Neuropathy in NIDDM Patients. A 4-Month Randomized Controlled Multicenter Trial (DEKAN Study). *Diabetes Care*. March 1997, volume 20, number 3, pages 369–373.

Chapter 11: Walking Away from Diabetes: Foot and Wound Care

American Diabetes Association. Consensus Development Conference on Diabetic Foot Wound Care: 7–8 April 1999, Boston, Massachusetts. *Diabetes Care*. 1999, volume 22, pages 1354–1360.

American Diabetes Association. DiabetesFacts. Complications of diabetes in the United States. www.libertymedical.com/pdf/diabetes-management/diabetes-complications-fact-sheet.pdf

Basu, T.K. Vitamin C-Aspirin Interactions. *International Journal of Vitamin and Nutrition Research Supplement*. 1982, volume 23, pages 83–90.

Boulton, A.J.M., Kirsner, R.S., Vileikyte, L. Neuropathic Diabetic Foot Ulcers. *New England Journal of Medicine*. 2004, volume 351, pages 48–55.

Caputo, G.M., Cavanagh, P.R., Ulbrecht, J.S., Gibbons, G.W., Karchmer, A.W. Assessment and Management of Foot Disease in Patients with Diabetes. *New England Journal of Medicine*. 1994, volume 331, pages 854–860.

Cereda, E., Gini, A., Pedrolli, C., Vanotti, A. Disease-Specific, Versus Standard, Nutritional Support for the Treatment of Pressure Ulcers in Institutionalized Older Adults: A Randomized Controlled Trial. *Journal of the American Geriatric Society*. June 25, 2009, volume 57, pages 1395–1402.

Chang, H. Neuropathic Diabetic Foot Ulcers [letter]. *New England Journal of Medicine*. October 14, 2004, volume 351, pages 1694–1697.

Cohen, S. *Drug Muggers*. Emmaus, Pennsylvania: Rodale, 2010.

The Diabetes Control and Complications Trial Research Group. The Effect of Intensive Treatment of Diabetes on the Development and Progression of Long-Term Complications in Insulin-Dependent Diabetes Mellitus. *New England Journal of Medicine*. 1993, volume 329, pages 977–986.

Litzelman, D.K., Slemenda, C.W., Langefeld, C.D., et al. Reduction of Lower Extremity Clinical Abnormalities in Patients with Non–Insulin-Dependent Diabetes Mellitus: A Randomized, Controlled Trial. *Annals of Internal Medicine*. 1993, volume 119, pages 36–41.

Malone, J.M., Snyder, M., Anderson, G., et al. Prevention of Amputation by Diabetic Education. *American Journal of Surgery*. 1989, volume 158, pages 520–524.

Mayfield, J.A., Reiber, G.E., Sanders, L.J., Janisse, D., Pogach, L.M. Preventive Foot Care in People with Diabetes. *Diabetes Care*. 2003, volume 26 (supplement), pages S78–S79.

National Diabetes Information Clearinghouse (NDIC): Prevent Diabetes Problems: Keep Your Feet and Skin Healthy. http://diabetes.niddk.nih.gov/dm/pubs/complications_feet/index.htm

Bio-Medicine. News. Two landmark papers on amputation prevention in diabetes unveiled. news.bio-medicine.org/medicine-news-3/Two-landmark-papers-on-amputation-prevention-in-diabetes-unveiled-7366-1.

Patout, C.A., Birke, J.A., Horswell, R., Williams, D., Cerise, F.P. Effectiveness of a Comprehensive Diabetes Lower-Extremity Amputation Prevention Program in a Predominantly Low-Income African-American population. *Diabetes Care*. 2000, volume 23, pages 1339–1342.

Reid, M.E., Duffield-Lillico, A.J., Slate, E., et al. The Nutritional Prevention of Cancer: 400 mcg per Day Selenium Treatment. *Nutrition and Cancer*. 2008, volume 60, number 2, pages 155–163.

Rith-Najarian, S., Branchaud, C., Beaulieu, O., et al. Reducing Lower-Extremity Amputations Due to Diabetes. *Journal of Family Practice*. 1998, volume 47, pages 127–132.

Rith-Najarian, S., Gohdes, D. Preventing Amputations Among Patients with Diabetes on Dialysis. *Diabetes Care*. 2000, volume 23, pages 1445–1446.

Suzana, S., Cham, B.G., Ahmad Rohi, G., et al. Relationship between Selenium and Breast Cancer: A Case-Control Study in the Klang Valley. *Singapore Medical Journal*. 2009, volume 50, number 3, pages 265–269.

Uccioli, L., Faglia, E., Monticone, G., et al. Manufactured Shoes in the Prevention of Diabetic Foot Ulcers. *Diabetes Care*. 1995, volume 18, pages 1376–1378.

WhereToFindCare.com. 3 in 20 short stay nursing home patients have pressure sores. (Based on the most recent Nursing Home Compare data from Medicare; see www.medicare.gov.) www.wheretofindcare.com/2009/04/3-in-20-short-stay-nursing-home.html

World Diabetes Foundation. www.worlddiabetesfoundation.org/composite-967.htm

Young, B.A., Maynard, C., Reiber, G., Boyko, E.J. Effects of Ethnicity and Nephropathy on Lower-Extremity Amputation Risk among Diabetic Veterans. *Diabetes Care*. February 2003, volume 26, number 2, pages 495–501.

PART 5: MOVING BEYOND DIABETES—YOUR PATH TO FULL RECOVERY

Chapter 12: Diabetes without Drugs: Steps 1, 2, and 3

Chapter 13: Natural Ways to Reduce Blood Sugar: Step 4

Chapter 14: The Magic of Minerals: Step 5

Abdel-Barry, J.A., Abdel-Hassan, I.A., Jawad, A.M., et al. Hypoglycaemic Effect of Aqueous Extract of the Leaves of Trigonella foenum-graecum in Healthy Volunteers. *Eastern Mediterranean Health Journal*. 2000, volume 6, pages 83–88.

Abudula, R., Jeppesen, P.B., Rolfsen, S.E., Xiao, J., Hermansen, K. Rebaudioside A Potently Stimulates Insulin Secretion from Isolated Mouse Islets: Studies on the Dose-, Glucose-, and Calcium-Dependency. *Metabolism: Clinical and Experimental*. October 2004, volume 53, number 10, pages 1378–1381.

Alarcon de la Lastra, C., Villegas, I. Resveratrol as an Anti-Inflammatory and Anti-Aging Agent: Mechanisms and Clinical Implications. *Molecular Nutrition and Food Research*. 2005, volume 49, number 5, pages 405–430.

Alfonso, B., Liao, E., Busta, A., Poretsky, L. Vitamin D in Diabetes Mellitus—A New Field of Knowledge Poised for D-velopment. *Diabetes Metabolism Research and Review*. June 29, 2009, volume 25, number 5, pages 417–419.

AmericanGrassFedBeef.com Scientific research on aphanizomenon flos-aqaue, blue green algae chlorophyll. (Includes many abstracts of peer-reviewed published studies.) www.americangrassfedbeef.com/e3live-research.asp

Babadzhanov, A.S., Abdusamatova, N., Yusupova, F.M., et al. Chemical Composition of Spirulina platensis Cultivated in Uzbekistan. *Chemistry of Natural Compounds*. 40, 3, 2004, pages 276–279.

Bagchi, D., Sen, C.K., Bagchi, M., Atalay, M. Anti-Angiogenic, Antioxidant, and Anti-Carcinogenic Properties of a Novel Anthocyanin-Rich Berry Extract Formula. *Biochemistry* (Moscow). January 2004, volume 69, number 1, pages 75–80.

Baskaran, K., Kizar Ahamath, B., Radha Shanmugasundaram, K., Shanmugasundarm, E.R.B. Antidiabetic Effect of a Leaf Extract from Gymnema sylvestre in Non Insulin-Dependent Diabetes Mellitus Patients. *Journal of Ethnopharmacology*. 1990, volume 30, pages 295–305.

Benford, D.J., DiNovi, M., Schlatter, J. Safety Evaluation of Certain Food Additives: Steviol Glycosides. WHO Food Additives Series (World Health Organization Joint FAO/WHO Expert Committee on Food Additives). 2006, volume 54, page 140.

Beppu, H., Shimpo, K., Chihara, T., et al. Antidiabetic Effects of Dietary Administration of Aloe arborescens Miller Components on Multiple Low-Dose Streptozotocin-Induced Diabetes in Mice: investigation on Hypoglycemic Action and Systemic Absorption Dynamics of Aloe Components. *Journal of Ethnopharmacology*. February 20, 2006, volume 103, number 3, pages 468–477.

Boocock, D.J., Faust, G.E., Patel, K.R., et al. Phase I Dose Escalation Pharmacokinetic Study in Healthy Volunteers of Resveratrol, a Potential Cancer Chemopreventive Agent. *Cancer Epidemiology, Biomarkers, and Prevention*. 2007, volume 16, pages 1246–1252.

Chatsudthipong, V., Muanprasat, C. Stevioside and Related Compounds: Therapeutic Benefits Beyond

Sweetness. *Pharmacology and Therapeutics.* January 2009, volume 121, number 1, pages 41–54.

Chiu, K.C., Chu, A., Go, V.L., Saad, M.F. Hypovitaminosis D Is Associated with Insulin Resistance and Beta Cell Dysfunction. *American Journal of Clinical Nutrition.* May 2004, volume 79, number 5, pages 820–825.

Cuzzolin, L., Benoni, G. Attitudes and Knowledge Toward Natural Products Safety in the Pharmacy Setting: An Italian Study. *Phytotherapy Research.* July 2009, volume 23, number 7, pages 1018–1023.

Delmas, D., Jannin, B., Latruffe, N. Resveratrol: Preventing Properties Against Vascular Alterations and Ageing. Molecular Nutrition & Food Research. 2005, volume 49, number 5, pages 377–395.

Emperor's Herbologist. www.emperorsherbologist.com

Ehrenbergerová, J., Brezinová Belcredi, N., Kopácek, J., et al. Antioxidant Enzymes in Barley Green Biomass. *Plant Foods for Human Nutrition.* June 2009, volume 64,number 2, pages 122–128.

Ferrazzano, G.F., Amato, I., Ingenito, A., De Natale, A., Pollio, A. Anti-Cariogenic Effects of Polyphenols from Plant Stimulant Beverages (Cocoa, Coffee, Tea). *Fitoterapia.* July 2009, volume 80, number 5, pages 255–262.

Gannagé-Yared, M.H., Chedid, R., Khalife, S., et al. Vitamin D in Relation to Metabolic Risk Factors, Insulin Sensitivity and Adiponectin in a Young Middle-Eastern Population. *European Journal of Endocrinology.* 2009, volume 160, pages 965–971.

Gharpurey, K.G. Natural Remedies for Diabetes Management. *Indian Medical Gazette.* 1926, volume 61, page 155.

Haas, E.M., Levin, B. *Staying Healthy with Nutrition: The Complete Guide to Diet and Nutritional Medicine.* Berkeley, California: Celestial Arts Publishing, 2006.

Hiremath, G., Cettomai, D., Baynes, M., et al Vitamin D Status and Effect of Low-Dose Cholecalciferol and High-Dose Ergocalciferol Supplementation in Multiple Sclerosis. *Multiple Sclerosis.* 2009, volume 15, pages 735–740.

Holick, M.F. Vitamin D Deficiency. *New England Journal of Medicine.* July 19, 2007, volume 357, number 3, pages 266–281.

Holick, M.F., Lim, R., Dighe, A.S. Case Records of the Massachusetts General Hospital. Case 3-2009. A 9-Month-Old Boy with Seizures. *New England Journal of Medicine.* January 22, 2009, volume 360, number 4, pages 398–407.

The Holistic Option. Adams M. FDA approves stevia. December 22, 2008. www.theholisticoption.com

Hsieh, M.H., Chan, P., Sue, Y.M., et al. Efficacy and Tolerability of Oral Stevioside in Patients with Mild Essential Hypertension: A Two-Year, Randomized, Placebo-Controlled Study. *Clinical Therapeutics.* November 2003, volume 25, number 11, pages 2797–2808.

Huemer, R.P. Chromium Keeps Blood Sugar in Check. Better Nutrition (1989–90). www.FindArticles.com. June 27, 2009.

Hui, H., Tang, G., Go, V.L. Hypoglycemic Herbs and Their Action Mechanisms. *Chinese Medicine.* June 12, 2009, volume 4, page 11.

Hussein, G., Nakagawa, T., Goto, H., et al. Astaxanthin Ameliorates Features of Metabolic Syndrome in SHR/NDmcr-cp. *Life Sciences.* 2007, volume 80, pages 522–529.

Inzucchi, S.E., Maggs, D.G., Spollett, G.R., et al, Efficacy and Metabolic Effects of Metformin and Troglitazone in Type II Diabetes Mellitus. *New England Journal of Medicine.* March 26, 1998, volume 338, number 13, pages 867–872.

Jani, R., Udipi, S.A., Ghugre, P.S. Mineral Content of Complementary Foods. *Indian Journal of Pediatrics.* January 2009, volume 76, number 1, pages 37–44.

Jeppesen, P.B., Gregersen, S., Rolfsen, S.E., et al. Antihyperglycemic and Blood Pressure-Reducing Effects of Stevioside in the Diabetic Goto-Kakizaki Rat. *Metabolism: Clinical and Experimental.* March 2003, volume 52, number 3, pages 372–378.

Jeppesen, P.B., Gregerson, S., Poulsen, C.R., Hermansen, K. Stevioside Acts Directly on Pancreatic Beta Cells to Secrete Insulin. *Metabolism.* February 2000, volume 49, number 2, pages 208–214.

Kaeberlein, M., McDonagh, T., Heltweg, B., et al. Substrate-Specific Activation of Sirtuins by Resveratrol. *Biological Chemistry.* April 29, 2005, volume 280, number 17, pages 17038–17045.

Kamenova, P. Improvement of Insulin Sensitivity in Patients with Type 2 Diabetes Mellitus after Oral Administration of Alpha-Lipoic Acid. *Hormones* (Athens). October–December 2006, volume 5, number 4, pages 251–258.

Kato, A., Minoshima, Y., Yamamoto, J., et al. Protective Effects of Dietary Chamomile Tea on Diabetic Complications. *Agricultural Food Chemistry.* September 10, 2008, volume 56, number 17, pages 8206–8211.

Kennel, K.A., Drake, M.T. Adverse Effects of Bisphosphonates: Implications for Osteoporosis Management. *Mayo Clinic Proceedings.* 2009, volume 84, pages 632–638.

Khajavi, M., Shiga, K., Wisniewski, W., et al. Oral Curcumin Mitigates the Clinical and Neuropathologic Phenotype of the Trembler-J Mouse: A Potential Therapy for Inherited Neuropathy. *American Journal of Human Genetics.* September 2007, volume 81, number 3, pages 438–453.

Khajavi, M., Inoue, K., Wiszniewski, W., et al. Curcumin Treatment Abrogates Endoplasmic Reticulum Retention and Aggregation-Induced Apoptosis Associated with Neuropathy-Causing Myelin Protein Zero-Truncating Mutants. *American Journal of Human Genetics.* November 2005, volume 77, number 5, pages 841–850.

Khan, Z., Bhadouria, P., Bisen, P.S. Nutritional and Therapeutic Potential of Spirulina. *Current Pharmaceutical Biotechnology.* October 2005, volume 6, number 5, pages 373–379.

Klein, G., Kullich, W. [Reducing Pain by Oral Enzyme Therapy in Rheumatic Diseases] [Article in German] *Wiener medizinische Wochenschrift.* 1999, volume 149, number 21–22, pages 577–580.

Kulshreshtha, A., Zacharia, A.J., Jarouliya, U., et al. Spirulina in Health Care Management. *Current Pharmaceutical Biotechnology.* October 2008, volume 9, number 5, pages 400–405.

Lairon, D., Arnault, N., Bertrais, S., et al. Dietary fiber intake and risk factors for cardiovascular disease in French adults. *American Journal of Clinical Nutrition.* December 2005, volume 82, number 6, pages 1185–1194.

Lajdova, I., Spustova, V., Oksa, A., et al. Intracellular Calcium Homeostasis in Patients with Early Stages of Chronic Kidney Disease: Effects of Vitamin D3 Supplementation. *Nephrology, Dialysis, Transplantation.* June 16, 2009. [Epub ahead of print].

Lampe, J.W., Peterson, S. Brassica, Biotransformation and Cancer Risk: Genetic Polymorphisms Alter the Preventive Effects of Cruciferous Vegetables. *Journal of Nutrition.* 2002, volume 132, number 10, pages 2991–2994.

Leipner, J., Iten, F., Saller, R. Therapy with Proteolytic Enzymes in Rheumatic Disorders. *BioDrugs.* 2001, volume 15, number 12, pages 779–789.

Li, M., Ding, W., Smee, J.J., et al. Anti-diabetic Effects of Vanadium(III, IV, V)-Chlorodipicolinate Complexes in Streptozotocin-Induced Diabetic Rats. *Biometals.* April 29, 2009. [Epub ahead of print].

Love to Know. Dangers of stevia. www.safety.lovetoknow.com/Dangers_of_Stevia

Markus, M.A., Morris, B.J. Resveratrol in Prevention and Treatment of Common Clinical Conditions of Aging. *Clinical Interventions in Aging.* 2008, volume 3, pages 331–339.

Marques, F.Z., Markus, M.A., Morris, B.J. Resveratrol: Cellular Actions of a Potent Natural Chemical That Confers a Diversity of Health Benefits. *International Journal of Biochemistry & Cell Biology.* June 13, 2009. [Epub ahead of print]

Melis, M.S. Effects of Chronic Administration of Stevia rebaudiana on Fertility in Rats. *Journal of Ethnopharmacology.* November 1, 1999, volume 67, number 2, pages 157–161.

Nakajima, S., Hagiwara, Y., Hagiwara, H., Shibamoto, T. Effect of the Antioxidant 2''-O-Glycosylisovitexin from Young Green Barley Leaves on Acetaldehyde Formation in Beer Stored at 50 Degrees C for 90 days. *Journal of Agriculture and Food Chemistry.* 1998, volume 46, number 4, pages 1529–1531.

Nakajima, Y., Inokuchi, Y., Shimazawa, M., et al. Astaxanthin, a Dietary Carotenoid, Protects Retinal Cells against Oxidative Stress in-vitro and in Mice in-vivo. *Journal of Pharmacy and Pharmacology.* October 2008, volume 60, number 10, pages 1365–1374.

Nohr, L.A., Rasmussen, L.B., Straand, J. Resin from the Mukul Myrrh Tree, Guggul: Can It Be Used for Treating Hypercholesterolemia? A Randomized, Controlled Study. *Complementary Therapies in Medicine.* January 2009, volume 17, number 1, pages 16–22.

Nöthlings, U., Murphy, S.P., Wilkens, L.R., et al. Flavonols and Pancreatic Cancer Risk. *American Journal of Epidemiology.* 2007, volume 166, number 8, pages 924–931.

Osawa, T. Nephroprotective and Hepatoprotective Effects of Curcuminoids. *Advances in Experimental Medicine and Biology.* 2007, volume 595, pages 407–423.

Osawa, T., Kato, Y. Protective Role of Antioxidative Food Factors in Oxidative Stress Caused by Hyperglycemia. *Annals of the New York Academy of Sciences.* June 2005, volume 1043, pages 440–451.

The Pakistan Agricultural Research Council. Sugar leaf—a new breed of "sweetener." www.parc.gov.pk/articles/sugar_leaf.htm

Parikh, P., Mani, U., Iyer, U. Role of Spirulina in the Control of Glycemia and Lipidemia in Type 2 Diabetes Mellitus. *Journal of Medicinal Food.* Winter 2001, volume 4, number 4, pages 193–199.

Pham, P.C., Pham, P.M., Pham, P.T., et al. The Link between Lower Serum Magnesium and Kidney Function in Patients with Diabetes Mellitus Type 2 Deserves a Closer Look. *Clinical Nephrology.* April 2009, volume 71, number 4, pages 375–379.

Prasanna, M. Hypolipidemic Effect of Fenugreek: A Clinical Study. *Indian Journal of Pharmacology.* 2000, volume 32, pages 34–36.

Riccardi, G., Rivellese, A.A. Effects of Dietary Fiber and Carbohydrate on Glucose and Lipoprotein Metabolism in Diabetic Patients. *Diabetes Care.* December 1991, volume 14, number 12, pages 1115–1125.

Rehman, H.U. Persistently Raised Alkaline Phosphatase in a Woman with Osteomalacia. *British Medical Journal.* 2009, volume 338, page b1874.

Roy, S., Khanna, S., Alessio, H.M., et al. Anti-angioneic Property of Edible Berries. *Free Radical Research.* 2002, volume 36, pages 1023–1031.

Satoskar, R.R., Shah, S.J., Shenoy, S.G. Evaluation of Anti-Inflammatory Property of Curcumin (Diferuloyl Methane) in Patients with Postoperative Inflammation. *International Journal of Clinical Pharmacology, Therapy, and Toxicology.* 1986, volume 24, number 12, pages 651–654.

Seo, K.I., Choi, M.S., Jung, U.J. et al. Effect of Curcumin Supplementation on Blood Glucose, Plasma Insulin, and Glucose Homeostasis Related Enzyme Activities in Diabetic db/db Mice. *Molecular Nutrition and Food Research.* April 8, 2008, volume 52, pages 995–1004.

Shabbeer, S., Sobolewski, M., Anchoori, R.K., et al. Fenugreek: A Naturally Occurring Edible Spice as an Anticancer Agent. *Cancer Biology & Therapy.* February 18, 2009, volume 8, number 3. [Epub ahead of print]

Shakibaei, M., Harikumar, K.B., Aggarwal, B.B. Resveratrol Addiction: to Die or Not To Die. *Molecular Nutrition and Food Research.* 2009, volume 53, pages 115–128.

Shanmugasundaram, E.R., Rajeswari, G., Baskaran, K., et al. Use of *Gymnema sylvestre* Leaf Extract in the Control of Blood Glucose in Insulin Dependent Diabetes Mellitus. *Journal of Ethnopharmacology.* 1990, volume 30, pages 281–294.

Shanmugasundaram, E.R., Venkatasubramanyam, M., Vijendran, M., Shanmugasundara, K.R. Effect of an Isolate of Gymnema sylvestre R.Br. in the Control of Diabetes Mellitus and the Associated Pathological Changes. *Ancient Science of Life.* 1988, volume 8, pages 183–194.

Sharma, R.D., Raghuram, T.C. Hypoglycaemic Effect of Fenugreek Seeds in Non-Insulin Dependent Diabetic Subjects. *Nutrition Research.* 1990, volume 10, pages 731–739.

Sharma, R.D., Raghuram, T.C., Rao, N.S. Effect of Fenugreek Seeds on Blood Glucose and Serum Lipids in Type I Diabetes. *European Journal of Clinical Nutrition.* 1990, volume 44, pages 301–306.

Shishodia, S., Harikumar, K.B, Dass, S., et al. The Guggul for Chronic Diseases: Ancient Medicine, Modern Targets. *Anticancer Research.* November-December 2008, volume 28, number 6A, pages 3647–3664.

Singh, R.B., Niaz, M.A., Rastogi, V., et al. Hypolipidemic and Antioxidant Effects of Fenugreek Seeds and Triphala as Adjuncts to Dietary Therapy in Patients with Mild to Moderate Hypercholesterolaemia. *Perfusion.* 1998, volume 11, pages 124–130.

Skinner, H.G., Michaud, D.S., Giovannucci, E., et al. Cancer Epidemiology Biomarkers & Vitamin D Intake and the Risk for Pancreatic Cancer in Two Cohort Studies. *Prevention.* September 2006, volume 15, pages 1688–1695.

Stevia Info. www.steviainfo.com

Switzer, L. Spirulina. In: *The Whole Food Revolution.* New York: Bantam Books, 1982.

Szapary, P.O., Wolfe, M.L., Bloedon, L.T., et al. Guggul and Cholesterol: Guggulipid for the Treatment of Hypercholesterolemia: A Randomized Controlled Trial. *Journal of the American Medical Association.* August 13, 2003, volume 290, number 6, pages 765–772.

Taylor, L. *The Healing Power of Natural Herbs.* Garden City Park, New York: Square One Publishers, 2005.

Teegarden, D., Donkin, S.S. Vitamin D: Emerging New Roles in Insulin Sensitivity. *Nutrition Research and Review.* June 2009, volume 22, number 1, pages 82–92.

Tokusoglu, O., Unal, M.K. Biomass Nutrient Profiles of Three Microalgae: Spirulina platensis, Chlorella vulgaris, and Isochrisis galbana. *Journal of Food Science.* 2003, volume 68, page 4.

Vonshak, A. (ed.) *Spirulina platensis* (Arthrospira). Physiology, Cell-biology and Biotechnology. Philadelphia: Taylor & Francis, 1997.

Wang, J., Wang, Y., Wang, Z., et al Vitamin A Equivalence of Spirulina Beta-Carotene in Chinese Adults as Assessed by Using a Stable-Isotope Reference Method. *American Journal of Clinical Nutrition.* June 2008, volume 87, number 6, pages 1730–1737.

Yu, Y.M., Chang, W.C., Liu, C.S., Tsai, C.M. Effect of Young Barley Leaf Extract and Adlay on Plasma Lipids and LDL Oxidation in Hyperlipidemic Smokers. *Biological and Pharmaceutical Bulletin.* June 2004, volume 27, number 6, pages 802–805.

Zafra-Stone, S., Yasmin, T., Bagchi, M., et al. Berry Anthocyanins as Novel Antioxidants in Human Health and Disease Prevention. *Molecular Nutrition and Food Research.* June 2007, volume 51, number 6, pages 675–683.

Zheng, S., Yumei, F., Chen, A. De Novo Synthesis of Glutathione Is a Prerequisite for Curcumin to Inhibit Hepatic Stellate Cell (HSC) Activation. *Free Radical Biology and Medicine.* 2007, volume 43, number 3, pages 444–453.

Ziegler, D., Gries, F.A. Alpha-Lipoic Acid in the Treatment of Diabetic Peripheral and Cardiac Autonomic Neuropathy. *Diabetes.* September 1997, volume 46 (supplement 2), pages S62–S66.

PART 6: RECIPES AND KITCHEN TIPS

Chapter 15: Eat Sweets without Suffering

American Chemical Society. Soda Warning? New Study Supports Link Between Diabetes, High-fructose Corn Syrup Libraries. Released: Mon 13-Aug-2007, 16:30 ET.

Bray, G.A., Nielsen, S.J., Popkin, B.M. Consumption of High-Fructose Corn Syrup in Beverages May Play a Role in the Epidemic of Obesity [letter]. *American Journal of Clinical Nutrition.* October 2004, volume 80, number 4, page 1081.

Collison, K.S., Saleh, S.M., Bakheet, R.H., et al. Diabetes of the Liver: The Link Between Nonalcoholic Fatty Liver Disease and HFCS-55. *Obesity* (Silver Spring). March 12, 2009. [Epub ahead of print]

Corn Syrup Soda Warning? High-fructose Corn Syrup Linked to Diabetes, New Study Suggests. *ScienceDaily.* August 23, 2007.

Engber, D. Dark Sugar. The Decline and Fall of High-Fructose Corn Syrup. Slate.com. April 28, 2009. www.slate.com/id/2216796/

Fowler, S.P., Williams, K., Resendez, R.G., et al. Fueling the Obesity Epidemic? Artificially Sweetened Beverage Use and Long-Term Weight Gain. *Obesity* (Silver Spring). April 2009, volume 17, number 4, page 628.

Jenkins, D.A., Kendall, C.W., McKeown-Eyssen, G., et al. Effect of a Low–Glycemic Index or a High–Cereal Fiber Diet on Type 2 Diabetes, A Randomized Trial. *Journal of the American Medical Association.* 2008, volume 300, number 23, pages 2742–2753.

Mezitis, N.H.E., Maggio, C.A., Koch, P., et al. Glycemic Effect of a Single High Oral Dose of the Novel Sweetener Sucralose in Patients with Diabetes. *Diabetes Care.* 1996, volume 19, ages 1004–1005.

Molan, P.C., Brett, M. Honey Has Potential as a Dressing for Wounds Infected with MRSA. A paper presented at the 2nd Australian Wound Management Association Conference, Brisbane, Australia, 1998.

Soffritti, M., Belpoggi, F., Degli Esposti, D., et al. First Experimental Demonstration of the Multipotential Carcinogenic Effects of Aspartame Administered in the Feed to Sprague-Dawley Rats. *Environmental Health Perspectives.* 2006, volume 114, number 3, pages 379–385.

Teff, K.L., Elliott, S.S., Tschöp, M., et al. Dietary Fructose Reduces Circulating Insulin and Leptin, Attenuates Postprandial Suppression of Ghrelin, and Increases Triglycerides in Women. *Journal of Clinical Endocrinology & Metabolism.* 2004, volume 89, pages 2963–2972.

Wallinga, D., Sorenson, J., Mottl, P., Yablon, B. Not So Sweet: Missing Mercury and High Fructose Corn Syrup. Institute for Agriculture and Trade Policy. www.healthobservatory.org/library.cfm?refid=105026

Westman, E.C., Yancy, W.S. Jr., Mavropoulos, J.C., Marquart, M., McDuffie, J.R. The Effect of a Low-Carbohydrate, Ketogenic Diet Versus a Low-Glycemic Index Diet on Glycemic Control in Type 2 Diabetes Mellitus. *Nutrition and Metabolism* (London). December 19, 2008, volume 5, page 5:36.

Zidan, J., Shetver, L., Gershuny, A., et al. Induced Neutropenia by Special Honey Intake. *Medical Oncology.* 2006, volume 23, number 4, pages 549–552.

Chapter 16: Construct a Healthy Kitchen

Barclay, A.W., Brand-Miller, J.C. Validity of Glycemic Index Estimates in the Insulin Resistance Atherosclerosis [letter]. Diabetes Care. July 2006, volume 29, number 7, pages 1718–1719.

Bazzano, L.A., Li, T.Y., Joshipura, K.J., Hu, F.B. Intake of Fruit, Vegetables, and Fruit Juices and Risk of Diabetes in Women. Diabetes Care. July 2008, volume 31, number 7, pages 1311–1317.

Colditz, G.A., Manson, J.E., Stampfer, M.J., et al. Diet and Risk of Clinical Diabetes in Women. *American Journal of Clinical Nutrition.* 1992, volume 55, pages 1018–1023.

Daher, G.C., Cooper, D.A., Zorich, N.L., et al. Olestra Ingestion and Retinyl Palmitate Ingestion in Humans. *Journal of Nutrition.* August 1997, volume 127, pages 1686S–1693S.

Feskens, E.J., Virtanen, S.M., Räsänen, L., et al. Dietary Factors Determining Diabetes and Impaired Glucose Tolerance: A 20-year Follow-up of the Finnish and Dutch Cohorts of the Seven Countries Study. *Diabetes Care.* 1995, volume 18, pages 1104–1112.

Ford, E.S., Mokdad, A.H. Fruit and Vegetable Consumption and Diabetes Mellitus Incidence among U. S. Adults. *Preventive Medicine.* 2001, volume 32, pages 33–39.

Jalil, A.M., Ismail, A., Pei, C.P., et al. Effects of Cocoa Extract on Glucometabolism, Oxidative Stress, and Antioxidant Enzymes in Obese-Diabetic (Ob-db) Rats. *Journal of Agriculture and Food Chemistry.* September 2008, volume 56, number 17, pages 7877–7884.

Liese, A.D., Schulz, M., Fang, F., et al. Dietary Glycemic Index and Glycemic Load, Carbohydrate and Fiber Intake, and Measures of Insulin Sensitivity, Secretion, and Adiposity in the Insulin Resistance Atherosclerosis Study. *Diabetes Care.* 2005, volume 28, pages 2832—2838.

Liu, S., Serdula, M., Janket, S.J., et al. A Prospective Study of Fruit and Vegetable Intake and the Risk of Type 2 Diabetes in Women. *Diabetes Care*. 2004, 27:2993–2996.

Meyer, K.A., Kushi, L.H., Jacobs, D.R. Jr., et al. Carbohydrates, Dietary Fiber, and Incident Type 2 Diabetes in Older Women. *American Journal of Clinical Nutrition*. 2000, volume 71, pages 921–930.

Miller, D.L., Castellanos, V.H., Shide, D.J., Peters, J.C., Rolls, B.J. Effect of Fat-Free Potato Chips with and without Nutrition Labels on Fat and Energy Intakes. *American Journal of Clinical Nutrition*. August 1998, volume 68, number 2, pages 282–290.

Montonen, J., Jarvinen, R., Heliovaara, M., et al. Food Consumption and the Incidence of Type II Diabetes Mellitus. *European Journal of Clinical Nutrition*. 2005, volume 59, pages 441–448.

Navas-Acien, A., Silbergeld, E.K., Pastor-Barriuso, R., Guallar, E. Arsenic Exposure and Prevalence of Type 2 Diabetes in US Adults. *Journal of the American Medical Association*. August 20, 2008, volume 300, number 7, pages 814–822.

Peters, J.C., Lawson, K.D., Middleton, S.J., Treibwasser, K.C. Assessment of the Nutitional Effects of Olestra, a Nonabsorbed Fat Replacement: Introduction and Overview. *Journal of Nutrition*. August 1997, volume 127, number 8, pages 1539S–1546S.

Robinson, T.N., Borzekowski, D.L., Matheson, D.M., Kraemer, H.C. Effects of Fast Food Branding on Young Children's Taste Preferences. *Archives of Pediatriatric and Adolescent Medicine*. August 2007, volume 161, number 8, pages 792–797.

Schlagheck, T.G., Kesler, J.M., Jones, M.B., et al. Olestras Effect on Viramins D and E in Humans Can Be Offset by Increasing Dietary Levels of These Vitamins. *Journal of Nutrition*. August 1997, volume 127, number 8, pages 1666S–1685S.

Tomaru, M., Takano, H., Osakabe, N., et al. Dietary Supplementation with Cacao Liquor Proanthocyanidins Prevents Elevation of Blood Glucose Levels in Diabetic Obese Mice. *Nutrition*. April 2007, volume 23, number 4, pages 351–355.

U.S. Food and Drug Administration. FDA and Monosodium Glutamate (MSG). August 31, 1995.

Weststrate, J., Vanherhof, K.H. Sucrose Polyester and Plasma Carotenoid Concentrations in Healthy Subjects. *American Journal of Clinical Nutrition*. September 1995, volume 62, number 3, pages 591–597.

World Health Organization. WHO Expert Committee on Drug Dependence. Sixteenth report. (Technical report series. No. 407). Geneva, Switzerland: World Health Organization; 1969.

Chapter 17: Recipes to Save Your Life and Limbs

No citations/references applicable

Index

Underscored page references indicate boxed text.

About the Author

Suzy Cohen, RPh, has been a pharmacist for over 2 decades. She is also a syndicated columnist, speaker, and author of three other books, *The 24-Hour Pharmacist, Drug Muggers: How to Keep Your Medicine from Stealing the Life Out of You!,* and *Real Solutions from Head to Toe.* Suzy is a graduate of the University of Florida and a member of the Institute of Functional Medicine, the Academy of Anti-Aging Medicine, the American College for Advancement in Medicine, and the American Pharmaceutical Association.

To receive Suzy's free weekly health newsletter, or to ask your own health question, visit her Web site at www.DearPharmacist.com.